# Handbook of Gastroenterologic Procedures

## Fourth Edition

# Handbook of Gastroenterologic Procedures

## Fourth Edition

## SENIOR EDITOR

### Douglas A. Drossman, M.D.

Professor
Division of Gastroenterology and Hepatology
University of North Carolina School of Medicine
Chapel Hill, North Carolina

## ASSOCIATE EDITORS

### Ian S. Grimm, M.D.

Associate Professor
Division of Gastroenterology and Hepatology
University of North Carolina School of Medicine
Chapel Hill, North Carolina

### Nicholas J. Shaheen M.D., M.P.H.

Associate Professor
Division of Gastroenterology and Hepatology
University of North Carolina School of Medicine
Chapel Hill, North Carolina

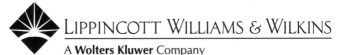

LIPPINCOTT WILLIAMS & WILKINS
A **Wolters Kluwer** Company

Philadelphia · Baltimore · New York · London
Buenos Aires · Hong Kong · Sydney · Tokyo

Acquisitions Editor: Charley Mitchell
Developmental Editor: Nicole Dernoski
Project Manager: Alicia Jackson
Senior Manufacturing Manager: Benjamin Rivera
Marketing Manager: Kathy Neely
Designer: Larry Didona
Production Service: Publishing Solutions for Retail, Book, ar
Schawk Inc.
Printer: RR Donnelley, Crawfordsville

WI
39
H23535
2005

**Library of Congress Cataloging-in-Publication Data**
Handbook of gastroenterologic procedures / senior editor, Douglas A. Drossman; associate
editors, Ian S. Grimm, Nicholas J. Shaheen.— 4th ed.
    p. ; cm.
    Rev. ed. of: Manual of gastroenterologic procedures / editor, Douglas A. Drossman. 3rd ed.
c1993.
    Includes bibliographical references and index.
    ISBN 0-7817-5008-3 (alk. paper)
    1. Gastroenterology—Handbooks, manuals, etc. I. Drossman, Douglas A. II. Grimm, Ian
S. III. Shaheen, Nicholas J. IV. Manual of gastroenterologic procedures.
    [DNLM: 1. Digestive System Surgical Procedures—Handbooks.    2. Diagnostic
Techniques, Digestive System—Handbooks. 3. Digestive System Diseases—Handbooks. 4.
Gastroenterology—methods—Handbooks. ]
RC801.H275 2005
616.3'3—dc22
                                                                            2004030551

10 9 8 7 6 5 4 3 2 1

*In honor of John T. Sessions, Jr., MD, the distinguished founder of our division. In recognition of Eugene M. Bozymski, MD, William D. Heizer, MD, and Henry T. Lesesne, MD for their commitment to our division through teaching and patient care and of Don W. Powell, MD for his support, leadership, and mentoring.*

# Contents

Contributing Authors .......................... xiii
Preface ..................................... xix
Preface to the Third Edition ................... xxi
Acknowledgment ............................. xxiii

## I. Preparation of the Patient

1.  Preprocedure Assessment of Patients
    Undergoing Gastrointestinal Procedures
    *Douglas J. Robertson*                              3

2.  Bowel Preps
    *Alphonso Brown*                                   10

3.  Analgesia and Sedation
    *Henning Gerke and John Baillie*                   13

## II. Basic Techniques

4.  Oral and Nasal Gastrointestinal Intubation
    *David M.S. Grunkemeier*                           21

5.  Esophagogastroduodenoscopy (EGD)
    *Kim L. Isaacs*                                    30

6.  Small Bowel Enteroscopy
    *Sauyu Lin and Michael A. Shetzline*               38

7.  Endoscopic Retrograde Pancreatography
    *Nina Phatak and Michael L. Kochman*               47

8.  Colonoscopy
    *Jerome D. Waye*                                   56

9.  Anoscopy and Rigid Sigmoidoscopy
    *Kim L. Isaacs*                                    64

10. Abdominal Paracentesis
    *Kimberly L. Beavers*                              72

11. Percutaneous Liver Biopsy
    *Kimberly L. Beavers*                              78

## III. Advanced and/or Secondary Techniques

12. Injection Therapy for Hemostasis and Anal Fissures
    *Lisa M. Gangarosa*                                87

13. Bipolar Electrocautery and Heater Probe
    *Lisa M. Gangarosa*                                93

14. Clips and Loops
    *Emad M. Abu-Hamda and Todd H. Baron*                97

15. Injection Therapy of Esophageal and Gastric
    Varices: Sclerosis and Cyanoacrylate
    *Stephen H. Caldwell, Vanessa M. Shami, and
    Elizabeth E. Hespenheide*                            103

16. Endoscopic Variceal Ligation
    *Jason D. Conway and Roshan Shrestha*                112

17. Balloon Tamponade
    *Kim L. Isaacs*                                      119

18. Polypectomy, Endoscopic Muscosal Resection,
    and Tattooing
    *Gregory G. Ginsberg and Nina Phatak*               127

19. Feeding Tubes (Nasoduodenal, Nasojejunal)
    *William D. Heizer*                                  138

20. Percutaneous Endoscopic Gastrostomy (PEG) and
    Percutaneous Endoscopic Jejunostomy (PEJ)
    *Todd H. Baron*                                      147

21. Colonic Decompression
    *Jeffrey T. Wei and Nicholas J. Shaheen*            156

22. Dilation of the Esophagus: Mercury-Filled
    Bougies (Hurst Maloney)
    *Douglas Morgan*                                     160

23. Dilatation of the Esophagus: Wire-Guided Bougies
    (Savary and American Endoscopy)
    *Nicholas J. Shaheen*                                164

24. Pneumatic Dilation for Achalasia
    *Joel E. Richter*                                    168

25. Through-the-Scope Balloon Dilation
    *Elena I. Sidorenko and Prateek Sharma*             176

26. Stenting of Esophageal Cancers: Placement of
    Expandable Stents
    *Kenneth K. Wang*                                    183

27. Biliary Sludge Analysis
    *Jason D. Conway*                                    191

28. Endoscopic Sphincterotomy (Including Precut)
    *John S. Goff*                                       194

29. Management of Lithiasis: Balloon and Basket
    Extraction, Endoprosthesis, and Lithotripsy
    *David Horwhat and M. Stanley Branch*               201

30. Management of Biliary and Pancreatic Ductal
    Obstruction: Endoprosthesis and
    Nasobiliary/Nasopancreatic Drain Placement
    *Nalini M. Guda and Martin L. Freeman*     214

31. Management of Fluid Collections
    *Richard A. Kozarek*     229

32. Argon Plasma Coagulation
    *Ian S. Grimm*     235

33. Photodynamic Therapy for Barrett's
    High-grade Dysplasia
    *Bergein F. Overholt, Masoud Panjehpour, and
    Mary Phan*     239

34. Infrared Coagulation of Hemorrhoids
    *Sidney E. Levinson*     246

35. Endoscopic Management of Foreign Bodies of the
    Upper Gastrointestinal Tract
    *Craig J. Cender*     251

36. Capsule Endoscopy
    *Blair S. Lewis*     263

37. Stretta
    *Douglas Corley*     270

38. Enteryx Injection for Gastroesophageal
    Reflux Disease
    *David A. Johnson*     277

39. Endoscopic Sewing—EndoCinch
    *David A. Johnson*     283

## IV. Tests of GI Function

40. Esophageal Manometry
    *Janice Freeman and Donald O. Castell*     291

41. Ambulatory 24-hour Esophageal pH Monitoring
    *Ronnie Fass, Leslie Eidelman, and Wilder
    Garcia-Calderaon*     299

42. Gastric Secretory Testing
    *Robert S. Bulat and Roy C. Orlando*     306

43. Secretin Test
    *Alphonso Brown*     313

44. Sphincter of Oddi Manometry
    *Daniel J. Geenen*     317

45.  Small Bowel Motility and the Role of
     Scintigraphy in Small Bowel Motility
     *Jonathan Gonenne and Michael Camilleri*          322

46.  Breath Hydrogen Text for Lactose Intolerance
     and Bacterial Overgrowth
     *Syed I.M. Thiwan and William E. Whitehead*        333

47.  Anorectal Manometry and Biofeedback
     *Yolanda V. Scarlett*                              341

## V. Endoscopic Ultrasound

48.  Endoscopic Ultrasound
     *Poonputt Chotiprasidhi and James M. Scheiman*     349

49.  Endosonography-guided Fine Needle
     Aspiration Biopsy
     *Maurits J. Wiersema and Michael J. Levy*          357

50.  Endosonography-guided Celiac Plexus Neurolysis
     *Maurits J. Wiersema and Michael J. Levy*          364

## Appendices

A.   The Procedure Unit
     *Melissa C. Brennen*                               371

B.   Handling of Specimens
     *Jason D. Conway*                                  378

C.   Doses of Common GI Drugs Used in GI Procedures
     *Sanjib Mohanty*                                   380

D.   Guidelines for Endoscopic Screening and
     Surveillace
     *Jason D. Conway*                                  382

E.   DDW Cards/Useful Websites
     *Sanjib P. Mohanty*                                387

F.   CPT Modifiers
     *Sanjib P. Mohanty*                                393

G.   Complete Listing of CPT Codes                      394

Index                                                   405

# Contributing Authors

**Emad M. Abu-Hamda, M. D.** *Advanced Endoscopy Fellow, Clinical Instructor of Medicine, Gastroenterology and Hepatology, Mayo Clinic, College of Medicine, Rochester, Minnesota*

**John Baillie, F. R. C. P., M. B., Ch. B.** *Professor, Medicine and Gastoenterology, Director, Billary Service, Division of Gastroenterology, Duke University Medical Center, Durham, North Carolina*

**Todd H. Baron, M. D.** *Professor of Medicine, Division of Gastroenterology and Hepatology, Mayo Clinic College of Medicine; Consultant, Division of Gastroenterology and Hepatology, Mayo Clinic, Rochester, Minnesota*

**Kimberly L. Beavers, M. D., M. P. H.** *Asheville Gastroenterology Associates, Asheville, North Carolina*

**M. Stanley Branch, M. D.** *Associate Professor, Department of Medicine, Duke University; Clinical Chief of Gastroenterology, Department of Medicine, Duke University Medical Center, Durham, North Carolina*

**Melissa C. Brennen, C.G.R.N., B. S. N.** *Clinical Nurse Supervisor II, GI Procedures, University North Carolina Health Care, Chapel Hill, North Carolina*

**Alphonso Brown, M. D., M. P. H.** *Assitant Professor of Medicine, Division of Gastroenterology and Hepatology, Department of Medicine, University of North Carolina-Chapel Hill, Chapel Hill, North Carolina*

**Robert S. Bulat, M. D., Ph. D.** *Assistant Professor, Department of Medicine, Tulane University; Director, GI Motility Service, Tulane University Health Sciences Center, New Orleans, Louisiana*

**Stephen H. Caldwell, M. D.** *Associate Professor, GI / Hepatology, University of Virginia, Charlottesville, Virginia*

**Michael Camilleri, M. D.** *Professor of Medicine and Physiology, Atherton and Winifred W. Bean Professor, Mayo Clinic College of Medicine; Consultant, Division of Gastroenterology, Department of Medicine, Mayo Clinic, Rochester, Minnesota*

**Donald O. Castell, M. D.** *Professor, Department of Medicine, Medical University of South Carolina; Director, Esophageal Disorders Program, Gastroenterology Division, Medical University of South Carolina Hospital, Charleston, South Carolina*

**Craig J. Cender, M. D.**  *Asheville Gastroenterology Associates, Asheville, North Carolina*

**Poonputt Chotiprasidhi, M. D.**  *Clinical Assistant Professor, Department of Internal Medicine, University of Michigan; Attending Physician, Department of Internal Medicine, University of Michigan Medical Center, Ann Arbor, Michigan*

**Jason D. Conway, M. D.**  *Fellow, Division of Gastroenterology and Hepatology, University of North Carolina at Chapel Hill, Chapel Hill, North Carolina*

**Douglas Corley, M. D., M. P. H., Ph. D.**  *Research Scientist, Kaiser Permanente, Division of Research, Oakland, California; Assistant Clinical Professor, Department of Medicine, University of California, San Francisco, San Francisco, California*

**Douglas A. Drossman, M. D.**  *Professor, Division of Gastroenterology and Hepatology, Co-director UNC Center for Functional GI and Motility Disorders, University of North Carolina School of Medicine, Chapel Hill, North Carolina*

**Leslie Eidelman, M. D.**  *Visiting Scholar, Department of Medicine, University of Arizona, Tucson, Arizona*

**Ronnie Fass, M. D.**  *Associate Professor of Medicine, Department of Medicine, University of Arizona; Director, GI Motility Laboratories, Department of Medicine, Southern Arizona VA Health Care System and University of Arizona Health Science Center, Tucson, Arizona*

**Janice Freeman, R.N., B. S. N.**  *Clinical and Research Coordinator, Esophageal Function Laboratory, Digestive Disease Center, Medical University of South Carolina, Charleston, South Carolina*

**Martin L. Freeman, M. D.**  *Professor, Department of Medicine, University of Minnesota, Gastroenterology Division, Hennepin County Medical Center, Minneapolis, Minnesota*

**Lisa M. Gangarosa, M. D.**  *Assistant Professor of Medicine, Department of Medicine, University of North Carolina - Chapel Hill, Chapel Hill, North Carolina*

**Wilder Garcia-Calderon, M. D.**  *Medical Resident, Department of Medicine, University of Arizona, Tucson, Arizona*

**Daniel J. Geenen, M. D.**  *Active Staff, Department of Gastroenterology, St. Luke's Medical Center, Milwaukee, Wisconsin*

**Henning Gerke, M. D.**  *Assistant Professor (Clinical), Department of Internal Medicine, University of Iowa, Iowa City, Iowa*

**Gregory G. Ginsberg, M. D.**   *Associate Professor, Department of Medicine, University of Pennsylvania; Director, Endoscopic Services, Hospital of the University of Pennsylvania, Philadelphia, Pennsylvania*

**John S. Goff, M. D.**   *Clinical Professor of Medicine, Gastroenterology, University of Colorado, Denver, Colorado; Rocky Mountain Gastroenterology Associates, Lakewood, Colorado*

**Jonathan Gonenne, M. D.**   *Fellow, Division of Gastroenterology, Department of Medicine, Mayo Clinic, Rochester, Minnesota*

**Ian S. Grimm, M. D.**   *Associate Professor, Division of Gastroenterology and Hepatology, University of North Carolina School of Medicine, Chapel Hill, North Carolina*

**David M. S. Grunkemeier, M. D.**   *Gastroenterology Fellow, Department of Medicine, University of North Carolina at Chapel Hill, Chapel Hill, North Carolina*

**Nalini M. Guda, M. D.**   *Gastroenterology Division, Hennepin County Medical Center, University of Minnesota, Minneapolis, Minnesota*

**William D. Heizer, M. D.**   *Clinical Professor of Medicine, Department of Medicine, University of North Carolina, Chapel Hill, North Carolina*

**Elizabeth E. Hespenheide, R.N., B. S. N.**   *Nurse Coordinator / Research Coordinator, Digestive Health Center of Excellence, University of Virginia, Charlottesville, Virginia*

**David Horwhat, M. D.**   *Associate in Medicine, Department of Medicine, Division of Gastroenterology, Duke University Health System; Advanced Endoscopy Fellow, Department of Medicine, Duke University Health System, Durham, North Carolina*

**Kim L. Isaacs, M. D., Ph. D.**   *Associate Professor of Medicine, Division of Gastroenterology and Hepatology, University of North Carolina; Attending Physician, Department of Medicine, University of North Carolina Hospitals, Chapel Hill, North Carolina*

**David A. Johnson, M. D., F. A. C. P., F. A. C. G.**   *Division Chief, Division of Gastroenterology, Department of Internal Medicine, Eastern Virginia Medical School, Norfolk, Virginia*

**Michael L. Kochman, M. D., F. A. C. P.**   *Professor of Medicine, Gastroenterology Division, University of Pennsylvania Health System; Co-Director, Gastrointestinal Oncology, Gastroenterology Division, Hospital of the University of Pennsylvania, Philadelphia, Pennsylvania*

**Richard A. Kozarek, M. D.**   *Clinical Professor of Medicine, University of Washington; Chief of Gastroenterology, Virginia Mason Medical Center, Seattle, Washington*

**Sidney E. Levinson, M. D.**   *Clinical Associate Professor, Department of Medicine, University of North Carolina; Attending Physician, Department of Medicine, UNC Hospitals, Chapel Hill, North Carolina*

**Michael J. Levy, M. D.**   *Assistant Professor, Division of Gastroenterology, Mayo Clinic College of Medicine, Rochester, Minnesota*

**Blair S. Lewis, M. D.**   *Clinical Professor, Department of Medicine, The Mount Sinai School of Medicine; Attending, Department of Medicine, The Mount Sinai Hospital, New York, New York*

**Sauyu Lin, M. D.**   *Fellow, Division of Gastroenterology, Duke University Medical Center, Durham, North Carolina*

**Sanjib P. Mohanty, M. D.**   *Fellow, Division of Gastroenterology and Hepatology, Department of Medicine, University of North Carolina-Chapel Hill, Chapel Hill, North Carolina*

**Douglas R. Morgan, M. D., M. P. H.**   *Assistant Professor of Medicine, Division of Gastroenterology and Hepatology, Department of Medicine, University of North Carolina-Chapel Hill, Chapel Hill, North Carolina*

**Roy C. Orlando, M. D.**   *Professor of Medicine, Adjunct Professor of Physiology, Department of Medicine, Tulane University; Chief, Section of Gastroenterology and Hepatology, Tulane University, New Orleans, Louisiana*

**Bergein F. Overholt, M. D., M. S.**   *Medical Director, Laser Center, Thompson Cancer Survival Center, Knoxville, Tennessee*

**Masoud Panjehpour, Ph. D.**   *Director, Laser Center, Thompson Cancer Survival Center, Knoxville, Tennessee*

**Mary Phan, B.S.**   *Research Associate, Laser Center, Thompson Cancer Survival Center, Knoxville, Tennessee*

**Nina Phatak, M. D.**   *Physician, Department of Medicine, University of Pennsylvania; Fellow, Gastroenterology Division, Hospital of the University of Pennsylvania, Philadelphia, Pennsylvania*

**Joel E. Richter, M. D., M. A. C. G.**   *Professor of Medicine, Cleveland Clinic Lerner College of Medicine of Case Western Reserve University; Chairman, Department of Gastroenterology and Hepatology, Cleveland Clinic Foundation, Cleveland, Ohio*

**Douglas Robertson, M. D.**  *Assistant Professor of Medicine, Department of Medicine, Dartmouth Medical School, Hanover, New Hampshire; Chief, Section of Gastroenterology, White River Junction Veterans Affairs Medical Center, White River Junction, Vermont*

**Yolanda V. Scarlett, M. D.**  *Assitant Professor of Medicine, Division of Gastroenterology and Hepatology, Department of Medicine, University of North Carolina-Chapel Hill, Chapel Hill, North Carolina*

**James M. Scheiman, M. D.**  *Professor, Division of Gastroenterology, Department of Internal Medicine, University of Michigan; Director, EUS Program, Division of Gastroenterology, Department of Internal Medicine, University of Michigan Health System, Ann Arbor, Michigan*

**Nicholas J. Shaheen, M. D., M. P. H.**  *Associate Professor, Division of Gastroenterology and Hepatology, University of North Carolina School of Medicine, Chapel Hill, North Carolina*

**Vanessa M. Shami, M. D.**  *Assistant Professor, Gastroenterology and Hepatology, University of Virginia, Charlottesville, Virginia*

**Prateek Sharma, M. D.**  *Associate Professor of Medicine, Division of Gastroenterology and Hepatology, University of Kansas School of Medicine and VA Medical Center; Director of Gastroenterology Fellowship Program, Division of Gastroenterology and Hepatology, Veterans Affairs Medical Center, Kansas City, Missouri; Supported by the Veterans Affairs Medical Center, Kansas City, MO and The American Gastroenterological Association (AGA) Castell Esophageal Clinical Research Award*

**Michael A. Shetzline, M. D., Ph. D.**  *Senior Medical Director, Department of Gastroenterology, Novartis Pharmaceuticals Corporation, East Hanover, New Jersey*

**Roshan Shrestha, M. D.**  *Professor of Medicine, Division of Gastroenterology and Hepatology, Department of Medicine, University of North Carolina-Chapel Hill, Chapel Hill, North Carolina*

**Elena I. Sidorenko, M. D.**  *Gastroenterology Fellow, Department of Gastroenterology, Kansas University, Kansas University Medical Center, Kansas City, Missouri*

**Syed I. M. Thiwan, M. D.**  *Instructor in Medicine, Division of Gastroenterology and Hepatology, University of North Carolina, School of Medicine, Chapel Hill, North Carolina*

**Kenneth K. Wang, M. D.**  *Associate Professor of Medicine, Department of Gastroenterology and Hepatology, Mayo Clinic, Rochester, Minnesota*

**Jerome D. Waye, M. D.**   *Clinical Professor of Medicine, Department of Gastroenterology, Mt. Sinai Medical Center; Director of Endoscopic Education, GI Department, Mt. Sinai Hospital, New York, New York*

**Jeffrey T. Wei, M. D.**   *Fellow, Department of Gastroenterology, University of North Carolina, Chapel Hill, North Carolina*

**William E. Whitehead, Ph. D.**   *Professor of Medicine, Division of Gasteroenterology and Hepatology, University of North Carolina School of Medicine*

**Maurits J. Wiersema, M. D.**   *Gastroenterologist, Fort Wayne, Indiana*

# Preface

We are most pleased to offer this fourth edition of our *Handbook of Gastroenterologic Procedures* (originally titled *Manual of Gastroenterologic Procedures*).Created more than two decades ago by our Division of Gastroenterology and Hepatology at the University of North Carolina School of Medicine, this handbook has maintained its uniqueness as a reliable and concise resource for almost all of the gastroenterological (GI) procedures commonly used in clinical practice and academic training programs. The handbook has also been noted for its broad readership. In the past, gastroenterologists have ordered multiple copies for personal use and for their staff in the procedure unit. Those physicians, nurses, technicians, and students have attested to the value of having "just the facts" at their level of interest and expertise - a collection of a wide range of procedures not easy to find elsewhere and in a standardized format. Thus, we have maintained the basic format for the chapters, with section headings relating to indications, contraindications, patient preparation, procedure, and complications; we also have relied on simple line drawings to illustrate key concepts.

Although this new, updated edition retains all these qualities, because so much has changed in the 12 years since the third edition was published, we have also made important enhancements and modifications. First, the rapid growth in imaging technology coupled with the maturation of endoscopy as a therapeutic discipline has produced an unprecedented increase in the range of diagnostic and therapeutic procedures now available. Thus we have taken care to include newer procedures that are only of high utility, that are of relatively low risk for the practicing gastroenterologist, and that are commonly used or are growing rapidly in their application frequency. However, we now have 50 chapters (fully a 25% increase from the third edition) and as a result have abandoned the previous spiral-bound handbook format but have retained the smaller book size. Second, the complexity of some of the procedural methods now requires that for some chapters, we include more details of the technique in exchange for brevity. However, we have kept the text as concise as possible within the basic outline structure. Third, the field has advanced to the point that expertise for these procedures can no longer be provided within one GI division. Therefore, we have recruited recognized experts outside our institution to write chapters for many of the newer procedures, and many of the techniques were actually developed by the authors.

The handbook is not intended, nor is it sufficient to provide complete endoscopic information; rather it serves as a supplement to more comprehensive endoscopy textbooks by providing a "quick look" at essential information and helpful tips (for example, what to do when the sphincterotome will not advance into the common duct). All previous chapters have been extensively revised from the previous edition. Furthermore, we have added new diagnostic (e.g., endoscopic ultrasound, capsule endoscopy, fine needle aspiration biopsy) and many therapeutic endoscopy chapters that cover celiac plexus neurolysis, injection therapy, the use of clips and loops bleeding and band ligation for varices and hemorrhoids, self-expandable metal stents for obstructing lesions, argon plasma, infrared and photodynamic therapy, and emerging techniques for gastroesophageal reflux such as the Stretta, Enteryx and sewing devices.

Perhaps one of the most unique aspects to this handbook is the inclusion of chapters devoted to nonendoscopic procedures, such as the insertion of the Minnesota tube for refractory variceal bleeding; esophageal, small bowel, and anorectal manometry; liver biopsy; the management of fluid collections including biliary crystal analysis; paracentesis; feeding tube placement; and breath $H_2$ testing for disaccharidase deficiency or bacterial overgrowth. This compendium of information is not easily found in any one resource.

Finally, we include chapters that contain generic information relating to the organization and function of the endoscopy unit, preprocedure planning and bowel preps, analgesia and sedation (including the use of propofol), handling of specimens and their analysis, and dosages of GI drugs. We also include appendices containing information on CPT codes for procedures, scoring systems, and the locations of outside resources when additional help is needed.

We hope that this fourth edition will continue to serve many purposes for all of us involved in the diagnosis, treatment, and care of patients with gastrointestinal disorders.

*Douglas A. Drossman, M.D.*
*Ian S. Grimm, M.D.*
*Nicholas W. Shaheen, M.D.*

# Preface to the Third Edition

It is with great pleasure that we offer this third edition of *Manual of Gastroenterologic Procedures* from the Division of Digestive Diseases at the University of North Carolina School of Medicine. As with the previous editions, our goal is to provide a resource for physicians, nurses, technicians, and students in most of the gastroenterological procedures. The information is presented in a standardized, yet straightforward format that highlights the indications, contraindications, patient preparation, techniques, and complications for 40 procedures. In addition to a section on the organization and function of the procedure unit itself, the chapters are conveniently organized into sections on tubes, needles, diagnostic endoscopy, therapeutic endoscopy, and pediatric procedures.

The manual can serve as a supplement to more comprehensive endoscopy manuals. Here, the endoscopic sections provide a "quick look," with essential information and helpful tips (for example, what to do when the sphincterotome will not advance into the common duct). In addition, about half of the chapters are devoted to important nonendoscopic procedures (e.g., insertion of Minnesota tube, esophageal and rectal manometry, liver biopsy, paracentesis, and feeding tube intubation) that are not easily found in one book.

Several changes have been made to reflect the advances in gastroenterological practice over the past five years. New chapters include ambulatory intraesophageal pH monitoring, laser therapy, and a section devoted to medications used in the procedure unit (conscious sedation, topical anesthetics, motility/antimotility drugs, antibiotics for bacterial endocarditis prophylaxis, and biliary tract manipulation). Several chapters have been extensively revised. We have updated the section on naso/gastrointestinal intubation to include newer devices, and we describe the endoscopic rather than capsule technique for small bowel biopsy (the capsule technique is included in the pediatric section). We have also added injection therapy to the chapter on ablation of bleeding gastrointestinal lesions, have described both the one-step and three-step methods for balloon dilatation of strictures, and have included a discussion on the use of dual (radiologic/endoscopic) biliary stent placement.

We trust that this third edition will continue to serve many purposes for all of us involved in the diagnosis and care of patients with gastrointestinal disorders.

*Douglas A. Drossman, M.D.*

The editors would like to thank Jerry Schoendorf for the accompanying illustrations and Susan Schneck for her support and technical assistance.

# Handbook of
# Gastroenterologic Procedures

## Fourth Edition

# Preparation of the Patient

# Preprocedure Assessment of Patients Undergoing Gastrointestinal Procedures

## Douglas J. Robertson

Prior to performing any gastrointestinal procedure, the clinician should carefully consider factors affecting the appropriateness and safety of the test. Determining the need for the procedure is based on a careful assessment of the potential risks and benefits of the intervention. A clear understanding of these issues both verbally and in writing constitutes the basis for informed consent. If a decision to proceed with testing is made, the clinician then considers factors such as the patient's preexisting medical conditions that may complicate the safe completion of the study. This chapter will review the basics of informed consent and special circumstances (e.g., diseases, medications) that need to be addressed prior to initiating the procedure.

### INFORMED CONSENT

At its core, informed consent is a process of *disclosure* (1). Central to the informed consent process is the discussion and deliberation that takes place *prior* to the patient's written authorization. The signed document simply verifies that the process occurred. The key components for informed consent are

1. Description of the procedure
2. Indication for the procedure
3. Risks and complications of the procedure
4. Alternatives to the procedure

Discussion and a written description of these items should be at a level appropriate to the patient's general education. Finally, patients should specifically be encouraged to ask questions to ensure full understanding of the material presented to them.

### ASSESSMENT OF THE PATIENT

After the informed decision to proceed with testing is made, the focus shifts to performing that procedure safely and comfortably. To that end, all patients should undergo a brief history with careful review of current medications and allergies. Cardiopulmonary assessment should also be completed prior to undertaking sedated endoscopy. The information summarizing the history and examination should be readily available to both the endoscopist and the assistants at the time of the procedure.

Certain subgroups of patients pose particular challenges for the gastroenterologist because of preexisting medical conditions. The following sections outline the general approach to these patient subgroups.

### Diabetes

Patients with long-standing diabetes frequently develop complications including nausea, vomiting, and alteration in bowel habits that may prompt the need for procedural evaluation. Because sedated endoscopy is performed on an empty stomach, glucose control and medication management are particular challenges. The following guidelines are suggested (2):

1.  Colonoscopy preparation generally requires that the patient take only clear liquids the day *prior* to the procedure. Diabetic patients should be reminded to check their glucose throughout this day (e.g., 4 times per day) and adjust their insulin dosage accordingly.

2.  All sedated procedures require that the patient be NPO on the day of the procedure. General recommendations for this period include the following:

    a.  For a.m. procedures, oral hypoglycemics can be held until after completion of the test; for p.m. procedures, oral medications may be taken early in the morning with a sip of water.
    b.  Insulin-requiring diabetics should take half of their routine daily NPH or 70/30-insulin dose. They need not take any routine regular insulin.
    c.  Upon arrival at the endoscopy unit, a preprocedural glucose level should be checked and a maintenance infusion of 5% dextrose started.
    d.  Postprocedural testing of glucose should also occur, with evaluation by the physician for abnormally high or low readings.

### Cardiac and Pulmonary Disease

Significant cardiac and pulmonary diseases are important comorbidities to consider prior to initiating endoscopic procedures. The risk of endoscopy increases for those with significant systemic disease. The American Society of Anesthesiologists (ASA) classification is one commonly used scale to assess general physical status (Table 1.1).(3). Prior studies have shown that increasing ASA class is associated with oxygen desaturation (4) and complications (5) during endoscopy. Therefore, for patients

**Table 1.1.    ASA classification (3)**

|         | Definition                                              |
| ------- | ------------------------------------------------------- |
| Class 1 | Healthy patient without medical problems                |
| Class 2 | Mild systemic disease                                   |
| Class 3 | Severe systemic disease, but not incapacitating         |
| Class 4 | Severe systemic disease that is a constant threat to life |
| Class 5 | Moribund; not expected to live 24 hrs                   |

with significant heart or lung disease, the following recommendations can be made:

1. Continuous monitoring of pulse, blood pressure, and oxygen saturation is generally recommended for all patients receiving conscious sedation. For patients with cardiopulmonary illness, such monitoring is *mandatory*.

2. Supplemental oxygen by nasal cannula is warranted. Close evaluation of respiratory effort during oxygen administration is essential for those with chronic obstructive lung disease to avoid profound hypercapnia.

3. Consider continuous electrocardiogram (EKG) monitoring for those with a history of significant arrhythmias or cardiac dysfunction.

Cardiac patients with implanted devices such as pacemakers and internal cardioverter/defibrillators (ICDs) merit special consideration if electrocautery might be used. The electrical energy (particularly from monopolar current discharged near the heart) can damage the pulse generator of the pacemaker or lead to firing of an internal defibrillator. For these circumstances, the following recommendations have been made (6):

1. During the procedure, monitor the patient's cardiac rhythm.

2. Position the grounding pad on the buttock or thigh (distant from the pacemaker/ICD and its leads).

3. Deactivate any ICD preprocedure and recheck function postprocedure.

4. In patients with a pacemaker, avoid long continuous discharges of electrocautery that may inhibit the pacemaker's function.

**Liver Disease**

Patients with cirrhosis frequently suffer life-threatening gastrointestinal bleeding that requires endoscopy. Cirrhosis complicates the performance of endoscopy in a number of ways. First, liver dysfunction may alter drug metabolism. In a prospective study, the elimination half-life of midazolam was significantly longer in cirrhotic patients (3.9 hours) when compared to controls (1.6 hours) (7). Use of opioid narcotics may also be more complicated in these patients. Respiratory depression is a specific concern, particularly in those with tense ascites, hepatic hydrothorax, or hepatopulmonary syndrome. Given these considerations, the following precautions have been advised (8):

1. Decrease the initial dose of sedative agents by one-half of that for a standard healthy patient of the same weight and age.

2. Administer sedation in small increments.

3. Reversal agents for both benzodiazepines (Romazicon) and narcotics (Narcan) should be readily available. The responsible physician should be familiar with the use of these drugs and their standard doses.

Second, cirrhosis of the liver predisposes the patient to increased bleeding risk via a number of mechanisms. Inadequate synthesis of clotting factors may prolong bleeding times. Furthermore, portal hypertension is associated with thrombocytopenia. For those with *active bleeding* that occurs while therapeutic endoscopy is being undertaken, correction of the clotting abnormalities needs to be rapid. To achieve correction, fresh frozen plasma (FFP) is used. The goal is to achieve an international normalized ratio (INR) of less than 1.5. If the platelet count of the patient is less than 50,000, transfusion of this product should be considered. For *elective* endoscopy in nonbleeding cirrhotic patients, such aggressive correction of clotting abnormalities is generally not necessary. If the patient's INR is less than 2.5 and the platelet count is greater than 20,000, the risk of a significant bleeding complication is minimal.

## APPROACH TO ANTICOAGULANTS AND ASPIRIN PRODUCTS

### Anticoagulants

Patients on chronic anticoagulation pose a particular challenge because bleeding may complicate many commonly performed endoscopic procedures. The American Society for Gastrointestinal Endoscopy (ASGE) recommends (9) the following when deciding whether to discontinue/reverse anticoagulation:

1. The urgency of the endoscopic procedure being considered

    a. If the procedure is *elective* and the indication for anticoagulation is temporary (e.g., deep vein thrombosis), then the procedure should be delayed until the patient is off anticoagulation.

    b. If the indication for the procedure is an *emergency* (e.g., gastrointestinal bleeding), then FFP to reverse anticoagulation should be used (target INR of 1.5).

2. The bleeding risk of the endoscopic procedure being considered

    a. *Diagnostic* endoscopic procedures (with or without pinch biopsy), including esophogogastroduodenoscopy (EGD), endoscopic ultrasound (EUS), endoscopic retrograde cholangiopancreatography (ERCP) without sphincterotomy, enteroscopy, colonoscopy, and flexible sigmoidoscopy, can generally be performed *without* changing the patient's anticoagulation.

    b. *Therapeutic* endoscopic procedures, including polypectomy, sphincterotomy, esophageal dilation, variceal sclerotherapy/banding, and feeding tube placement, generally require the interruption of oral anticoagulation.

3. The underlying medical disease prompting the need for chronic anticoagulation

    a. If the indication for anticoagulation is *low risk* for thromboembolism (Table 1.2), oral anticoagulation may be stopped for 3 to 5 days prior to the *therapeutic* procedure.

**Table 1.2.  Patient risk for thromboembolism (9)**

| Low risk: consider stopping anticoagulation 3 to 5 days prior to procedure | High risk: consider heparin as a bridge periprocedure |
| --- | --- |
| Nonvalvular atrial fibrillation | Atrial fibrillation with valvular heart disease |
| Mechanical heart valve in aortic position | Mechanical heart valve in mitral position |
| Bioprosthetic heart valve | Mechanical valve and prior thromboembolic event |
| Mechanical heart valve in aortic position | |
| Deep vein thrombosis | |

From Eisen GM, Baron TH, Dominitz JA, et al. Guideline on the management of anticoagulation and antiplatelet therapy for endoscopic procedures. *Gastrointest Endosc* 2002; 55(7):775-779, with permission from Elsevier.

   b.  If the indication for anticoagulation is *high risk* for thromboembolism (Table 1.2), then either unfractionated intravenous heparin or subcutaneous low-molecular-weight heparin should be considered to "bridge" the patient through a *therapeutic* procedure.

## Aspirin/Nonsteroidal Antiinflammatory Drugs

There is good evidence to suggest that endoscopic procedures can be carried out in patients on aspirin products or nonsteroidal antiinflammatory drugs (NSAIDs). The current ASGE guidelines suggest that in the absence of a preexisting bleeding disorder, gastrointestinal procedures can be performed on patients taking these medications (9).

## PREPROCEDURE ANTIBIOTICS

### Subacute Bacterial Endocarditis Prophylaxis

The risk of infection from most gastrointestinal endoscopic procedures is small, and endoscopy has rarely been associated with episodes of bacterial endocarditis (10). Therefore, indiscriminate use of preprocedural antibiotics is discouraged. However, some endoscopic procedures are associated with significant rates of bacteremia, including (11)

Esophageal dilation (22.8%)

Variceal sclerotherapy (15.4%)

Variceal ligation (8.9%)

ERCP in the setting of duct obstruction (11%)

For these four procedures, both the ASGE (12) and the American Heart Association (AHA) (10) agree that *high-risk*

**Table 1.3.   Agents for SBE prophylaxis**

| Penicillin sensitivity | Route of administration | |
|---|---|---|
| | Oral (1 hr prior to exam) | Intravenous (30 min prior to exam) |
| No | Amoxicillin 2 g | Ampicillin 2 g |
| Yes | Azithromycin 500 mg | Clindamycin 600 mg |

patients for endocarditis merit prophylactic antibiotics. *High-risk* patients for endocarditis are those with the following conditions:

a.   Prosthetic cardiac valves

b.   A history of endocarditis

c.   Complex cyanotic heart disease

d.   Surgically constructed systemic-pulmonary shunts

Guidelines vary for patients who are at *moderate risk* for endocarditis and who may undergo one of the four high-risk endoscopic procedures. The ASGE states that there is insufficient data to make a recommendation regarding prophylaxis in these patients. However, the AHA does recommend prophylaxis for those at moderate risk for endocarditis as a result of the following:

1.   Rheumatic valvular disease

2.   Mitral valve prolapse with insufficiency

3.   Hypertrophic cardiomyopathy

4.   Most congenital cardiac malformations

For low-risk procedures (e.g., EGD, colonoscopy, flexible sigmoidoscopy with or without biopsy), both organizations agree that antibiotic prophylaxis is not recommended.

For those patients requiring antibiotics, the choice of regimen depends on whether the patient can take oral medication and whether he or she is allergic to penicillin (Table 1.3).

**Prophylaxis for Percutaneous Endoscopic Gastrostomy**

Infectious complications after percutaneous endoscopic gastrostomy (PEG) placement are well described. Peristomal wound infection is the most common complication, occurring in 4% to 30% of procedures (13). More serious infectious complications (e.g., abscess, necrotizing fasciitis) can also occur. A meta-analysis suggested that antibiotics reduce the absolute risk of infection by 17.5% (number needed to treat = 5.7) (14). The ASGE recommends (12) that all patients receive prophylaxis for this procedure.

Suggested regimen:

Cefazolin 1 g IV (30 minutes prior to the procedure).

**REFERENCES**
1. Informed consent for gastrointestinal endoscopy. *Gastrointest Endosc* 1988;34(3 Suppl):26S–27S.
2. Hermann J. Planning for a safe preparation, endoscopic procedure, and follow-up for patients with diabetes. *Gastroenterol Nurs* 1997;20(6):198–202.
3. Keats AS. The ASA classification of physical statusa recapitulation. *Anesthesiology* 1978;49(4):233–236.
4. Alcain G, Guillen P, Escolar A, et al. Predictive factors of oxygen desaturation during upper gastrointestinal endoscopy in nonsedated patients. Gastrointest Endosc 1998;48(2):143–147.
5. Eisen G, de Garmo P, Brodner R, et al. Can the ASA grade predict the risk of endoscopic complications? *Gastrointest Endosc* 2000;51:AB142.
6. Kimmey M, Al-Kawas F, Burnett D, et al. Electrocautery use in patients with implanted cardiac devices. *Gastrointest Endosc* 1994;40(6):794–795.
7. MacGilchrist AJ, Birnie GG, Cook A, et al. Pharmacokinetics and pharmacodynamics of intravenous midazolam in patients with severe alcoholic cirrhosis. *Gut* 1986;27(2):190–195.
8. McGuire BM. Safety of endoscopy in patients with end-stage liver disease. *Gastrointest Endosc Clin N Am* 2001;11(1):111–130.
9. Eisen GM, Baron TH, Dominitz JA, et al. Guideline on the management of anticoagulation and antiplatelet therapy for endoscopic procedures. *Gastrointest Endosc* 2002;55(7):775–779.
10. Dajani AS, Taubert KA, Wilson W, et al. Prevention of bacterial endocarditis. Recommendations by the American Heart Association. *JAMA* 1997;277(22):1794–1801.
11. Nelson DB. Infection control during gastrointestinal endoscopy. *J Lab Clin Med* 2003;141(3):159–167.
12. Antibiotic prophylaxis for gastrointestinal endoscopy. *Gastrointest Endosc* 1995;42(6):630–635.
13. Safadi BY, Marks JM, Ponsky JL. Percutaneous endoscopic gastrostomy. *Gastrointest Endosc Clin N Am* 1998;8(3):551–568.
14. Sharma VK, Howden CW. Meta-analysis of randomized, controlled trials of antibiotic prophylaxis before percutaneous endoscopic gastrostomy. *Am J Gastroenterol* 2000;95(11):3133–3136.

# Bowel Preps

## Alphonso Brown

Adequate bowel preparation is necessary for all endoscopic procedures. Furthermore, ease of patient administration and adequate patient compliance with the prep instructions are important to achieve successful bowel cleansing. This chapter will provide an overview of the various bowel preparatory regimens utilized in current gastrointestinal (GI) practice.

### INDICATIONS

1. Flexible sigmoidoscopy: The preparation of the bowel for sigmoidoscopy is determined by the indication for procedure. If the sigmoidoscopy is being used to evaluate chronic diarrhea, then the procedure is often performed on an unprepped colon. If the procedure is being performed for colorectal cancer screening or as a diagnostic tool, then a colonic preparation is necessary. If the sigmoidoscopy is being performed in conjunction with a barium enema as a screening tool, then a colonic prep is also required.

2. Colonoscopy: Bowel cleansing is a prerequisite for all colonoscopic evaluations, except when it is unsafe due to obstruction or risk of perforation.

3. Upper endoscopy: Fasting prior to upper endoscopy is required for nearly all elective cases.

4. Physiology studies: The preparation for the performance of physiologic studies also depends upon the indication for the procedure. Individuals undergoing 24-hour pH studies may need to discontinue all acid suppressive medicines or may need to be tested while on their standard dose. Subjects should refrain from taking motility altering agents such as narcotics prior to undergoing esophageal, gastric, or small bowel motility studies.

5. Capsule endoscopy: The preparation for capsule endoscopy is similar to upper endoscopy.

### CONTRAINDICATIONS

1. Flexible sigmoidoscopy/colonoscopy: Use sodium phosphate enemas with caution in individuals with renal impairment, partial colonic obstruction, or ileus because of the risk of fatal hyperphosphatemia. Orally administered colonic cleansing regimens are contraindicated in subjects with high-grade obstruction, ileus, or a known bowel perforation.

2. Upper endoscopy: Upper endoscopy is contraindicated in subjects with known esophageal, gastric, or duodenal perforation. Relative contraindications include severe strictures and tortuosity of the esophagus and large diverticula involving the cervical esophagus.

3. Physiology studies: There are no absolute contraindications to the performance of motility studies. Relative contraindications include patient anxiety and an inability to cooperate with the procedure.

4. Capsule endoscopy: A high-grade stricture or obstruction is a contraindication to capsule endoscopy, and severe motility disorders, such as scleroderma, are relative contraindications.

**PREPARATION**

1. Flexible sigmoidoscopy: The preparation for sigmoidoscopy is determined by the indication. When a bowel prep is required, the patient takes nothing by mouth 6 hours prior to the procedure. Purgatory agents may consist of enemas or oral laxatives. Several studies have compared the efficacy of enema preparations to oral regimens. The results of these studies have been variable with regard to patient acceptance and quality of preparation.

2. Colonoscopy:

    a. Polyethylene glycol (e.g., GoLYTELY). Patients undergoing the GoLYTELY preparation and any other colonoscopy preparation should maintain a clear liquid diet the day before the procedure. This consists of water, strained fruit juices, clear broths, coffee, tea, and non-carbonated clear drinks such as Gatorade or Sprite. The subjects need to take at least 1 gal of the GoLYTELY prep on the day before the procedure by drinking 250 cc of prepared solution every 10 to 15 minutes until 1 gal is consumed. GoLYTELY is available in a plain flavor as well as in a cherry formulation (NuLYTELY). Although this method is often used, the poor taste of the prep and the volume required often make it difficult for patients to fully comply.

    b. Fleet's phospho-soda. The Fleet's phospho-soda prep is similar to the GoLYTELY prep except that only two 1.5-oz doses of the laxative are required. Subjects take the first 1.5-oz dose at about 7 p.m. on the night before their colonoscopy. After consuming the first dose of the prep, they consume at least 10 oz of clear liquid immediately and at least three to five additional glasses of clear liquids (10 oz or greater) before going to bed. On the morning of the procedure at some time between 3 a.m. and 6 a.m. the subject should take the second 1.5-oz dose of the Fleet's phospho-soda followed by the recommended clear liquid consumption. Several studies have shown that the Fleet's prep is well-tolerated, and it has the advantage of requiring smaller volume. For these reasons, the Fleet's bowel prep has replaced the GoLYTELY prep as the preferred method for outpatient bowel preparation in many centers.

    c. Pill-based prep. The oral agent Visicol is a new pill-based prep that requires the subject to take 20 pills over a 1-hour period the night before the procedure. As with the Fleet's prep the subject must also drink copious amounts of clear liquid concomitantly. On the morning of the procedure, the patient takes four Dulcolax tablets to complete the bowel cleansing regimen. Earlier studies using a slightly different variation of the Visicol preparation had efficacy rates equivalent to those of Fleet's phospho-soda and GoLYTELY. Fatal seizures due to prep-induced electrolyte abnormalities have occurred with Visicol.

3.  Upper endoscopy: Preparation for upper endoscopy consists of nothing by mouth 6 hours before the procedure. Occasionally when a large blood clot or bezoar is located in the stomach, a promotility agent such as metoclopramide 10- to 20-mg IV or erythromycin 250-mg IV may be given in advance of the procedure. Large bore orogastric lavage may also be beneficial in those situations.

4.  Physiology studies: Most physiology studies require that the patient take nothing by mouth 6 hours before the procedure. Subjects are also usually required to refrain from taking any medicines which may alter motility such as narcotics and antidiarrheals.

5.  Capsule endoscopy: Individuals undergoing capsule endoscopy are instructed to take nothing by mouth 6 hours before the procedure.

## POSTPROCEDURE

For all of the procedures mentioned above, subjects are free to eat without restriction after recovery from sedation unless their condition prohibits this.

## COMPLICATIONS

The two major complications associated with bowel preps are fluid overload and electrolyte disturbances. Subjects with a history of congestive heart failure or renal failure should be made aware of the possibility of fluid overload. Bowel preps should not be performed on individuals with a known high-grade obstruction, peritonitis, toxic or fulminant colitis, or acute diverticulitis.

## SUGGESTED READINGS

ASGE guidelines. Patient preparation for gastrointestinal endoscopy. *Gastrointest Endosc* 1998;48(6):691–694.

Bell GD. Premedication, preparation, and surveillance. *Endoscopy* 2000;32(2):92–100.

Lazzaroni M, Bianchi PG. Preparation, medication and surveillance. *Endoscopy* 1996;28:6.

# Analgesia and Sedation

## Henning Gerke and John Baillie

It is standard in most countries to perform endoscopic procedures under sedation. Objectives of sedation are to increase patient comfort and to allow a technically successful procedure. These goals can usually be achieved with moderate sedation (formerly named "conscious sedation"), in which the patient responds to verbal contact or light tactile stimulation. Airway patency is maintained, and spontaneous ventilation is adequate. Prolonged procedures (e.g., endoscopic ultrasound, endoscopic retrograde cholangiopancreatography [ERCP]) might require deeper levels of sedation (1,2), but this increases the risks of adverse events. The endoscopy team should be able to detect and manage cardiorespiratory complications and to rescue patients from a deeper level of sedation than that intended. General anesthesia might be indicated if intolerance to sedation or problems in managing respiratory or cardiovascular instability is anticipated.

The following recommendations give guidance on how to perform moderate to deep sedation.

### LEVELS OF SEDATION

1. Minimal sedation (anxiolysis): The patient responds normally to verbal commands. Ventilatory and cardiovascular functions are unaffected.

2. Moderate ("conscious") sedation: The patient is able to respond purposefully to verbal and light tactile stimuli. Ventilatory and cardiovascular functions are maintained.

3. Deep sedation: The patient cannot easily be aroused but responds purposefully to repeated or painful stimuli. Airway support may be required. Spontaneous ventilation may be inadequate.

4. General anesthesia: The patient is not arousable, even after painful stimuli. The ability to independently maintain ventilatory function may be impaired. Cardiovascular function may also be impaired.

### INDICATIONS

1. Rigid and flexible (procto)sigmoidoscopies, rectal endosonography: Sedation is not routinely required. Moderate sedation is optional for anxious patients, anticipation of pain, or therapeutic procedures.

2. Diagnostic and uncomplicated therapeutic upper endoscopies and colonoscopies: Moderate sedation is required.

3. Prolonged or complex procedures (e.g., ERCP, endosonography): Deeper levels of sedation may be required.

## CONTRAINDICATIONS FOR MODERATE TO DEEP SEDATION

### Absolute

1. Unstable patient: Resuscitate first

### Relative

2. Children

3. Uncooperative patients (i.e., incompetent, mentally ill)

4. Severe comorbidity

5. Difficult airway

6. Anticipated intolerance to standard sedatives (see "Pre-procedure Evaluation" under "Preparation")

For contraindications 2 through 6 consider anesthesiology assistance.


## PREPARATION

### Preprocedure Evaluation

1. Obtain a medical history and perform a physical examination including vital signs, auscultation of heart and lungs, and airway assessment. Consider the following patient factors that might alter the response to sedation and analgesia or indicate difficulties in airway management.

   | | |
   |---|---|
   | Morbidity: | Abnormalities of major organ systems |
   | Difficult airways: | Sleep apnea, marked obesity, short neck, reduced mouth opening, large tongue (Mallampati classification), anatomical abnormalities |
   | Risks of aspiration: | Acute upper gastrointestinal bleeding, gastric outlet obstruction, delayed gastric emptying, achalasia |
   | Reduced tolerance/ paradoxical reactions to standard sedatives: | Tobacco/alcohol/substance abuse, previous adverse experience with sedation, neuropsychiatric disorder, allergies, and drug interactions |

2. Consider procedure-related factors that might influence the target level of sedation/analgesia: degree of pain involved, expected findings, and interventions.

3. Require preprocedure fasting (at least 2 hours for clear liquids, 6 hours for meals).

4. Obtain written consent.

5. Establish a vascular access, which should be maintained throughout the procedure and until the patient is no longer at risk for cardiorespiratory depression.

6. Document baseline vital signs and oxygenation.

## SEDATIVE/ANALGESIC AGENTS, EQUIPMENT, AND PERSONNEL

### Sedative/Analgesic Agents

1. Benzodiazepines (midazolam, diazepam): Midazolam is often preferred over diazepam because of its shorter duration of action, lack of active metabolites, and better amnestic properties. Midazolam is also much less likely than diazepam to cause chemical phlebitis.

2. Opioids (meperidine, fentanyl, morphine, hydromorphone) are added for an additional sedative effect and for analgesia. Meperidine can produce seizures and accumulates in patients with renal impairment. It has been withdrawn from use in many U.S. centers. Fentanyl has a more rapid onset of action and shorter half-life and is therefore easier to titrate. Hydromorphone can be used as a replacement for patients in whom meperidine and fentanyl show limited effect.

## ALTERNATIVES FOR PATIENTS WHO ARE DIFFICULT TO SEDATE

1. Adjuncts to benzodiazepine/opioid combinations: These drugs should be reserved for selected cases due to the risk of oversedation and adverse effects.

   a. Droperidol: Neuroleptic agent with sedative and antiemetic effects. Caveat: Droperidol has been associated with QT prolongation and life-threatening arrhythmias. Its use should be limited to selected cases and requires special precautions including preprocedural electrocardiogram (ECG) evaluation and ECG monitoring (1). Give 2.5 mg to 5 mg intravenously (IV) prior to the procedure as an adjunct to benzodiazepine/opioid combinations.

   b. Promethazine: 25 mg to 50 mg IV.

2. Propofol: Short-acting hypnotic for inducing general anesthesia. In subhypnotic doses it is used for moderate to deep sedation. It can be combined with midazolam or short-acting opioids (fentanyl). High patient satisfaction, extremely rapid onset, short duration of action, and fast patient recovery are attractive properties of propofol. Caveat: Oversedation resulting in a state of general anesthesia with impairment of respiratory and cardiovascular function can easily occur. No specific antagonist is available. The effects of propofol are usually short lasting due to the rapid clearance. Yet, concerns about the safety in the hands of nonanesthesiologists remain (3,4). Current guidelines require special training under anesthesiologist supervision and advanced cardiac life support (ACLS) certification. Therefore, propofol is not yet in widespread use.

## EQUIPMENT

1. Suction equipment, equipment to administer oxygen, emergency airway equipment, and resuscitation medications

2. Specific antagonists (naloxone, flumazenil) whenever benzo-diazepines and opioids are given

3. A defibrillator immediately available for all patients during deep sedation and for patients with cardiovascular disease during moderate sedation

**PERSONNEL**

1. An individual is dedicated to administering sedative drugs and monitoring the patient throughout the procedure. This individual may assist with minor interruptible tasks during moderate sedation but should not be involved in the procedure during deep sedation.

2. At least one qualified individual trained in basic life support (BLS certification) must be present in the procedure room.

3. An individual with advanced life support skills (tracheal intubation, defibrillation, use of resuscitation medication, ACLS certification) has to be immediately available (within 5 minutes) for moderate sedation and present within the procedure room for deep sedation or sedation with propofol.

**PROCEDURE**

**Application of Sedatives/Analgesics**

1. Titration to the desired level of sedation and analgesia with small incremental doses is preferable to a single dose. Start with a small dose based on the patient's size, age, weight, and comorbidity (i.e., midazolam: 1 mg to 2.5 mg or diazepam: 2.5 mg to 5 mg).

2. Allow sufficient time between doses (at least 2 minutes for midazolam and 3 to 4 minutes for diazepam).

3. Give incremental doses as necessary to reach and maintain the desired level of sedation (midazolam: 1 mg to 2 mg, diazepam: 2.5 mg).

4. Combine benzodiazepines with opioids as necessary for additional sedative effect and/or analgesia (fentanyl: initial dose 25 mcg to 50 mcg, peak effect after 3 to 5 minutes, incremental doses 25 mcg to 50 mcg; meperidine: 25 mg to 50 mg, peak effect after 5 to 7 minutes, repeat infrequently as necessary; morphine: 1- to 2-mg boluses, repeat as necessary).

5. Propofol sedation: Special demands on personnel, training, and monitoring apply because the risk of inducing general anesthesia and apnea is increased. In most U.S. centers propofol is administered by anesthesiologists only. Bolus titration: Give initial bolus of 30 mg to 50 mg over 5 to 10 seconds (caveat: painful injection). Give decreasing incremental doses in minute intervals until the desired level of sedation is reached. Maintenance is with 10- to 20-mg boluses 30 to 60 seconds apart.

**Monitoring During Sedation**

1. Monitor oxygenation and heart rate continuously by pulse oximetry. Pulse oximetry does not substitute for monitoring of ventilation (see below).

2. Monitor respiratory frequency and ventilation (thoracic palpation, observation of abdominal/chest excursions/sensation of exhaled air).

3. Consider capnography during deep sedation/propofol sedation.

4. Give supplemental oxygen during deep sedation (optional during moderate sedation). Rate: 2 to 4 L/min via nasal cannula (reduced rate in patients with severe chronic obstructive pulmonary disease [COPD] or history of hypercapnia).

   Monitor blood pressure at least every 10 minutes and every 2 minutes three times after each dose of IV sedative.

5. Monitor ECG during deep sedation and in selected patients (with significant cardiovascular disease or dysrhythmia) during moderate sedation.

6. Monitor level of consciousness periodically with response to verbal commands and light tactile stimuli (moderate sedation) and response to more profound stimuli (deep sedation).

## POSTPROCEDURE

1. Monitor the patient in a designated recovery area until the consciousness has returned to baseline or close to baseline and the vital signs are stable and within acceptable limits.

2. Resuscitation equipment and an individual capable of managing complications should be immediately available.

3. Prolonged observation (up to 2 hours) after administration of reversal agents is required to ensure that the patient does not become resedated after the effect of the reversal agent has worn off.

## COMPLICATIONS

1. Hypoxia (respiratory depression and/or upper airway obstruction)

2. Hypotension (vasodilation, vagal response, hypovolemia)

3. Aspiration (loss of protective airway reflexes)

4. Allergic reaction

**Management of Hypoxia Unresponsive to Verbal or Tactile Stimulation**

1. Give oxygen/increase flow rate of supplemental oxygen.

2. Assess for upper airway obstruction and perform maneuver accordingly: head tilt, chin lift, jaw thrust, placement of nasal/oral airway.

3.   Administer reversal agents: naloxone (0.4 mg to 2.0 mg, may be repeated in 3 to 5 minutes) to counteract opioid effect, flumazenil (0.2 mg, may be repeated at 1-minute intervals up to a cumulative dose of 1 mg) to counteract benzodiazepine effect. Caution: Reversal of benzodiazepine-induced ventilation might be incomplete.

4.   Perform manual bag ventilation, endotracheal intubation.

**CPT Codes**

**99141** – Moderate (conscious) sedation.

**REFERENCES**

1.   American Society of Gastrointestinal Endoscopy. Guidelines for the use of deep sedation and anesthesia for GI endoscopy. *Gastrointest Endosc* 2002;56(5):613–617.
2.   American Society of Anesthesiologists. Task force on sedation and analgesia by non-anesthesiologists: Practice guidelines for sedation and analgesia by non-anesthesiologists. *Anaesthesiology* 2002;96:1004–1017.
3.   Graber R. Propofol in the endoscopy suite: an anesthesiologist's perspective. *Endoscopy* 1999;49(6):803–806.
4.   Bell GD. Premedication, preparation, surveillance. *Endoscopy* 2002;34(1):2–12.

# Basic Techniques

# Oral and Nasal Gastrointestinal Intubation

## David M. S. Grunkemeier

An increasing variety of gastrointestinal tubes are available. The type of tube selected is determined by its intended use, efficacy, and cost-effectiveness. Due to their tendency to stiffen with time and to produce tissue irritation or necrosis, polyvinyl chloride tubes should generally be relegated to decompression and drainage, gastric lavage, and diagnostic sampling. Pliable small-bore silicone or polyurethane tubes are best for long-term infusion and feeding. In addition, silicone tubes may produce less patient discomfort (1), but reduced clogging and enhanced feeding flow have been reported with polyurethane tubes. Large-bore orogastric tubes are most effective for removing clots.

Indicated below are general features of oral and nasogastric tubes, followed by specific details for each type of tube.

**GENERAL INDICATIONS**

1. Gastric lavage

2. Gastrointestinal feeding and administration of medicines

3. Gastrointestinal decompression

4. Gastrointestinal diagnostic sampling and testing

**GENERAL CONTRAINDICATIONS**

1. Luminal obstruction

2. Severe maxillofacial trauma and/or basilar skull fracture

3. Severe uncontrolled coagulopathy

4. Esophageal varices and severe esophagitis are contraindications to prolonged use of large-bore polyvinyl chloride tubes. More pliable, small-diameter tubes reduce trauma but do not abolish the reflux acid upstream along the exterior surface of the tube ("wick effect").

5. Bulbous disorders of the esophageal mucosa

**GENERAL COMPLICATIONS**

**During Intubation**

1. Nasal or pharyngeal trauma

2. Laryngeal trauma

3. Laryngotracheal obstruction

4. Nasotracheal intubation or transbronchial perforation (2,3)

5.  Esophageal or gastric trauma or perforation (4)
6.  Intracranial penetration, especially in setting of maxillo-facial trauma (5)

**During Use**
1.  Pulmonary aspiration
2.  Gastroesophageal reflux
3.  Mucosal injury, ulceration (1), and, rarely, stricture
4.  Chronic irritation causing rhinitis, sinusitis (6), pharyngitis, otitis media, and, rarely, vocal cord paralysis
5.  Metabolic derangements from loss of electrolytes and fluids

**During Extubation**
1.  Mucosal damage
2.  Entrapment (7)

## GENERAL PATIENT PREPARATION
1.  Give nothing by mouth for several hours.
2.  Explain the procedure to the patient, including route, purpose, and anticipated duration of intubation.
3.  Have the patient sit upright, or raise the head of the bed. If this is not possible, passing the tube with the patient in the left lateral decubitus position has less risk of aspiration than if the patient is supine.
4.  Check for nasal obstruction or maxillofacial trauma. Have the patient inhale briskly through each nostril and use the more patent nostril for intubation.
5.  Test the gag reflex. Patients unable to gag are at increased risk of pulmonary aspiration.

## GENERAL EQUIPMENT
1.  Gastrointestinal tube of choice
2.  A water-soluble lubricant, such as K-Y jelly, is often enough to facilitate passage. However, for topical anesthesia, 1.5 mL of atomized lidocaine may be atomized into the nasopharynx, with 3 mL applied to the oropharynx and swallowed, or 5 ml of 2% lidocaine jelly can be injected into the nostril. Do not use oil-based lubricant.
3.  Cup of water and straw
4.  Emesis basin and towel
5.  Tongue blade and flashlight
6.  Aspirating and irrigating syringes
7.  Tincture of benzoin, scissors, and tape or semipermeable transparent membrane dressing
8.  Stethoscope

## SPECIFIC TUBES
### Styleted Feeding Tubes (e.g., Corpak, Dobhoff)
Review the intended destination of the feeding tube. These tubes are improperly positioned if the feeding ports are located in the respiratory tract or esophagus, past the pylorus for tubes intended for gastric feedings, or in the stomach for feedings intended to be given into the intestine. Postpyloric tube feedings are of no proven clinical benefit compared to gastric tube feedings in most critically ill patients, and waiting for duodenal passage may delay necessary nutrient administration.

*Characteristics*
1. These are long silicone or polyurethane tubes, generally 91 cm to 109 cm in length. Transpyloric feedings require 109-cm tubes.
2. Intraluminal diameter of 5 to 12 Fr
3. Distal tip weighted by a tungsten bolus
4. Placement stylet packaged with tubes
5. Delivery ports encased in nonperforable material for safer reuse of stylet, when necessary
6. Radiopaque markings to aid in fluoroscopic placement
7. Y port to minimize touch contamination and encourage tube flushing
8. Increased pliability, to reduce tissue irritation and increase taping options to the face

*Special Indications*
1. Inability to ingest sufficient nutrients and/or prescribed medications
2. Impaired swallowing or gastric emptying
3. Transition from parenteral to oral alimentation or adjunctive use with limited oral feeding
4. Reduction (but not elimination) of pancreatic or biliary stimulation

*Equipment*
See also "General Equipment."
1. Small-bore feeding tube and stylet
2. 3-cc syringe for aspirating
3. Water and 10-cc syringe to activate hydromer lubricant
4. Liquid silicone lubricant
5. pH testing supplies
6. Metoclopramide, 10 mg to 20 mg for intravenous (IV) or intramuscular (IM) administration to promote passage beyond pyloris
7. Contrast material, if needed

*Procedure for Direct Placement*

1.  Estimate the proper length of tube to be inserted. For 90% confidence of placing the tip 1 cm to 10 cm beyond the cardia in adults, use Hanson's formula (8): (NEX − 50)/2 + 50 cm. Mark the tube 50 cm from its tip. Then, with the patient's head in a neutral position, hold the tip of the tube on the patient's nose and lay the tube along the shortest path from the nose (N) to the earlobe (E) to the xyphoid (X) process. Mark the tube where it reaches the end of the xyphoid. The length of insertion should be halfway between 50 cm and the xyphoid mark. Conventional insertion to the NEX distance placed more than 10 cm of tube in the stomach in 26% of subjects studied. Unless it traverses the pylorus, excess tube in the stomach often loops, pushing the tip into the fundus or cardia.

2.  Lubricate the tube or activate hydromer lubricant, and examine the tube for rough edges or blocked holes. The tube should be emptied of any liquid that might trickle into the trachea. Fix the stylet in place, if packaged separately. In more distal placements, removal of the stylet is easier when it has been previously lubricated with liquid silicone.

3.  With the patient's head tilted down, gently push the tube through the nares, aiming it horizontally. If pointed too high, the tip will abrade the turbinates.

4.  As the tip reaches the posterior pharyngeal wall, have the patient sip water through a straw or initiate dry swallows as the tip is advanced. This is the most uncomfortable part of the procedure. If resistance is met, retract and try again. Do not force the tube. If the patient coughs or is unable to speak, remove the tube as it may be in the trachea. However, smaller tubes do not always elicit these signs. In the unconscious patient, cyanosis may be the first sign of tracheal intubation. Refer to Chapter 19 for methods to prevent inadvertent placement of feeding tubes into the airway.

5.  Pass the tube to the predetermined length, checking that it is not coiled in the patient's pharynx and mouth. Remove the stylet slowly with a slight jiggling motion to reduce adherence to the lumen.

6.  Confirm the tube's placement in the stomach by radiographic imaging. Alternatively, gently aspirate gastric contents with a 3-cc syringe, and check the pH. A pH < 4 suggests the tip is in a gastric location. A pH > 5 does not reliably predict location because the respiratory system and intestinal tract distal to the pylorus often have a pH > 5. Additionally, patients on proton pump inhibitors may not have an accurate pH test. Verifying tube position by auscultation alone is not as helpful because the sounds of air in the bronchial tree can be mistaken for gastric insufflation.

7.  If small bowel placement is desired, after gastric placement is verified, place the patient on his or her right side for

several hours. Maintain 20 cm to 30 cm of tube slack between the taping location on the cheek and the nares, in order to allow further passage of the tube into the duodenum.

8. When the slack has disappeared, have the patient lie on his or her back and then on the left side, to promote the tube's passage into the jejunum. If it has not passed through the pyloris, metoclopramide 10- to 20-mg IV or IM can be helpful. Secure the tube to the nose.

9. Check the tube position fluoroscopically, if necessary. Irrigate with water after using contrast material to avoid clogging.

*Procedure for Endoscopically Guided Placement (9,10)*

Endoscopically guided placement is advantageous in the presence of esophageal diverticula, strictures, tortuosity, and obstructing lesions. This method is also useful for transpyloric placement in the presence of surgical alterations, gastroparesis, and pyloric obstruction.

1. Tie a small loop of umbilical tape to the distal tip of the tube.

2. Pass the lubricated, styleted feeding tube via the nose, into the esophagus.

3. Pass the endoscope into the esophagus.

4. Pass biopsy forceps through the endoscope and grasp the loop of tape on the end of the tube. Guide the feeding tube to the appropriate position.

5. Keep the stylet in place until the endoscope is removed. This prevents backwards displacement of the tube by friction with the endoscope.

6. Confirm tube placement by radiographic imaging (i.e., x-ray) or, if needed, fluoroscopically.

7. Remove the stylet with a gentle jiggling motion.

*Procedure for Endoscopic Wire-guided Tube Placement (e.g., Endo-tube)*

This method is often successful, even in the presence of duodenal stenosis through which an endoscope cannot pass. One disadvantage is the large diameter of the stainless-steel weighted tip of the feeding tube, which must be passed through the nostril.

1. Perform endoscopy to the second or third portion of the duodenum if possible.

2. Using fluoroscopic guidance, advance the guidewire through the endoscope deep into the jejunum. This is facilitated by use of a hydrophilic biliary guidewire (0.035 in.) placed through a standard endoscopic retrograde cholangiopancreatography catheter.

3. With fluoroscopic guidance, remove the endoscope while feeding the guidewire through the channel to maintain a considerable length of guidewire in the jejunum.

4. Using the 8-Fr polyurethane cannula provided, transfer the guidewire from the oral to a nasal exit.

5. Using fluoroscopic guidance, withdraw the guidewire to reduce any gastric looping.

6. Activate the hydromer lubricant by flushing the feeding tube with 20 cc of water.

7. Using fluoroscopic control, pass the feeding tube over the guidewire. Repeated removal of gastric loops may be required for advancement of the tube into the jejunum. Slight withdrawal of the guidewire through the tube may facilitate advancement of the tube.

8. Recheck the tube placement fluoroscopically before feeding.

*Special Complications*
1. Vomiting or aspiration due to displacement of the tube from the small bowel to the stomach, or from the stomach to the esophagus

2. Perforation of the gut because of misuse or reuse of the stylet, or as a result of overzealous use of the stylet to unclog the tube

3. Clogging of the tube due to inadequate irrigation or improper medication instillation techniques (11)

4. Tube rupture as a result of too much irrigation pressure, or the use of an irrigating syringe smaller than 50 cc in size

**Gastric Decompression Tubes (e.g., Salem Sump Tube)**

*Characteristics*
1. Polyvinyl chloride tubes 109 cm to 122 cm long in 12-, 14-, 16-, and 18-Fr diameter (also available in pediatric sizes)

2. Double lumen, one for suction drainage and one for sump vent

3. Radiopaque sentinel line and periodic markings

*Specific Indications*
1. Decompression due to gastric atony, ileus, or bowel obstruction

2. Routinely used to predict high-risk lesions in patients with acute upper gastrointestinal bleeding, though the value of this remains controversial (12)

*Equipment*
See "General Equipment."

*Specific Procedure*
1. Soften the polyvinyl chloride tube in warm water before passing it.

2. Place the tube in the same manner as for feeding tubes except that no stylet is needed.

3. Tube position can be verified by radiographic imaging (i.e., x-ray) or aspiration of gastric contents.

*Specific Complications*
1. Clogging of either or both lumens because of inadequate irrigation
2. Loss of patency of small lumen because of crushing by a clamp
3. Tissue damage because of improper taping at nostril

**Gastric Lavage Tubes (e.g., Edlich, Ewald, Code Blue)**

*Characteristics*
1. Polyvinyl chloride or rubber tubes 91 cm long with 34-Fr outer diameter
2. Large ports

*Specific Indications*
1. To empty the esophagus or stomach of particulate material (i.e., soft bezoars)
2. To irrigate blood clots, toxins, or other substances requiring large-volume lavage

*Equipment*
   See "General Equipment."
1. Overbed table and two large basins. Alternately, use the large water bags provided in the Code Blue kit.
2. Water-resistant covering for the patient's upper body
3. Extra-large lavage syringe (save, wash, and disinfect as per endoscopic equipment)
4. Clamp (large hemostats are more effective than the sliding clamp that is provided)

*Specific Procedure*
1. Pass the well-lubricated tube orally with the head partially flexed.
2. Check position by aspiration and auscultation before initiating lavage.
3. Keep the patient warm if an iced lavage solution is used.

*Specific Complications*
1. Mucosal trauma during insertion or during removal if suction is not released
2. Aspiration if tube is not clamped during removal

**Intestinal Decompression Tubes**

*Characteristics*
1. Andersen Miller-Abbott–type intestinal tube (*AN 22*) 18 Fr, 8 ft (244 cm) with a tungsten-weighted, inflatable latex balloon tip. This is designed for situations when aspiration of liquid and air from the gastrointestinal tract is of therapeutic importance, as in management of early

mechanical obstruction of the small or large intestines. Twenty-four uniquely designed aspiration ports screen out tube-blocking matter. The invaginated tip facilitates easy transnasal passage.

2. Andersen long-weighted sump tube (*AN 20*) 8 ft (244 cm), 16 Fr with a tungsten-weighted distal capsule tip that relies on peristalsis to advance the tube. Designed to be passed transnasally, it can offer an alternative to the Rhefus and Einhorn tubes for diagnostic duodenal aspirations. Low intermittent wall suction diminishes likelihood of damage to the intestinal mucosa. The weighted capsule is easily identified on x-ray for fluoroscopic intubation.

3. The Andersen-type tubes have replaced the older, mercury-based Cantor and Miller-Abbott tubes because of safety issues.

*Specific Indications*
1. To decompress the small bowel

*Equipment*
See "General Equipment."
1. No. 21-gauge needle and 10-cc syringe, for balloon inflation
2. Umbilical tape, which may be used to form a support loop for the tube during its advancement

*Specific Procedures*
1. Read the package insert and retain it in the patient's chart.
2. Do not affix the tube to the nostril until full passage is achieved.
3. Advance the tube according to package insert instructions.

*Specific Complications*
1. Knotting of the tube in the stomach due to premature advance of excess tubing
2. Failure to reach the desired location due to obstruction or motility disorder
3. Tissue damage or necrosis due to inadequate slack during advancement of the tube
4. Passage of the weighted capsule through the anus (rare). If this occurs, cut off the capsule section of the tube and remove the tube according to instructions.

**CPT Codes**

**43752** – Nasogastric or orogastric tube placement, requiring physician's skill and fluoroscopic guidance (includes fluoroscopy, image documentation and report).

**44500** – Introduction of long gastrointestinal tube (e.g., Miller-Abbott) (separate procedure).

## REFERENCES

1. Herrman ME, Lyehr RM, Tanhoefner H, et al. Subjective distress during continuous enteral alimentation: superiority of silicone rubber to polyurethane. *JPEN* 1989;13:281–285.
2. Wendell GD, Lenchner GS, Promisloff RA. Pneumothorax complicating small small-bore feeding tube placement. *Arch Intern Med* 1991;151:599–602.
3. Carey TS, Holcombe BJ. Endotrachial intubation as a risk factor for complications of nasoenteric tube insertion. *Crit Care Med* 1991;19:427–429.
4. Jackson RH, Payne DK, Bacon BR. Esophageal perforation due to naso-gastric intubation. *Am J Gastroenterol* 1990;85: 439–442.
5. Koch KJ, Becker GJ, Edwards MK, Hoover RL. Intracranial placement of a naso-gastric tube. *AJNR* 1989;10(2):443–444.
6. Bos AP, Tibboel D, Hazebroek PW, et al. Sinusitis: hidden source of sepsis in post-operative pediatric intensive care patients. *Crit Care Med* 1989;17:886–888.
7. Jones M. The knotted naso/gastric tube: a simple solution. *Br J Clin Pract* 1989;43:183–184.
8. Hanson RL. Predictive criteria for length of naso/gastric tube insertion for tube feeding. *JPEN* 1979;3:160–163.
9. Stark SP, Sharpe JN, Larson GM. Endoscopically placed nasoenteral feeding tubes. Indications and techniques. *Am Surg* 1991;57:203–205.
10. Rives DA, LeRoy JL, Hawkins ML, Bowden TA Jr. Endoscopically assisted naso/jejunal feeding tube placement. *Am Surg* 1989;55:88–91.
11. Marcuard SP, Stegall KS. Unclogging feeding tubes with pancreatic enzyme. *JPEN* 1990;14:198–200.
12. Abdulrahman M, Fallone Carlo A, Barkun AN. Nasogastric aspirate predicts high risk endoscopic lesions in patients with acute upper-GI bleeding. *Gastrointest Endosc* 2004;59(2): 172–178.

# Esophagogastroduodenoscopy (EGD)

## Kim L. Isaacs

Upper gastrointestinal (GI) endoscopy provides a means for accurate diagnosis and therapy of upper gastrointestinal diseases. The purpose of this chapter is to provide an overview of upper GI endoscopy. It is not intended to be a comprehensive source of instruction. Endoscopic technique and interpretation are best taught by an experienced endoscopist, supplemented by a review of recent inclusive texts (1–4) that outline technique and pathology in detail. Training guidelines have been established by professional societies (5).

## INDICATIONS

### Diagnostic

1. To establish the site of upper GI bleeding
2. To visually define biopsy abnormalities seen on radiological studies (ulcers, filling defects, and cancers)
3. To evaluate healing of medically treated gastric ulcers
4. To evaluate dysphagia, dyspepsia, abdominal pain, gastric outlet obstruction; chest pain after negative cardiac evaluation; and iron deficiency anemia after negative colonoscopy
5. To evaluate odynophagia
6. To determine the extent of damage after a caustic ingestion
7. To sample for infection (e.g., cytomegalovirus) or disease (e.g., graft versus host response) in an immunocompromised host

### Therapeutic

1. Gastric, duodenal, and esophageal polypectomy
2. Removal of foreign bodies
3. Disintegration of bezoars and food impactions
4. Treatment of bleeding lesions with directed thermal or injection therapy
5. Treatment of esophageal varices (banding and/or sclerotherapy)
6. Placement of guidewires or balloons for esophageal and gastric dilatation
7. Placement of small intestinal feeding tubes and percutaneous gastrostomy tubes
8. Palliation of esophageal tumors with tissue vaporization and/or esophageal stent placement

## CONTRAINDICATIONS

### Absolute
1. Shock (unless used as a preoperative to guide emergent surgical therapy)
2. Acute myocardial infarction
3. Severe dyspnea with hypoxemia
4. Coma (unless patient is intubated)
5. Seizures
6. Acutely perforated ulcer or perforated esophagus
7. Atlantoaxial subluxation

### Relative
1. Uncooperative patient
2. Coagulopathy
   a. Prothrombin time 3 seconds over control
   b. Partial thromboplastin time (PTT) 20 seconds over control
   c. Bleeding time > 10 minutes
   d. Platelet count < 50,000/mm$^3$
3. Myocardial ischemia
4. Thoracic aortic aneurysm

## PREPARATION
1. The patient should have nothing by mouth for 6 to 8 hours prior to the procedure. If this is not possible due to the need for emergent EGD, the stomach should be evacuated by means of an orogastric lavage. Intubation for airway protection should be considered in patients who are having vigorous upper gastrointestinal bleeding in which it is not possible to completely evacuate the stomach, such as in variceal bleeding.
2. Review the patient's chart, including x-rays and coagulation studies.
3. See the patient prior to the procedure. Be certain the study is indicated and that the patient understands the risks and benefits and agrees to the procedure. Obtain written informed consent from the patient or his or her legal proxy.
4. Write a preprocedure note that documents cardiovascular and airway assessment, comorbidities, and informed consent.
5. Start an intravenous (IV) line; anesthetize the patient's throat with a topical agent, and attach the pulse oximeter. Oxygen saturation, blood pressure, and pulse rate are routinely monitored during procedures requiring conscious sedation.
6. Administer a short-acting narcotic such as fentanyl through the intravenous line.

7. If needed, slowly administer midazolam (0.75 mg to 2 mg) intravenously until an appropriate level of sedation is reached. Watch the patient carefully for respiratory depression and give preoperative medication cautiously in elderly or malnourished patients. Many patients undergoing diagnostic endoscopy with small-caliber scopes need little if any sedation.

## EQUIPMENT

1. Endoscope of choice. A small-caliber endoscope is routinely used. The endoscope diameters for adult endoscopes typically range from 8.6 mm to 11 mm. Larger endoscopes with multiple channels are used when more complex therapeutic procedures are anticipated. Comparisons of the technical details of commercially available endoscopes have been published (6).

2. Fiber optic light source or video processing monitor depending on the type of the endoscope used

3. Video monitor for video endoscopy or a video adaptor or camera for fiber-optic imaging

4. Biopsy forceps

5. Cytology brush

6. Washing cannula and syringe

7. Computer disc for image storage for video endoscopy or camera

## PROCEDURE

### Passing the Endoscope

1. Administer medication so that patient is sedated but alert enough to assist in swallowing.

2. Place the recumbent patient in the left lateral position with the bite block in place.

3. Hold the scope with the left hand on the controls and the right hand on the shaft at the 25- to 30-cm mark in a partially flexed (60°) configuration.

4. With the patient's neck partially flexed, pass the endoscope through the hypopharynx. Under direct visualization using light pressure, slowly guide the tip of the scope past the epiglottis to rest on the cricopharyngeus, which is located in the midline posterior to the larynx and between the pyriform sinuses, 15 cm to 18 cm from the incisors (Fig. 5.1). Gently insert the endoscope into the esophageal lumen during relaxation of the cricopharyngeus as the patient swallows. Be certain to keep the scope in the midline, out of the pyriform sinuses, and posterior to the larynx.

5. Once the scope has passed the upper esophageal sphincter (20 cm), advance it under *direct vision* at all times and with only enough air insufflation to permit visualization.

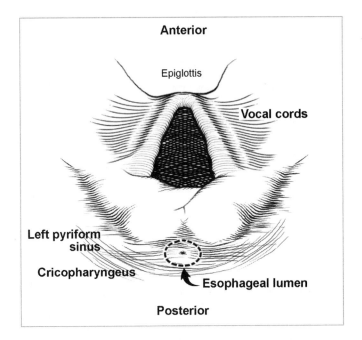

**Fig. 5.1.  View of the hypopharynx and laryngeal structures during endoscopic intubation. The cricopharyngeus is posterior at the 6 o'clock position.**

### Visualization of Esophagus, Stomach, and Duodenum

1.  Advance the scope through the distal esophagus, identifying the gastroesophageal junction by the change from white to coral-colored mucosa ("Z" line) and the lower esophageal sphincter. The level of the diaphragm can be determined by asking the patient to sniff. A hiatal hernia is present if the gastroesophageal junction and gastric folds are above the level of the diaphragm. Barrett's esophagus is identified by an irregular Z line with fingers or islands of pink gastric epithelium extending into the whitish esophageal mucosa.

2.  Observe the motility of the stomach, particularly the antrum, for asymmetry and fixation, as subtle invasive lesions are sometimes suspected from damping of gastric contractions.

3.  Insert the scope through the pyloric channel into the duodenal bulb, then into the second portion of the duodenum by torquing clockwise and turning the tip posteriorly (to the right).

4.  The duodenal bulb and pyloric channel are visualized best by slowly withdrawing the scope while rotating the tip by

torquing the shaft from side to side. Pay particular attention to the superior and posterior portions of the duodenal bulb.

5.  Returning to the stomach, pay special attention to the angulus and the gastroesophageal junction, visualizing both by retroflexion as well as by forward viewing. The endoscope is retroflexed by maximally turning the tip upward so that it is in a J shape. By rotating the retroflexed scope, the entire gastric cardia can be thoroughly visualized.

6.  After thoroughly evaluating the stomach, by slowly withdrawing the scope while rotating the tip in a 360° fashion, remove the excess air from the stomach by suction to minimize abdominal distension.

**Biopsy**

1.  To obtain adequate depth of sampling, gently compress the open biopsy forceps against the mucosa.

2.  It is not necessary to perform a biopsy on a routine duodenal bulbar ulcer unless lymphoma is suspected or if nodularity or a mass is seen.

3.  Always perform a biopsy on a gastric ulcer, unless it is a pyloric channel ulcer or prepyloric erosion that is clearly benign. Biopsies should be performed to include the *margin* of the ulcer in all four quadrants, the base several times, and the mucosa next to the ulcer (i.e., at least six to eight biopsies). Avoid performing a biopsy in an area where there is evidence of active or recent bleeding from the ulcer (clot on the base or visible vessel).

4.  In the case of ulcer disease a biopsy should be taken of the antral mucosa to assess for the presence of *H. pylori*. Take another biopsy from the fundus if the patient is taking a proton pump inhibitor. The biopsy may be used for a rapid urease test (Clotest) or sent for histologic assessment of the presence of *H. pylori*.

5.  Do not perform a biopsy of the esophageal mucosa in a stricture or ring if the patient is to have an esophageal dilatation within a week of the endoscopy. Use the brush for cytology only. However, biopsies can be safely performed *after* dilatation.

6.  Esophageal biopsies can be obtained more easily by turning the tip of the scope toward the mucosa, then partially deflating the lumen.

7.  If the biopsy forceps do not pass through the distal channel, straighten the endoscope and try again.

8.  Larger biopsies of polypoid lesions can be obtained with a snare cautery or "hot" biopsy technique.

**Cytology**

Cytologic examination of possible malignant lesions will complement biopsies by increasing the yield of positive results.

1. Obtain cytologic specimens before biopsies to diminish dilution of cells by blood. Brush suspicious areas (gastric ulcers, mucosal masses) to obtain adequate cellular material. The use of a disposable, retractable brush protected by a plastic sheath will protect the sample from being lost in the biopsy channel of the endoscope.

2. Stroke the brush over a glass slide moistened with normal saline.

3. Place the slide in preservative in a Pap smear bottle.

4. Submucosal cytologic specimens can be obtained from mass lesions by aspiration of saline through a sclerotherapy needle inserted into the lesion.

5. Lesions to be brushed should be cleansed of surface mucus, blood, and exudate by a jet of water through the biopsy channel.

**Subacute Bacterial Endocarditis Prophylaxis**

Subacute bacterial endocarditis (SBE) prophylaxis is not routinely recommended in routine diagnostic upper endoscopy. Limited data is available for patients with high-risk cardiac lesions such as prosthetic valves. With upper endoscopic procedures that increase the risk of bacteremia such as esophageal dilatation and sclerotherapy, routine antibiotic prophylaxis is recommended in high-risk individuals such as those with prosthetic valves. Antibiotic prophylaxis for intermediate-risk patients should be addressed on an individual basis. Complete guidelines, including antibiotic regimens, are available from the American Society of Gastrointestinal Endoscopy (7). These guidelines should be available in a procedure and policy manual in the procedure unit for quick reference.

**MISCELLANEOUS**

1. In patients with achalasia, the esophagus should be emptied of retained food prior to endoscopy with a large-diameter tube and lavage. This will permit better visualization and reduce the risk of aspiration.

2. If esophageal varices are encountered and are not clinically suspected, make sure they are *carefully* documented by multiple observers and photographs.

3. Endoscopic images should be attached to the procedure note to allow the referring physician to visualize the morphologic findings.

**POSTPROCEDURE**

1. Perform vital signs every 3 to 5 minutes immediately following the procedure.

2. Document the procedure with a note that includes the indications for the procedure, the details of procedure performed, medications administered, findings, and recommendations.

3.  Give nothing by mouth until the gag reflex and sensation in the throat return.

4.  The patient should not drive for 6 to 8 hours after conscious sedation. Detailed instructions should be given since many patients do not recall verbal discussions after sedation.

## COMPLICATIONS

Overall complication rates of the procedure and the medications are estimated at 0.13% with mortality in the range of 0.014% (8).

1.  Drug-induced
    a.  Respiratory arrest (0.07%)
    b.  Phlebitis

2.  Perforation (0.033% to 0.1%). The most common sites are the pharynx, upper esophagus, and stomach.

3.  Bleeding (0.03%). This is from biopsies, dislodging clots from bleeding points, and Mallory-Weiss tears induced by retching during endoscopy.

4.  Aspiration (0.08%). The risk can be decreased by giving the patient nothing by mouth, lavaging patients with bleeding or achalasia, and using minimum air insufflation.

5.  Retropharyngeal hematomas and crush injuries

6.  Infection
    a.  Transient bacteremia (5%). There are approximately seven reported cases of bacterial endocarditis temporally associated with upper endoscopy (9).
    b.  There is no evidence of HIV being transmitted by properly cleaned endoscopes and equipment (10).

7.  Complications to the endoscopist
    a.  Bitten finger
    b.  Herpetic conjunctivitis
    c.  Because of the potential transmission of hepatitis and HIV viruses, gloves, gown, and mask should be worn at all times, and all specimens should be handled in accordance with universal precaution guidelines.

## CPT Codes

**43200** – Esophagoscopy, rigid or flexible; diagnostic, with or without collection of specimen(s) by brushing or washing (separate procedure).

**43202** – With biopsy, single or multiple.

**43215** – With removal of foreign body.

**43235** – Upper gastrointestinal endoscopy including esophagus, stomach, and either the duodenum and/or jejunum as appropriate; diagnostic, with or without collection of specimen(s) by brushing or washing (separate procedure).

**43239** – With biopsy, single or multiple.

**43241** – With transendoscopic intraluminal tube or catheter placement.

**43248** – With insertion of guidewire followed by dilation of esophagus over guidewire.

**43255** – With control of bleeding, any method.

**43258** – With ablation of tumor(s), polyp(s), or other lesion(s) not amenable to removal by hot biopsy forceps, bipolar cautery or snare technique.

## REFERENCES

1.  DiMarino A. *Gastrointestinal disease: an endoscopic approach*, 2nd ed. Slack Incorporated, 2002.
2.  Sivak M, Schleutermann D, Zorab R. *Gastroenterologic endoscopy*, 2nd ed. Philadelphia: WB Saunders, 2000.
3.  Nagasako K, Fujimori T, Hoshihara Y, Tabuchi M. *Atlas of gastroenterologic endoscopy: by high-resolution video-endoscope*. Lippincott Williams & Wilkins, 1998.
4.  Cotton P. *Practical gastrointestinal endoscopy: the fundamentals*, 5th ed. Blackwell Publishing, 2003.
5.  Vennes J, Ament M, Boyce H, Cotton P, et al. Principles of training in gastrointestinal endoscopy. *Gastrointest Endosc* 1999;49(6):846–853.
6.  Bosco J, Barkun A, Isenberg G, et al. *SER – Technology status evaluation report gastrointestinal endoscopes*. Oak Brook, Illinois: American Society for Gastrointestinal Endoscopy, 2003.
7.  Hirota W, Petersen K, Baron T, et al. Guidelines for antibiotic prophylaxis for gastrointestinal endoscopy. *Gastrointest Endosc* 2003;58:475–482.
8.  Eisen G, Baron T, Dominitz J, et al. Complications of upper GI endoscopy. *Gastrointest Endosc* 2002;55(7):784–793.
9.  Nelson D. Infectious disease complications of GI endoscopy: Part I, endogenous infections. *Gastrointest Endosc* 2003;57(4): 546–556.
10. Nelson D. Infectious disease complications of GI endoscopy: Part II, exogenous infections. *Gastrointest Endosc* 2003;57(6): 695–711.

# Small Bowel Enteroscopy

## Includes Stoma and Pouch Endoscopy CPT Codes

### Sauyu Lin and Michael A. Shetzline

The evaluation of small bowel diseases has long been a diagnostic dilemma for gastroenterologists. Unlike examinations of the colon or upper gastrointestinal (GI) tract, evaluation of the small bowel is more difficult and complex. The average length of the small bowel (6 m to 7 m), its free intraperitoneal location, and its active contractile pattern make endoscopic exams challenging. Given this endoscopic challenge, physicians have often resorted to radiologic contrast imaging to evaluate the small bowel; however, the multiple overlying loops of bowel make contrast studies less than optimal. Studies such as small bowel follow-through and enteroclysis have diagnostic yields as low as 5% to 10% in the evaluation of patients with obscure gastrointestinal bleeding (1,2). This experience has made endoscopic visualization a critical component of the workup of small bowel disorders. With the appropriate expertise, adequate visualization of the small bowel mucosa can be safely achieved by the use of small bowel enteroscopy (3,4). Thus small bowel enteroscopy has been used increasingly for investigation and treatment of small bowel disorders.

There are currently three different approaches to small bowel enteroscopy: push enteroscopy, sonde enteroscopy, and intraoperative enteroscopy. Compared to the regular upper endoscope, the standard push enteroscope is longer and more rigid, allowing for deeper intubation into the small intestine. The push method is currently the most commonly used method because the procedure itself is not distinctly different from that of conventional upper endoscopy. The prolonged procedure time and the inability to perform therapeutic intervention or diagnostic biopsies have made sonde enteroscopy a rarely performed intervention. Intraoperative enteroscopy, as its name implies, is invasive and used only in selected cases.

## PUSH ENTEROSCOPY

### Indications

1. Obscure overt gastrointestinal bleeding
2. Obscure occult gastrointestinal bleeding
3. Iron deficiency anemia with a negative upper endoscopy and colonoscopy
4. Radiographic abnormalities found in the proximal and/or mid-small bowel
5. Evaluation of patients with polyposis syndrome
6. Placement of a percutaneous jejunostomy tube

**Note:** Indications such as anemia not otherwise specified, chronic abdominal pain, and chronic diarrhea with malabsorption have been found to have conflicting diagnostic yields. The utility for these indications is unknown (5).

## Contraindications (Similar to Those of Upper Endoscopy)

*Absolute*

1.  Bowel perforation, known or suspected
2.  Bowel obstruction, known or suspected
3.  Severe respiratory distress (unless the patient is on mechanical ventilation)
4.  Atlanto-axial subluxation
5.  Hemodynamic instability
6.  Inability to provide adequate sedation

*Relative*

1.  Uncooperative patient
2.  Acute myocardial infarction
3.  Small bowel ileus
4.  Coagulopathy
    a.  Prothrombin time 3 seconds over control
    b.  Partial thromboplastin time (PTT) 20 seconds over control
    c.  Bleeding time >10 minutes
    d.  Platelet count < 50,000/mm$^3$

## Equipment

1.  A dedicated push enteroscope (available from various manufacturers) should be used; however, a pediatric colonoscope may be substituted based on availability. The length of the average small bowel enteroscope is approximately 200 cm to 220 cm.
2.  Light source and video system
3.  Air and water supply
4.  Lubricating jelly, gloves, eye protection, protective gown, shoe covers, and washcloth
5.  60-cc syringe for flushes, biopsy forceps, cautery equipment/epinephrine injections as indicated for hemostasis
6.  Continuous electrocardiogram and pulse oximetry monitoring

## Preparation (Similar to Upper Endoscopy)

1.  Have the patient fast overnight (NPO for at least 8 hours).
2.  The patient should stop taking aspirin, nonsteroidal antiinflammatory drugs (NSAIDs), antiplatelet medications, and warfarin for one week.
3.  Informed consent should be performed in writing prior to initiation of the procedure.

4.   Place an intravenous line for administration of sedation.

5.   Antibiotic indications are the same for small bowel enteroscopy as for upper endoscopy.

6.   Sedation medications: a combination of midazolam and fentanyl. It is important for the endoscopist to realize that there are two parts of the exam in which patients may experience difficulty: first, passage through the upper esophageal sphincter (UES) and second, deep intubation into the proximal jejunum. During conventional upper endoscopy, passage through the UES elicits the most discomfort due to the more limited flexibility of the scope tip. The rest of the endoscopic exam is usually uncomplicated, and in the absence of therapeutic intervention, patients rarely require further sedation. During push enteroscopy, a detailed examination of the small bowel mucosa may require significantly more time, and patients may need additional sedation.

7.   Procedure times for push enteroscopy are often longer than standard endoscopy because of deeper intubation into the small bowel. Thus a deeper level of sedation is recommended for patient comfort. Close attention must be paid to respiratory and blood pressure status.

8.   Place the patient in the left lateral decubitus position similar to that of a routine upper endoscopy. Gently flex the patient's head toward the chest prior to insertion of push enteroscope.

**Procedure**

1.   Under direct visualization, pass the scope over the tongue and across the epiglottis to the cricopharyngeous muscle. This should be approximately 20 cm. With gentle pressure, traverse the upper esophageal sphincter, esophagus, and stomach slowly, closely examining the mucosal for abnormalities. Up to 46% of patients with a prior upper endoscopy for obscure gastrointestinal blood loss were found to have a diagnostic lesion within reach of the standard endoscope on push enteroscopy exam; therefore, a complete examination of this region must be performed (5).

2.   When performing small bowel enteroscopy, a complete view of the stomach, including retroflex visualization of the cardia and lower esophageal sphincter (LES) should occur prior to enteroscope passage through the pylorus. With deep intubation of the small bowel, the cardia and LES may experience "scope trauma." Differentiating this trauma from true pathology may be difficult. Also, finding a significant lesion, such as a Cameron's erosion in the setting of obscure GI blood loss, may be diagnostic.

3.   Use of an overtube may reduce significant gastric looping. Small bowel studies have suggested that intubation may be deeper with the use of the overtube, although diagnostic yield was not statistically higher in the overtube group (6,7). However, most enteroscopy complications have been related to use of an overtube, and patient intolerance may

be increased (7,8). For these reasons, as well as improved enteroscope stiffness, the use of the overtube has lost favor over the past several years (5).

4. Once in the duodenum, the scope should be slowly advanced. Always keep the tip of the scope centered in the bowel lumen. Advancement should be taken slowly, oftentimes waiting for the bowel to relax prior to navigating around flexures. Insufflation should be kept to a minimum. Excessive small bowel air not only increases patient discomfort, but also makes the procedure more difficult.

5. Inspection of the mucosa should be done during intubation as well as during withdrawal of the endoscope.

6. Intravenous (IV) glucagon (0.5 mg to 1 mg) may be given to reduce small bowel motility, thus improving mucosal examination; however, the timing of administration should be carefully selected, since IV glucagon has a very short half-life (minutes). Early administration will also slow peristalsis and may make intubation more difficult (8).

7. Working channels are present for diagnostic biopsies and therapeutic hemostasis. Cautery should be performed at lower energy settings because of the thinner wall of the small intestine.

8. Gastric and small bowel loops may cause difficulty in passing instruments through the channel. Early insertion of the biopsy forceps or heater probe into the scope prior to intubation of the small bowel may prevent this situation. In addition, "shortening" of the enteroscope prior to passing instruments may also help. Shortening occurs by pulling the enteroscope back and thus removing redundant loops while maintaining deep intubation.

9. Estimating the depth of insertion is difficult because of looping, which occurs in the small bowel and stomach. To minimize the inclusion of gastric loops in the calculation of the total length of the small bowel examined, the length of intubation may be measured as centimeters from the ligament of Trietz. A good push enteroscopy exam should reach the midjejunum. Accurate notation of enteroscope intubation can only be defined by passage beyond the ligament of Trietz under fluoroscopic view. It is important to note that fluoroscopic views have confirmed that complete 150- to 160-cm enteroscope insertion may not result in passage beyond the ligament of Trietz.

10. Average procedure time should be longer than a routine upper endoscopy. A well-performed push enteroscopy should reasonably take approximately 15 minutes.

11. Diagnostic yield is dependent on the indication for the procedure. Push enteroscopy has a yield of approximately 40% to 60% for obscure gastrointestinal bleeding, 41% to 78% for abnormal radiographic studies, 6% to 42% for iron deficiency anemia, and 0% to 45% for chronic diarrhea. Chronic abdominal pain and nonspecific anemia have yields of $\leq 25\%$ (5).

**Complications (5,9,10)**

1. Discomfort
2. Bleeding (<1%)
3. Perforation (<1%)
4. Aspiration
5. Medication reactions
6. Mucosal damage
7. Oversedation
8. Hypotension
9. Tachycardia
10. Procedure intolerance
11. Hypoxia
12. Drug reaction
13. Major complications, which include perforation, bleeding, infection, and significant cardiovascular collapse such as arrhythmias and shock, may occur in 0.64% to 1% of procedures.
14. Other complications reported in the literature, such as mucosal stripping, acute pancreatitis, and pharyngeal tears, are very rare and have been related to the use of the stiffening overtube.

**SONDE ENTEROSCOPY**

Sonde enteroscopy was introduced in 1977 as a method of visualizing the entire small bowel. The longest sonde enteroscope measured 400 cm, although the average length is approximately 270 cm. The main indication for the use of sonde enteroscope is the evaluation of obscure gastrointestinal bleeding. The sonde enteroscope is much less rigid than standard endoscopes, has minimal tip deflection (up and down only), and does not have working channels for biopsy or hemostasis equipment. The sonde procedure is also time-intensive and labor-intensive, and the diagnostic yield is comparable to push methods (11). For these reasons, and because of the availability of capsule endoscopy (see Chapter 36), sonde enteroscopy has fallen out of favor for evaluation of the small bowel.

**Preparation**

1. Video equipment to document the endoscope withdrawal is advised because bowel looping and lack of endoscope control result in rapid withdrawal periods, and review of a video at slow speed may result in improved diagnostic frequency.
2. The balloon is tied to the end of the endoscope and inflated prior to insertion to ensure no tears or problems with inflation are present. A prolene suture is tied to the distal tip of the endoscope.

3.  Appropriately trained endoscopic staff should be available to monitor the patient during sonde passage (up to 6 to 8 hours).

4.  Medications such as metoclopramide should be available to enhance peristalsis.

**Procedure**

1.  Advance the sonde enteroscope through the nose into the stomach. Once it is in the stomach, a standard endoscope or enteroscope (called the carrier scope) is passed orally. The tip of the sonde enteroscope carries an inflatable balloon and a prolene suture. Forceps from the carrier scope grasp the suture, and the sonde enteroscope is "carried" into the duodenum. Once in the distal duodenum, the balloon is inflated, and the sonde scope is allowed to move via peristalsis into the small bowel. Metoclopramide 10-mg IV may assist movement of the scope down the small intestine. The progress of the scope is followed by fluoroscopy.

2.  Average time for the sonde endoscope to reach the ileum is 6 to 8 hours.

3.  Careful mucosal inspection of the small bowel occurs during withdrawal of the enteroscope; unfortunately, withdrawal is complicated by rapid movement around loops. A nurse or assistant performing dedicated abdominal pressure during the withdrawal phase may improve mucosal visualization.

4.  Success rate for intubation of the terminal ileum is approximately 80%.

5.  Due to small bowel anatomy and limited control of tip deflection, only 40% to 70% of small bowel mucosa is adequately examined, even when the terminal ileum is reached.

6.  Complications occur in approximately 10% of patients with epistaxis being the most common. Perforation of small bowel ulcers has also been reported.

7.  Diagnostic yield is approximately 40% to 50%, comparable to push methods (12).

## INTRAOPERATIVE ENTEROSCOPY

Intraoperative enteroscopy is the most compete, as well as the most invasive, method of evaluating the small bowel. Indications are similar to those of push enteroscopy. All patients undergoing this procedure should have had an extensive negative standard workup, including a negative push enteroscopy and capsule endoscopy (see Chapter 36).

**Procedure**

1.  An open laparotomy is the most common surgical procedure, and the surgeon should perform a meticulous inspection of the entire gastrointestinal tract at that time. If gross inspection does not localize a lesion, a total small bowel enteroscopy is performed in a darkened room to better define vascular lesions through transillumination of the bowel by the enteroscope light source.

2.  A standard push enteroscope or sonde enteroscope is the best instrument for this procedure. The gastroenterologist commonly introduces the scope orally, although intubation via a surgical enterotomy or via the anus has been performed. Once in the stomach, the surgeon slowly guides the bowel over the scope. An assistant isolates a 15-cm segment of the bowel and pinches the distal portion, trapping air within the segment and allowing careful mucosal inspection by the gastroenterologist without over-distention (air-trapping technique) (13).

3.  Use of longer enteroscopes, primarily the sonde instrument, may allow for complete visualization of the entire small bowel from oral intubation. If length or extensive air trapping hampers complete visualization of the small bowel from the oral route, retrograde views of the distal ileum via anal intubation should be performed.

4.  Unlike standard endoscopy procedures, careful mucosal examination is performed during intubation because trauma (tactile and endoscopic) will be induced during endoscope insertion and bowel manipulation. Regions of iatrogenic trauma should not be mistaken for the etiology of the bleeding during withdrawal of the endoscope.

5.  Complications related to endoscopy are relatively rare. Small bowel ileus and mucosal tears have been reported.

6.  Diagnostic yields may be as high as 70%. Unfortunately, a large percentage of these patients (over 50%) have recurrence of bleeding even after initial surgical intervention (14).

## CPT Codes

**44360** – Small intestinal endoscopy, enteroscopy beyond second portion of duodenum, not including ileum; diagnostic, with or without collection of specimen(s) by brushing or washing (separate procedure).

**44361** – Small intestinal endoscopy, enteroscopy beyond second portion of duodenum, not including ileum; with biopsy, single or multiple.

**44363** – Small intestinal endoscopy, enteroscopy beyond second portion of duodenum, not including ileum; with removal of foreign body.

**44364** – Small intestinal endoscopy, enteroscopy beyond second portion of duodenum, not including ileum; with removal of tumor(s), polyp(s), or other lesion(s) by snare technique.

**44365** – Small intestinal endoscopy, enteroscopy beyond second portion of duodenum, not including ileum; with removal of tumor(s), polyp(s), or other lesion(s) by hot biopsy forceps or bipolar cautery.

**44366** – Small intestinal endoscopy, enteroscopy beyond second portion of duodenum, not including ileum; with control of bleeding, any method.

**44369** – Small intestinal endoscopy, enteroscopy beyond second portion of duodenum, not including ileum; with ablation of tumor(s), polyp(s), or other lesion(s) not amenable to removal by hot biopsy forceps, bipolar cautery, or snare technique.

**44372** – Small intestinal endoscopy, enteroscopy beyond second portion of duodenum, not including ileum; with placement of percutaneous jejunostomy tube.

**44373** – Small intestinal endoscopy, enteroscopy beyond second portion of duodenum, not including ileum; with conversion of percutaneous gastrostomy tube to percutaneous jejunostomy tube.

**44376** – Small intestinal endoscopy, enteroscopy beyond second portion of duodenum, including ileum; diagnostic, with or without collection of specimen(s) by brushing or washing (separate procedure).

**44377** – Small intestinal endoscopy, enteroscopy beyond second portion of duodenum, including ileum; with biopsy, single or multiple.

**44378** – Small intestinal endoscopy, enteroscopy beyond second portion of duodenum, including ileum; with control of bleeding, any method.

**44380** – Ileoscopy, through stoma; diagnostic, with or without collection of specimen(s) by brushing or washing (separate procedure).

**44382** – Ileoscopy, through stoma; with biopsy, single or multiple.

**44385** – Endoscopic evaluation of small intestinal (abdominal or pelvic) pouch; diagnostic, with or without collection of specimen(s) by brushing or washing (separate procedure).

**44386** – Endoscopic evaluation of small intestinal (abdominal or pelvic) pouch; with biopsy, single or multiple.

## REFERENCES

1. Rabe FE, Becker GJ, Besozzi MJ, et al. Efficacy study of the small bowel examination. *Radiology* 1981;140:47–50.
2. Rex DK, Lappas JC, Maglinte DD, et al. Enteroclysis in the evaluation of suspected small intestinal bleeding. *Gastroenterology* 1989;97:58–60.
3. Standards of Practice Committee. Complications of upper GI endoscopy. *Gastrointest Endosc* 2002;55:784–793.
4. Standards of Practice Committee. Enteroscopy. *Gastrointest Endosc* 2001;53:871–873.
5. Lin S, Branch MS, Shetzline M. The importance of indication in the diagnostic value of push enteroscopy. *Endoscopy* 2003;35:315–321.
6. Taylor ACF, Chem RYM, Desmond PV. Use of an overtube for enteroscopy—does it increase depth of insertion? A prospective study of enteroscopy with and without an overtube. *Endoscopy* 2001;33:227–230.
7. Benz C, Jakobs R, Riemann JF. Do we need the overtube for push-enteroscopy? *Endoscopy* 2001;33:658–661.
8. Cotton P, Williams C. *Practical gastrointestinal endoscopy.* Oxford: Blackwell Science, 1996.
9. Wilmer A, Rutgeerts P. Push enteroscopy. Technique, depth, and yield of insertion. *Gastrointest Endosc Clin North Am* 1996;6:759–776.
10. Yang R, Laine L. Mucosal stripping: a complication of push enteroscopy. *Gastrointest Endosc* 1995;41:156–158.

11. Seensalu R. The sonde examination. *Gastrointest Endosc Clin North Am* 1999;9:37–59.
12. Berner J, Mauer K, Lewis B. Push and sonde enteroscopy for the diagnosis of obscure gastrointestinal bleeding. *Am J Gastroenterol* 1994;89:2139–2142.
13. Delmotte J, Gay G, Houcke P, et al. Intraoperative endoscopy. *Gastrointest Endosc Clin North Am* 1999;9:61–69.
14. Ress AM, Benacci JC, Sarr MG, et al. Efficacy of intra-operative enteroscopy in diagnosis and prevention of recurrent, occult gastrointestinal bleeding. *Am J Surg* 1992;163:94–98.

# Endoscopic Retrograde Pancreatography

## Nina Phatak and Michael L. Kochman

Endoscopic retrograde cholangiopancreatography (ERCP) is an endoscopic procedure in which fluoroscopy is employed to allow visualization of endoscopically placed contrast in the pancreatic and biliary ductal systems. Since the introduction of magnetic resonance cholangiopancreatography (MRCP) nearly a decade ago, the focus of ERCP has begun to shift from both a diagnostic and therapeutic modality to a mostly therapeutic interventional method (1,2). However, diagnostic utility of ERCP remains an essential cornerstone in the repertoire of use of this technique. It allows for the evaluation of acute and chronic processes, is often needed to assess pancreatic and ductal anatomy prior to operative and radiologic intervention, and is always a required portion of an endoscopic therapeutic intervention. Therefore, diagnostic ERCP should be performed by those who are capable of proceeding with and completing the required endoscopic therapeutic interventions and should not be performed as a separate procedure (3).

### INDICATIONS

1. Evaluation and therapy of selected patients with obstructive jaundice (4) and biliary strictures (including postoperative)
2. Evaluation and therapy of choledocholithiasis
3. Evaluation and therapy for recurrent pancreatitis of unknown origin
4. Evaluation and therapy of patients with suspected bile leaks
5. Evaluation and therapy of patients with suspected ampullary neoplasms
6. Evaluation and therapy of patients with suspected intrahepatic biliary tract disease
7. Evaluation and therapy of pancreatic ductal diseases
8. Evaluation and therapy of biliary and pancreatic trauma

### CONTRAINDICATIONS

1. Uncorrected coagulation abnormalities
2. Suspected visceral perforation
3. Uncomplicated acute pancreatitis

### EQUIPMENT

1. Side-viewing duodenoscope
2. Water-soluble lubricant to aid passage of duodenoscope

3.  Sterile ionic (or nonionic) contrast agent and syringes

4.  Sterile water and sterile water bottles. Infectious complications are well recognized due to the use of nonsterile water bottles.

5.  Various ERCP catheters. The catheter tip may be of any number of different designs; it is important that the tip be radio-opaque to aid in localization during fluoroscopy. The lumen of the catheter will typically permit the passage of a 0.035-in. guidewire, which is considered a standard size. Various catheter designs are available from a variety of manufacturers, including specialized catheters for minor duct cannulation and Bilroth II anatomy. A review of individual preferences and design differences is beyond the intended scope of this monograph.

6.  Guidewires (various). A number of different wires are typically stocked to aid in the successful completion of the intended procedure. Various wire designs and manufacturers are available. The individual preferences and design differences are beyond the intended scope of this monograph.

7.  Tilting fluoroscopy table (helps to distribute contrast material and to distinguish air bubbles from small stones).

8.  Dedicated fixed fluoroscopic unit or C-arm unit. Spot film ability, recording capability, and digital features are often present.

9.  Radiation shields for the patient and staff

10. Monitors and ancillary equipment as typical for upper endoscopy

Due to the risk of introducing infection in closed spaces, thorough processing of the equipment is mandatory. Single-use catheters and accessories help in this aspect, though exact costs vary unit to unit due to variable acquisition costs and reprocessing overhead.

### PREPARATION OF THE PATIENT

1.  Patients should be instructed to be NPO for 4 hours prior to elective procedures, except for required medications.

2.  Record allergies and daily medications. Dependent upon the nature and severity of the potential allergy, steroids or antihistamines may be given prior to the procedure, or nonionic dyes may need to be used. Though the contrast will be intraductal and rare reports of anaphylaxis to contrast are reported, local policy and custom will dictate the exact response to a reported intravenous (IV) contrast allergy (5). Obtain a social history including drug use and alcohol intake, as this may make conscious sedation difficult, and anesthesiology-assisted sedation may be required if not routinely utilized.

3.  Ascertain whether any recent study using contrast (e.g., computed tomography scan or barium study) was performed, as this may obscure the field and the procedure may best be deferred.

4.   Obtain informed, written consent; ERCP is one of the most litigious areas in gastroenterology (6).

5.   Robust IV access should be in place, with an easily accessible port for the administration of sedating medicine and antimotility agents.

6.   Typically the patient is placed in the left lateral decubitus position with his or her left arm behind the back (this facilitates rolling the patient into the prone position during the procedure). Some endoscopists will start the procedure in the prone position.

7.   Vital signs including heart rhythm, blood pressure, and pulse oximetry should be performed and documented during the procedure as per local standards. Occasionally, continuous monitoring during the procedure is warranted (sepsis, mechanical ventilation, etc.).

8.   If there is concern about cholangitis, or pancreatic or biliary tree infection, systemic antibiotics should be administered. The American Society for Gastrointestinal Endoscopy has recommendations for antibiotic prophylaxis, which are periodically updated (7). See Chapter 1.

**PROCEDURE**

1.   Place the patient in the chosen starting position and sedate in a fashion similar to upper endoscopy (see Chapter 5). Inadequate sedation may result in patient uncooperativeness and may ultimately result in a poor quality study.

2.   Take a baseline plain film of the abdomen to identify artifacts, problematic electrocardiogram (EKG) lead placement, incorrect placement of the groin shield, calcifications, or the presence of prior contrast material.

3.   Intubate the upper esophagus. Due to the rounded tips of the side-viewing duodenoscopes, passage is typically easier compared to an end-viewing upper endoscope. However, passage should be cautious because the region of the upper esophagus will be essentially blindly intubated. Therefore, use gentle pressure. If the scope does not pass easily, a preliminary evaluation with a regular endoscope may be necessary to exclude an unanticipated diverticulum or neoplasm.

4.   With the tip of the duodenoscope straightened (such that a clear view of the forward lumen is not visible), advance the duodenoscope into the stomach. There may be a slight lessening of resistance as it traverses the gastroesophageal junction into the cardia of the stomach.

5.   Examine the stomach by rotating the scope, orienting it to the lesser curve to the upper portion of the visual field, and following it to the antrum.

6.   Once in the antrum, deflect the tip down to view the pylorus. Then angle the tip up to straighten it, and rotate the duodenoscope so the duodenoscope's relationship to the pylorus is such that it is in the 6 o'clock position relative to the pylorus. At this point the tip is raised so that the pylorus

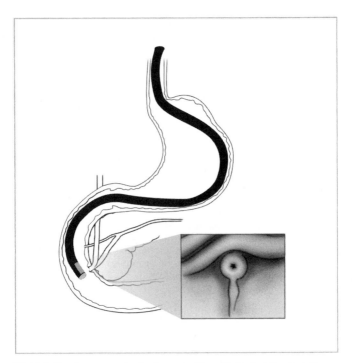

**Fig. 7.1. Duodenoscope in the long position. Reducing the gastric loop to bring the scope into the short position facilitates cannulation. The insert demonstrates an en-face view of the major ampulla, in position for cannulation. The minor ampulla would be approximately 1 cm up and to the right in the 2 o'clock position.**

is not visible, and the duodenoscope is advanced into the pylorus with an essentially blind maneuver.

7. Upon entering the pylorus, there may be slight resistance as the scope is advanced into the duodenum. A slight turn of the hand to the right and a gentle downward deflection of the tip will ease the transition from the bulb into the second portion of the duodenum. If there is altered anatomy or tumor compression, this maneuver may be difficult, and blindly forcing the duodenoscope forward may result in duodenal perforation.

8. Check the position by insufflating with a small amount of air. Slight withdrawal of the duodenoscope and deflecting the tip down and to the left will allow a clear view of the distal lumen.

9. Subsequent to the passage of the duodenoscope into the third portion of the duodenum, a shortening of the scope is required to eliminate the existing loop in the stomach.

10. Although working in the "long" position may appear easy, it can make cannulation and subsequent maneuvers difficult (Fig. 7.1). Shortening can be accomplished by first advancing

the duodenoscope so that it is in the proximal part of the third portion of the duodenum. Then angle the scope tip up so that the scope is in the neutral position and lies in the same longitudinal axis of the lumen. Use the right knob to deflect the tip of the duodenoscope, rotate the duodenoscope scope clockwise, and pull back, removing the loop in the stomach.

11. The papilla should be visible in the second portion of the duodenum. If it is not, then most likely the duodenoscope needs to be withdrawn and rotated further. Occasionally the duodenoscope may have to be advanced; a quick fluoroscopic check may aid in determining the correct secondary maneuver.

12. Once the papilla is identified, roll the patient to the prone position (if the patient was not in that position at the beginning) to facilitate cannulation and spot filming. As noted earlier, some physicians start with the patient in the prone position and only place the patient on his or her side if there is difficulty in entering the duodenum. Position the papilla so that it is at the 12 o'clock position. This positioning is the key to the success of cannulation (Fig. 7.2).

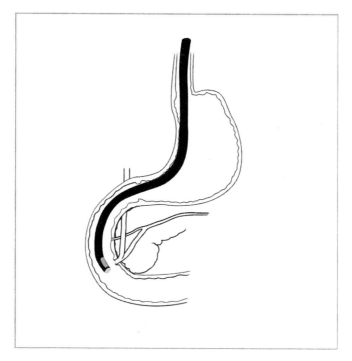

**Fig. 7.2. Duodenoscope in the short position, which generally favors cannulation.**

13. Remove any bubbles that are interfering with clear visualization with a simethicone flush or by adding simethicone to the water bottle. If excessive motility is present, glucagon (0.2-mg IV) or atropine may be used to control peristalsis.

14. Flush the ERCP catheter with the contrast solution in advance of cannulation. In addition to checking the catheter's function, this prevents air from being introduced into the biliary system (which confounds evaluation for choledocholithiasis). For stones, half-strength dye may allow smaller stones to be visualized.

15. The key to cannulation is to visualize the anatomic position of the ductal system and follow the direction of this with catheter insertion. Often the intraduodenal segment of the common bile duct (CBD) is easily identified. Place the catheter tip perpendicular to the orifice of the papilla, though often an approach from the lower right works better. Advancement of the catheter into the orifice aiming to the left upper side of the ampulla preferentially cannulates the CBD. Make smooth subtle movements of the big knob to move the duodenoscope closer to the papilla, and use the elevator to alter the cannulation angle. While small adjustments with the duodenoscope tip may be needed, frequent manipulations of the scope, such as advancing and retracting, may lead to patient discomfort and dislodgement of the duodenoscope from the duodenum and are best avoided.

16. Once cannulation occurs, inject small wisps of contrast or advance a wire to determine if the desired ductal system has been cannulated successfully. Often the biliary and pancreatic ductal systems have a shared segment.

17. Selectively investigate the pancreatic and biliary ductal systems to obtain the greatest amount of technical information. Injections from the common channel typically do not yield the required amount of contrast in the biliary tree, may increase the risk for pancreatitis, and will decrease the success rate for subsequent interventions.
    a. To access the common bile duct, approach the papillary orifice from the right and below, aiming up and towards the 11 o'clock position.
    b. To access the pancreatic duct, enter at a more head-on position and aim at the 5 o'clock position. A small amount of contrast is needed to opacify the pancreatic duct, while 15 cc to 30 cc may be needed for the biliary tree. Avoid overfilling of either ductal system, especially the pancreas, as this may increase the risk of postprocedure pancreatitis.

18. If contrast injection through the papilla does not adequately demonstrate the pancreatic ductal system and this is the desired duct, then consider cannulating the accessory or minor papilla. Minor papilla cannulation is best accomplished with a more fine-tipped or needle-tip catheter, with the scope in the long position. Secretin may be used to

stimulate the pancreas after methylene blue spraying of the area of the minor duct and may allow identification of the orifice if it is hard to visualize. However, once the pancreatic secretions begin to flow, it may be difficult to inject contrast.

19. Due to the risks of repeated radiation exposure, all personnel should wear lead aprons and thyroid shields. Female patients of child-bearing age should have an additional pelvic shield. A procedure should be in place for women who are pregnant to minimize radiation exposure and to record exposure to the fetus.

20. Use the bare minimum of fluoroscopy (individual hard copies cause less exposure than continuous fluoroscopy), stand as far from the radiation source as possible, use the shields provided with the equipment, and wear a dosimeter to accurately record exposure (8).

## POSTPROCEDURE

1. Keep the patient in the lateral position until he or she is able to control secretions.

2. Monitor vital signs, level of pain, and consciousness until the patient returns to baseline.

3. Once the patient is awake and there are no signs of immediate complications, the patient can begin clear liquids and advance his or her oral intake as tolerated. Some experts avoid giving a full meal until the following day.

4. If there is incomplete contrast drainage from the biliary system, consider giving antibiotics and an alternative drainage procedure (percutaneous transhepatic cholangiography versus repeat ERCP).

5. If there are signs of complications, consider taking appropriate steps such as radiographs, systemic antibiotics, surgical consultation, or hospital admission.

## COMPLICATIONS

1. Pancreatitis occurs in about 5% of most diagnostic procedures, but may approach 30% for sphincter of Oddi manometry (9). This relates both to patient characteristics (young age, normal bilirubin, history of ERCP pancreatitis) and endoscopic maneuvers (frequent pancreatic duct injection, repeated manipulation causing papillary trauma, sphincterotomy, or therapeutic techniques).

2. Hemorrhage is very rare in diagnostic ERCP (≤1%). Major risk factors include coagulopathy, initiation of anticoagulation, cholangitis before ERCP, and low ERCP case volume.

3. Perforation occurs in <1% of ERCPs, and there is increased risk with therapeutic procedures.

4. Cholangitis occurs in up to 6% of ERCPs, particularly if there is failed stone extraction without endoprosthesis placement or incomplete biliary drainage in patients with biliary obstruction.

5. At times it is difficult to determine whether cholecystitis is a direct result of ERCP or if it is due to the natural history of gallbladder stones.

6. Medication-related complications include contrast allergy, allergy to sedative drugs, phlebitis, or cardiopulmonary complications, including aspiration.

## CANNULATION CHALLENGES

Situations where ERCP cannulation is particularly difficult include the following:

1. Periampullary diverticula

2. Windsock deformity of the periampullary region

3. Local invasion of tumor involving the papilla or periampullary region

4. Impacted bile duct stone deforming ampullary landmarks and structures

5. Bilroth II gastrectomy making access into the afferent loop difficult and resulting in an "upside-down" approach to the ampulla, which may be disorienting for some

## ADJUNCTIVE PROCEDURES

1. Bile and pancreatic juice collection: Selective duct cannulation can yield specific ductal juice. Bile can yield information regarding microlithiasis and neoplasia, while pancreatic secretions can be evaluated for evidence of chronic pancreatitis and neoplasia. Intravenous Secretin may be used to stimulate pancreatic secretions, and cholecystokinin (CCK) may be used to aid bile flow. See Chapter 43.

2. Cytology: Using various brushes, biliary and pancreatic ductal specimens can be collected.

3. Papillary, biliary, and pancreatic ductal biopsies can be taken with a variety of forceps designs.

4. Needle aspiration of strictures may be obtained.

5. Remediation of strictures and pseudocysts may be undertaken, as can removal of biliary and pancreatic stones.

## CPT Codes

**43260** – Endoscopic retrograde cholangiopancreatography (ERCP); diagnostic, with or without collection of specimen(s) by brushing or washing (separate procedure).
**43261** – Endoscopic retrograde cholangiopancreatography (ERCP); with biopsy, single or multiple.

## REFERENCES

1. Schofl R. Diagnostic endoscopic cholangiopancreatography. *Endoscopy* 2001;33(2):147–157.
2. National Institutes of Health State-of-the-Science Conference Statement: Endoscopic Retrograde Cholangiopancreatography

(ERCP) for Diagnosis and Therapy. January 14-16, 2002. http://consensus.nih.gov/ta/020/020sos_intro.htm.

3. The Role of ERCP in Diseases of the Biliary Tract and Pancreas. *Gastrointest Endosc* 1999;50:915–920.

4. Baron TH, Mallery JS, Hirota WK, et al. Role of endoscopy in the evaluation and treatment of patients with pancreaticobiliary malignancy. *Gastrointest Endosc* 2003;58:643–649.

5. Kimmey MB, Al-Kawas FH, Carr-Locke DL, et al. Radiographic contrast media used in ERCP. *Gastrointest Endosc* 1996;43: 647–651.

6. Newton J, Hawes R, Jamidar P, et al. Survey of informed consent for endoscopic retrograde cholangiopancreatography. *Dig Dis Sci* 1994;39(8):1714–1718.

7. Hirota WK, Petersen K, Baron TH, et al. Guidelines for antibiotic prophylaxis for gastrointestinal endoscopy. *Gastrointest Endosc* 2003;58:475–482.

8. Larkin CJ, Workman A, Wright RER, Tham TCK. Radiation doses to patients during ERCP. *Gastrointest Endosc* 2001;53(2): 161–164.

9. Freeman M. Adverse Outcomes of ERCP. *Gastrointest Endosc* 2002;56(6 Suppl):S273–282.

# Colonoscopy

## Jerome D. Waye

Colonoscopy is the current standard for the diagnostic evaluation of the large intestine. Using fiberoptic or video versions of the long flexible instrument, every portion of the large bowel can be examined, and therapeutic maneuvers can be performed at any site. A coordinated series of manipulations permits safe intubation through the multiple turns and twists of the colon. An accessory channel allows passage of various instruments through the length of the colonoscope for biopsy or therapy.

### INDICATIONS

The two major categories of indications for colonoscopic examination of the colon are diagnostic and therapeutic.

#### Diagnostic

1. Screening for colorectal neoplasia, the most common indication for colonoscopy
2. Symptom Evaluation
    a. Bleeding, occult or gross, minimal or severe
    b. Change in bowel habits such as new onset constipation or unexplained chronic diarrhea
3. Preoperative/postoperative evaluation of patients with colon cancer
4. Abnormal barium enema examination
5. Screening or surveillance for neoplasia in high-risk patients
    a. Ulcerative colitis or Crohn's disease of long-standing duration that affects a significant portion of the colon
    b. Family history of polyps or cancer
    c. Polyposis syndromes such as familial adenomatous polyposis or hereditary nonpolyposis colon cancer
    d. Persons over 50 years of age

#### Therapeutic

1. Polypectomy, the most frequent therapeutic intervention during colonoscopy
2. Hemostasis of bleeding lesions
3. Stricture dilation
4. Removal of foreign bodies
5. Decompression (Ogilvie's syndrome or volvulus)

## CONTRAINDICATIONS

### Absolute

1. Peritonitis with or without bowel perforation
2. Acute diverticulitis
3. Recent myocardial infarction or pulmonary embolus
4. Fulminant colitis

### Relative

1. Torrential colonic bleeding
2. Cardiopulmonary instability
3. Poor bowel preparation
4. Uncooperative patient

## PREPARATION

1. Preparation of the patient: The procedure should be explained to the patient in simple terms, and the patient should be informed of the indications for the procedure, alternative therapy, possible complications, and the possibility of overlooking lesions.

2. Bowel preparation: A colon free of solid stool is the goal. See Chapter 2 on bowel preparation. Liquid effluent can be suctioned through the accessory channel of the colonoscope and does not usually pose a problem for visualization. Modern cathartics are such potent bowel cleansers that enemas are only infrequently used. A one-day liquid diet is usually prescribed. The two most commonly used regimens are

    a. Colon "washout": Ingestion of a 4-L balanced electrolyte solution usually provides an adequate preparation. It is taken the night before the procedure for morning examinations, or in the morning for procedures performed in the afternoon. Every 10 to 15 minutes, 250 mL (about 8 oz) of the solution is taken. The solution is iso-osmolar, so there is no shift in fluid or electrolytes providing that no source of sugar is added or taken during the drinking phase (this includes chewing gum, sucking candy, or adding flavors). Because there is little absorption of fluid or sodium, this preparation can be safely utilized in patients with renal disease, congestive heart failure, or other fluid retention syndromes. In the United States, this is available as GoLYTELY or Colyte.

    b. Phosphate of soda provides a clean colon, given in two separate doses of 45 mL taken the evening before and 4 hours before the procedure. Ingestion of fluids is encouraged during this preparation. Because of the possibility of absorption of sodium and phosphate, this is contraindicated in patients with fluid retention syndromes (congestive heart failure, ascites) or renal insufficiency. In spite of its taste (and the possibility of complications), the sodium phosphate preparation has been well accepted because of its small volume as compared to the 4 L required of the electrolyte solution.

3. Medication: Most colonoscopies in the United States are performed with a combination of sedative/analgesic agents. The medications most frequently used are meperidine (Demerol) (25 mg to 50 mg intravenously), or fentanyl (50 mcg to 100 mcg intravenously) in conjunction with a benzodiazepine, usually midazolam in doses of 1 mg to 3 mg intravenously. More potent anesthetic agents such as diprivan are occasionally employed (usually administered by an anesthesiologist).

## EQUIPMENT

1. Colonoscope, either 133 cm or 168 cm in length
2. Light source
3. Image processor
4. Monitoring equipment (pulse, blood pressure, with or without continuous electrocardiogram)
5. Ancillary equipment such as biopsy forceps, snares, electrosurgical unit, injector needle
6. Universal precautions with gloves, gowns, masks
7. Protective coverings for universal precautions: gloves, gowns, masks

## PROCEDURE

Most colonoscopic examinations are performed with the patient in the left lateral position using a one-person technique, although it is possible to perform the procedure with a two-person team. The performance of colonoscopy requires a combination of several maneuvers using a limited number of available options. The operator may inflate with air; deflate with suction; torque the instrument to the right or to the left; use angulation control wheels to manipulate the tip up/down or right/left; push the instrument in or withdraw it; change the patient's position; or use abdominal pressure. These are the only maneuvers that can be used, and the difference between a swift and a slow procedure is the rapidity with which the operator uses the various combinations.

1. After sedation, insert the instrument into the rectum following a digital rectal examination.
2. Use the left hand to control the up/down angulation knob, to provide adjustments of the instrument tip, and to depress buttons which provide suction or air insufflation.
3. Use the right hand to torque (twist) the instrument to provide directional changes while insertion or withdrawal of the shaft is performed simultaneously.
4. Move the right/left angulation knob with either hand.
5. Because of the spiral S-shape configuration of the sigmoid mesocolon, the instrument always tends to loop as it is

being advanced through the sigmoid and into the descending colon. Make frequent attempts to straighten the instrument by withdrawal, usually in a clockwise fashion. This removes the obligatory loop caused by the mesenteric attachments.

6. The colon can be pleated onto the instrument shaft by jiggling the scope with rapid in-and-out motions during intubation, usually with clockwise torque (Fig. 8.1).

7. Advance the colonoscope under direct vision, never blindly; pushing the scope is only done after the direction of the lumen has been visually identified.

8. A trained endoscopist can reach the cecum 90% to 95% of the time. Persons who have not been taught the specific techniques of colonoscopy have a much lower probability of cecal intubation.

9. Estimate scope position by identifying intraluminal landmarks. For example, the descending colon appears as a long

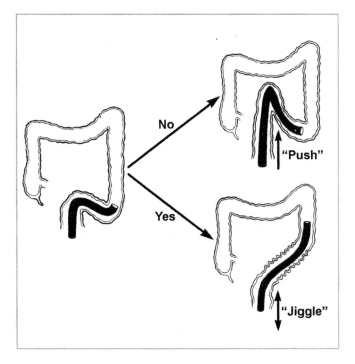

Fig. 8.1. Techniques for advancing the endoscope in difficult situations. Pushing the endoscope through areas of angulation tends to form loops. A series of gentle but rapid in-and-out motions sheaths the colon on the endoscope and tends to straighten the bowel, thus permitting advancement.

circular tube; the transverse colon has triangular folds; the ascending colon is large in diameter and usually has golden brown stool effluent; and the cecum is identified beyond the ileocecal valve by noting the appendiceal orifice. These are relatively gross approximations, with the only absolute positional markers being the rectum and cecum. Modern endoscopists only rarely use fluoroscopy during the course of colonoscopy. A positioning device is available that relies on electromagnets within a special instrument to create a computer-generated image of the colonoscope shaft on a dedicated monitor. The location and configuration of the shaft is extremely accurate, and it can be used as an aid during difficult colonoscopy, as well as for teaching purposes.

10. Obtain single or multiple biopsies at any site in the large bowel. Because of the inability to precisely localize a specific lesion in the colon, as well as the increasing popularity of laparoscopic colon operations (and the inability to palpate the bowel during surgery), it is often desirable to place a permanent marker in the colon wall at the site of a tumor that may need subsequent surgery or at an area that requires subsequent colonoscopic identification, such as for follow-up of a polypectomy. Accomplish this by injecting a solution of carbon particles into the sub-mucosa at the desired location, permitting lifelong visualization from both the mucosal and serosal aspects of the bowel.

11. Intubate the ileocecal valve during colonoscopy using withdrawal techniques, torque, and tip deflection simultaneously after reaching the cecal caput (Fig. 8.2).

12. Visualize the colon using withdrawal once the cecum has been intubated. This is the most important phase of the examination because the straightened instrument provides the ability to easily torque the instrument right or left, making it possible to visualize the large bowel's entire mucosal surface.

13. Perform a retroflexion maneuver in the rectum to completely visualize the distal-most portions of the rectal ampulla.

14. Even though colonoscopy is the best way of looking at the mucosal surfaces of the colon, lesions can possibly be overlooked during the examination. Inadequate preparation may cause this, but hasty withdrawal of the instrument or polyps hidden behind folds of the colon may cause this as well. Reports using tandem colonoscopies have demonstrated that 24% of lesions may be missed during routine colonoscopic examinations, but most of these are relatively small lesions, in the size range of 1 mm to 4 mm wide. It is unusual to miss any lesion equal to or more than 1 cm wide.

## THERAPEUTIC COLONOSCOPY

The most common therapeutic application during colonoscopy is the removal of colon polyps, which has been shown to decrease dramatically the incidence of colon cancer.

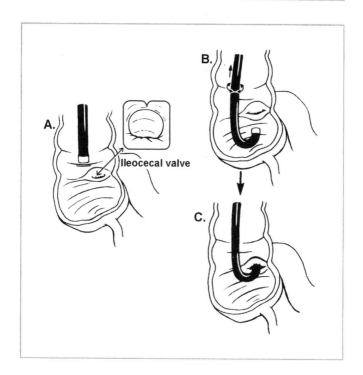

**Fig. 8.2. Cannulation of the ileocecal valve.** The valve orifice is directed downwards and away from the endoscope. Cannulation can be accomplished by (A) advancing the endoscope beyond the fold and (B) turning into the fold and slowly withdrawing the scope while gently torquing the shaft back and forth. The tip will "pop" through the valve and advance into the ileum (C).

1. Place a wire lasso (snare) over the polyp, and close it while applying electrocautery current. This usually results in severance of the polyp with complete hemostasis.

2. Note that the colon wall, distended with air, is quite thin (varying from 1.7 mm to 2.3 mm throughout its entire length), and removal of polyps with cautery current has the possibility of thermal damage to the full thickness of the colon wall.

3. Control of bleeding can be accomplished during emergency colonoscopy, which is usually done for acute diverticular bleeding or for bleeding from vascular ectasias.

4. Strictures (most often caused by anastomotic narrowing) can be dilated with rigid balloons passed through the colonoscope channel, and stents can be inserted through obstructing cancers to open the channel in inoperable patients.

## POSTPROCEDURE

Recovery from the sedative/analgesia takes 30 minutes to 2 hours. Because of the prolonged effects of medication, the patient should be informed beforehand that driving is not permitted for several hours and that someone should accompany the patient to the procedure in order to safely see him or her home. A brief note in the medical record should contain the following information:

1. Indication for procedure
2. Type of instrument used
3. Medication given and dosages
4. The most proximal portion of the intestinal tract intubated (e.g., cecum or terminal ileum)
5. Procedures performed (e.g., biopsy, polypectomy)
6. Detailed description of findings
7. Procedural difficulties (e.g., excessive pain, poor preparation, complications)
8. Postprocedure condition of the patient
9. Follow-up plan

## FOLLOW-UP

The American Cancer Society recommends a 10-year interval for repeat colonoscopy following a negative screening examination. Shorter intervals are required if symptoms develop, if adenomas have been removed, or if patients have an increased risk for colonoscopic neoplasia.

## COMPLICATIONS

1. Cardiopulmonary: The most common complications during colonoscopic examinations are related to the cardiopulmonary system, with bradycardia, hypotension, and reactions to various sedation medications.

2. Perforation: More serious complications such as perforation occur in less than two per thousand diagnostic examinations; however, the incidence of perforation is approximately doubled during therapeutic applications of colonoscopy. Almost all traumatic perforations occurring during the course of colonoscopic examinations will require surgery for repair. Laparoscopic surgery has been reported to be successful in the closure of traumatic perforations, most of which occur in the sigmoid colon because of expansile pressure on a loop in this region causing rupture of the bowel. It is unusual to actually place the tip of the instrument through the bowel wall during intubation. Perforations that may occur postpolypectomy can often be handled conservatively provided that the patient does not develop signs or symptoms of peritonitis.

3.  Bleeding: Bleeding can occur following polypectomy and has been reported in approximately 1% of patients from whom colon polyps are removed. Most bleeding can be controlled at the time of polypectomy, but late bleeding may occur up to 2 to 3 weeks following removal of a colon polyp.

## CPT Codes

**45378** – Colonoscopy, flexible, proximal to splenic flexure; diagnostic, with or without collection of specimen(s) by brushing or washing, with or without colon decompression (separate procedure).

**45380** – Colonoscopy, flexible, proximal to splenic flexure; with biopsy, single or multiple.

**45381** – Colonoscopy, flexible, proximal to splenic flexure; with directed submucosal injection(s), any substance.

**45383** – Colonoscopy, flexible, proximal to splenic flexure; with ablation of tumor(s), polyp(s), or other lesion(s) not amenable to removal by hot biopsy forceps, bipolar cautery, or snare technique.

**45384** – Colonoscopy, flexible, proximal to splenic flexure; with removal of tumor(s), polyp(s), or other lesion(s) by hot biopsy forceps, bipolar cautery, or snare technique.

**45385** – Colonoscopy, flexible, proximal to splenic flexure; with removal of tumor(s), polyp(s), or other lesion(s) by snare technique.

**45391** – Colonoscopy, flexible, proximal to splenic flexure; with endoscopic ultrasound examination, for colonoscopy with EUS.

**45392** – Colonoscopy, flexible, proximal to splenic flexure; with transendoscopic ultrasound guided intramural or transmural fine needle aspiration/biopsy(s), for colonoscopy with fine needle aspiration.

## REFERENCES

Askin MP, Waye JD, Fiedler L, Harpaz N. Tattoo of colonic neoplasms in 113 patients with a new sterile carbon compound. *Gastrointest Endosc* 2002;56:339–342.

Poon CM, Lee DW, Mak SK, et al. Two liters of polyethylene glycol-electrolyte lavage solution versus sodium phosphate as bowel cleansing regimen for colonoscopy: a prospective randomized controlled trial. *Endoscopy* 2002;34:560–563.

Rex DK, Bond JH, Winawer S, et al. U.S. Multi-Society Task Force on Colorectal Cancer. Quality in the technical performance of colonoscopy and the continuous quality improvement process for colonoscopy: recommendations of the U.S. Multi-Society Task Force on Colorectal Cancer. *Am J Gastroenterol* 2002;97:1296–1308.

Rex DK. Colonoscopic withdrawal technique is associated with adenoma miss rates. *Gastrointest Endosc* 2000;51:33–36.

Waye JD, Rex DK, Williams CB, eds. *Colonoscopy: Principles and Practice.* London: Blackwell Publishing, 2003.

Winawer S, Fletcher R, Rex D, et al. Gastrointestinal Consortium Panel. Colorectal cancer screening and surveillance: clinical guidelines and rationale—update based on new evidence. *Gastroenterology* 2003;124:544–560.

# Anoscopy and Rigid Sigmoidoscopy

## Kim L. Isaacs

The routine use of flexible sigmoidoscopy to examine the rectum and distal colon has not alleviated the need for physicians to become proficient in the use of the anoscope and the rigid sigmoidoscope. Most gastroenterologists believe that the anal canal is still most optimally evaluated with the anoscope. It allows for evaluating the anorectum for conditions such as fistula in ano, perirectal abscess, or fissure (1). The anoscope also allows for treatment of lesions in the anal canal and distal rectum. Rigid sigmoidoscopy has a role both in evaluating the distal colon and in certain types of therapeutic maneuvers in the distal colon that cannot be performed with the flexible instrument, such as the topical application of formalin in radiation proctopathy and the removal of foreign bodies. In addition, rigid sigmoidoscopy can be performed anywhere there is an electrical outlet, with largely disposable equipment that does not require expertise for cleaning or maintenance, and without the need for specially trained ancillary personnel. This section will cover the techniques of anoscopy and rigid sigmoidoscopy. Please refer to the section on colonoscopy (Chapter 8) for details related to flexible sigmoidoscopy.

## INDICATIONS (2–5)

1. Symptoms referable to the colon, rectum, or anus: bleeding, discharge, protrusions or swellings, abdominal or anorectal pain, diarrhea, constipation or a change in bowel habits, severe itching

2. Evaluation prior to anorectal surgery (flexible sigmoidoscopy is preferred)

3. To observe the progression or regression of colorectal disease

4. To obtain tissue for histologic study or stool and/or exudate for bacteriologic or parasitologic study

5. To remove foreign bodies from the rectum

6. For applying topical therapy such as formalin in cases of radiation proctopathy (6)

7. To allow for injection therapy such as botulinum toxin injection into the anal sphincter in the treatment of anal fissures

8. As a routine part of the physical examination in areas where flexible sigmoidoscopy or colonoscopy are not available for colorectal cancer screening

## CONTRAINDICATIONS

For anoscopy alone there are no absolute contraindications.

### Absolute
1. Suspected perforation of the rectum

### Relative
1. Acute peritonitis
2. Fulminant colitis/toxic megacolon
3. Acute, severe diverticulitis
4. Uncooperative patient

## PREPARATION
1. Obtain informed consent.
2. Patients with heart disease have an increase in ectopic beats with sigmoidoscopy. Cardiac monitoring and/or awareness of possible arrhythmias in these patients is advised (6).
3. Bacteremia may occur in up to 10% of patients undergoing sigmoidoscopy. Routine antibiotic prophylaxis is not recommended in low-risk to intermediate-risk patients but can be considered in high-risk individuals on a case-by-case basis (7).
4. Most patients can be examined with no prior bowel preparation.
5. If stool precludes an adequate examination, a bisacodyl suppository or Fleet (or other proprietary small volume hypertonic phosphate) enema can be given and the examination carried out following evacuation. Outpatients may take the enema at home 1 to 2 hours prior to procedure.
6. Very rarely, an oral preparation with polyethylene glycol electrolyte solution or phospho-soda will be required the day prior to the procedure.
7. Premedication (sedation) is rarely necessary, although intravenous fentanyl and/or midolazam can be useful in unusual circumstances. Severely painful conditions may require examination under anesthesia or with sedation.

## EQUIPMENT
### Minimal Equipment
1. Anoscope and rigid sigmoidoscope: An adult rigid sigmoidoscope is adequate for all but the infant. The disposable plastic anoscope allows for 360° visualization of the anal canal through the transparent plastic. Nondisposable anoscopes are available that have openings in the side to allow for side viewing as well as end viewing of the anal canal on withdrawal of the instrument (5).
2. Light source
3. Cotton swab sticks

4.  Examination table or bed

5.  Sheet to cover the patient

6.  Gloves, 4-x-4-in. gauze pads, lubricant (2% topical lidocaine may be useful as a lubricant in painful anorectal disease)

**Useful Equipment**

1.  Sigmoidoscopy table or routine exam table with availability of pillows/blankets to position the patient in knee-chest position if necessary

2.  Suction

3.  Air insufflator

4.  Sigmoidoscopy spoon

5.  Biopsy tools: either alligator-type (see "Procedure" section, "Rectal Biopsy with Alligator Forceps"), colonoscopic biopsy forceps taped to a stick, or suction-type biopsy capsule

6.  Epinephrine solution and silver nitrate sticks

**PROCEDURE**

Be gentle and reassuring throughout the procedure. Inform the patient what is to be done. Advise the patient that a few deep breaths during the examination will often relax muscles and sphincters.

**Position**

Position the patient for the examination (2,5).

*Left Lateral (Sims') Position*

This is best for bedridden or feeble patients or to assess anal pathology such as hemorrhoids. Be sure to get buttocks to the edge of the bed or table by placing the patient diagonally across the bed (Fig. 9.1A).

*Knee-chest Position*

This is adequate for most examinations. It requires more patient stamina and cooperation (Fig. 9.1B).

*Prone, Inverted (Jackknife) Position with Sigmoidoscopy Table*

This is the most comfortable position for the patient and the examiner (Fig. 9.1C). Place the patient's knee rest high enough so that the "broken" table does not compress the abdomen. This allows the pelvic organs to "fall away" when the sigmoidoscope is advanced. Elbow rests are preferred so that the patient does not slide off the end of the table.

**Digital Examination**

Inspect the perianal area, and perform a digital examination (5).

1.  If two gloves are worn on the examining hand, some decrease in sensitivity of touch is experienced; however, time is saved because the soiled glove can be stripped off, and one can proceed with anoscopy or sigmoidoscopy.

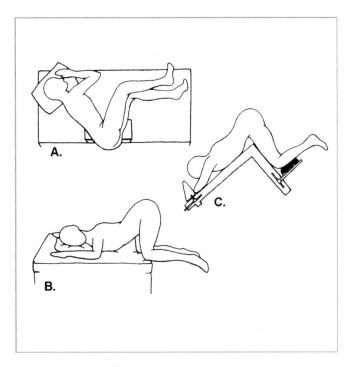

**Fig. 9.1. Three major positions for anoscopy and sigmoidoscopy. A: Left lateral (Sims') position. B: Knee-chest position. C: Prone, inverted (jackknife) position.**

2.  Spread the buttocks apart and inspect the perineum for cutaneous or anal pathology.

3.  Palpate the perianal and perineal tissues for abscesses or fistulae.

4.  Perform the digital exam with a well-lubricated finger. The digital exam relaxes the anal sphincters and facilitates insertion of the scope. Try to palpate any abnormalities you wish to visualize at anoscopy. Sweep the finger circumferentially around the anal canal; a blind spot to sigmoidoscopy is directly posterior and proximal to the anal ring. Examine anteriorly for cul-de-sac lesions; do not mistake the cervix for tumor. Stool from the examining finger can be checked for occult blood.

### Anoscopic Examination

Perform anoscopic examination. The anoscope is most useful to view fissures, fistula openings, internal hemorrhoids, papillitis and cryptitis, and neoplasm.

1.  Insert a clean plastic anoscope. It should be warm and well lubricated.

2. Stabilize the obturator with the thumb, and insert by aiming it toward the umbilicus.

3. After inserting 3 cm to 4 cm, move the tip posteriorly.

4. If anal spasm is encountered, ask the patient to bear down or breathe through the mouth.

5. Visual examination of hemorrhoids with the anoscope is facilitated by having the patient strain (Valsalva) as you remove the anoscope. This is particularly important in the knee-chest position, where internal hemorrhoids may collapse.

6. If there is access to a video-flexible sigmoidoscope, the end of the sigmoidoscope may be inserted into the anoscope with video evaluation (and magnification) on withdrawal of the instrument. This may increase diagnostic yield for small lesions (8).

**Sigmoidoscopy Examination**

Perform sigmoidoscopic examination (2,5).

1. Introduce the sigmoidoscope blindly only for the first 3 cm to 5 cm while stabilizing the obturator with the thumb. Aim toward the umbilicus (Fig. 9.2A). Remove the obturator and, from this point on, advance the sigmoidoscope under direct vision.

2. Swing the tip of the sigmoidoscope posteriorly to follow the curve of the sacrum (Fig. 9.2B). Advance the scope as far as possible.

3. If the lumen is lost, the end of the sigmoidoscope is probably occluded by a valve or the rectal wall or is at the rectosigmoid junction (Fig. 9.2C). Do not push forward! Pull back 2 cm to 3 cm, rotate the scope until the lumen reappears, and then advance (Fig. 9.2D). Often, the tip of the advancing scope can "iron out" a fold or curve and aid in passage. Some examiners insufflate air if the lumen cannot be visualized; however, this may produce some discomfort. The rectosigmoid junction is encountered at 12 cm to 15 cm, and many sigmoidoscopies will end here. Often, this point can be negotiated by straightening the bend with the end of the scope or by insufflating air.

4. Withdraw the scope slowly, rotating the tip circumferentially to observe the entire rectal wall. Check the stool from this point for occult blood. Also test the mucosa for friability. Twirl a swab on the mucosa; remove it and look for capillary bleeding. Look behind the rectal valves of Houston.

**Rectal Biopsy with Alligator Forceps**

1. Unless a specific lesion is to be biopsied, a biopsy of the posterior rectal mucosa should be obtained below the peritoneal reflection (within 7 cm to 10 cm of the anal verge) to lessen the chance of free peritoneal perforation.

2. Biopsies from the free edge of a valve technically are the easiest, but the large biopsy obtained increases the chance of bleeding or perforation. Biopsy from the base of the valve is probably safer.

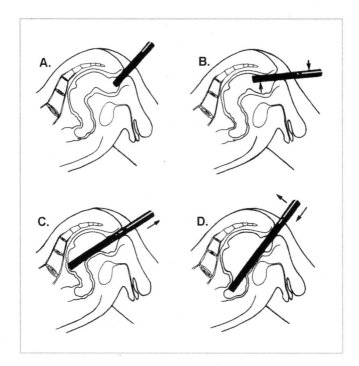

**Fig. 9.2. Sequence of steps of the sigmoidoscopy. A: Sigmoidoscope, with obturator, is inserted, aimed toward the umbilicus. B: With the obturator removed, the tip of the scope is rotated posteriorly and advanced. C: If the lumen is lost, the sigmoidoscope is retracted until the lumen is found. D: The sigmoidoscope is then advanced.**

3. Bleeding can usually be stopped by applying pressure with dry cotton or with epinephrine-soaked swabs (1 mL of 1:1,000 epinephrine diluted 1 to 10 with saline fluid).

4. After the bleeding has halted, the biopsy site may be cauterized with silver nitrate sticks.

**POSTPROCEDURE**

The patient may resume normal activity. Inform the patient that some "gas pains" may be experienced but to notify you if persistent pain or bleeding occurs.

**CPT Codes**

**45300** – Proctosigmoidoscopy, rigid; diagnostic, with or without collection of specimen(s) by brushing or washing (separate procedure).

**45303** – Proctosigmoidoscopy, rigid; with dilation, any method.

**45305** – Proctosigmoidoscopy, rigid; with biopsy, single or multiple.

**45307** – Proctosigmoidoscopy, rigid; with removal of foreign body.

**45308** – Proctosigmoidoscopy, rigid; with removal of single tumor, polyp, or other lesion by hot biopsy forceps or bipolar cautery.

**45309** – Proctosigmoidoscopy, rigid; with removal of single tumor, polyp, or other lesion by snare technique.

**45315** – Proctosigmoidoscopy, rigid; with removal of multiple tumors, polyps, or other lesions by hot biopsy forceps, bipolar cautery, or snare technique.

**45317** – Proctosigmoidoscopy, rigid; with control of bleeding, any method.

**45320** – Proctosigmoidoscopy, rigid; with ablation of tumor(s), polyp(s), or other lesion(s) not amenable to removal by hot biopsy forceps, bipolar cautery, or snare technique (e.g., laser).

**45321** – Proctosigmoidoscopy, rigid; with decompression of volvulus.

**45327** – Proctosigmoidoscopy, rigid; with transendoscopic stent placement.

**46600** – Anoscopy; diagnostic, with or without collection of specimen(s) by brushing or washing (separate procedure).

**46604** – Anoscopy; with dilation, any method.

**46606** – Anoscopy; with biopsy, single or multiple.

**46608** – Anoscopy; with removal of foreign body.

**46610** – Anoscopy; with removal of single tumor, polyp, or other lesion by hot biopsy forceps or bipolar cautery.

**46611** – Anoscopy; with removal of single tumor, polyp, or other lesion by snare technique.

**46612** – Anoscopy; with removal of multiple tumors, polyps, or other lesions by hot biopsy forceps, bipolar cautery, or snare technique.

**46614** – Anoscopy; with control of bleeding, any method.

**46615** – Anoscopy; with ablation of tumor(s), polyp(s), or other lesion(s) not amenable to removal by hot biopsy forceps, bipolar cautery, or snare technique.

**REFERENCES**

1.  Abcarian H, Alexander-Williams J, Christiansen J, et al. Benign anorectal disease: definition, characterization and analysis of treatment. *Am J Gastroenterol* 1994;89:S182–S193.
2.  Bateson M, Boucher I. *Clinical investigations in gastroenterology*, 2nd edition. Hingham, Massachusetts: Kluwer Academic Publishers, 1997.
3.  Goligher J, Duthie H, Nixon H. *Surgery of the anus, rectum and colon.* London: Baillier Tindall, 1980.
4.  Hull T. Examination and diseases of the anorectum. In: Sleisinger M, Fordtran J, eds. *Gastrointestinal disease: pathophysiology, diagnosis, management.* Philadelphia: WB Saunders Company, 2002.
5.  MacKeigan J, Cataldo P. Disorders of the Anorectum. In: DiMarino A, Benjamin S, eds. *Gastrointestinal disease: An endoscopic approach.* Malden, Massachusetts: Blackwell Scientific, 1997.

6. Parikh S, Hughes C, Salvati E, et al. Treatment of hemorrhagic radiation proctitis with 4 percent formalin. *Dis Colon Rectum* 2003;46:596–600.
7. Hirota W, Petersen K, Baron T, et al. Guidelines for antibiotic prophylaxis for GI endoscopy. *Gastrointest Endosc* 2003;58:475–482.
8. Lazas D, Moses F, Wong R. Videoendoscopic anoscopy: A new technique for examining the anal canal. *Gastrointest Endosc* 1995;42:351–354.

# Abdominal Paracentesis

Kimberly L. Beavers

Abdominal paracentesis with appropriate ascitic fluid analysis is probably the most rapid and cost-effective method of diagnosing the cause of ascites (1). Paracentesis is safely and routinely performed in both inpatient and outpatient settings.

## INDICATIONS

1. Evaluation of new onset ascites
2. Evaluation for spontaneous bacterial peritonitis in all patients with ascites and abdominal pain, fever, or unexplained encephalopathy
3. Evaluation for subclinical infection in all patients with ascites admitted to the hospital
4. Treatment of symptomatic ascites

## CONTRAINDICATIONS

Coagulopathy should preclude paracentesis only when there is clinically evident fibrinolysis or clinically evident disseminated intravascular coagulation (2). There is no data to suggest coagulation parameter cutoffs beyond which paracentesis should be avoided (2). Patients with cirrhosis without fibrinolysis or disseminated intravascular coagulation (DIC) do not bleed seriously from needle sticks unless a blood vessel is entered (3).

## PREPARATION OF PATIENT

1. Explain the risks, benefits, and details of the procedure to the patient.
2. Obtain written consent.
3. Ask the patient to empty his or her bladder.

## EQUIPMENT

1. Sterile gloves
2. Iodine solution; sterile gauze
3. Draping towels
4. Local anesthetic (lidocaine, 1%) and needles
5. Syringes: 10 cc, 50 cc
6. Paracentesis needles:
   a. No. 16, 18, 20, or 22 gauge
   b. Spinal needle (No. 18, 20 gauge) for obese patients
7. Sterile specimen tubes
8. Blood culture bottles for bedside inoculation, if infection suspected

## PROCEDURE

### Diagnostic Paracentesis

1. Position the patient in the bed with the head elevated 45° to 90° to allow fluid to accumulate in the lower abdomen.

2. Identify the point of aspiration on either flank, usually two finger breadths cephalad and two finger breadths medial to the anterior superior iliac spine. An alternative location is in the midline midway between the umbilicus and pubic bone. Although the midline is avascular, the abdominal wall in the left lower quadrant is thinner, and there is usually a larger pool of fluid than the midline (4). Be careful to avoid abdominal wall scars, as bowel may be fixed to the wall. The rectus muscles should also be avoided because the epigastric arteries travel within the rectus sheath (Fig. 10.1).

3. Confirm dullness to percussion in the site selected for needle entry.

4. Put on sterile gloves.

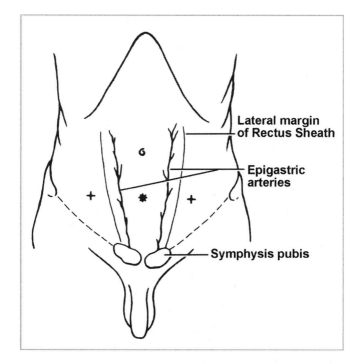

**Fig. 10.1. Various sites of paracentesis. (+) preferred; (*) secondary.**

5.  Sterilize the site with an iodine solution.

6.  Arrange sterile draping towels.

7.  Infiltrate the skin and subcutaneous tissue with a local anesthetic.

8.  Attach a 20- or 22-gauge needle to a 10-cc syringe. Spinal needles (3.5-in. needles) are needed only in the setting of a large panniculus.

9.  Insert the needle into the peritoneal cavity using a "Z-tract" to minimize leakage of ascites after the procedure. To create a Z-tract, use one gloved hand to move the skin approximately 2 cm in any direction in relation to the deep abdominal wall, and then insert the paracentesis needle. The skin is not released until the needle has penetrated the peritoneum and fluid flows. When the needle is removed, the skin slips back into its original position and seals the leak. Although not backed by data, the theory behind the Z-tract maneuver is that if the needle is inserted directly into the fluid without a Z-tract, the straight line of flow allows fluid to leak out more easily.

10. Advance the needle in 5-mm increments, with gentle aspiration of the syringe between needle advancements while the needle is stationary. If no fluid returns after several attempts, ultrasonography can be used to identify a site.

11. When fluid is flowing, stabilize the needle to ensure a steady flow, and attach a larger syringe to the needle. It is not unusual for flow to stop as bowel or omentum are suctioned over the bevel of the needle. When flow stops, twist the needle 90° and reinsert in 1- to 2-mm increments.

12. For a diagnostic paracentesis, at least 25 mL of ascites is required.

13. Remove the needle, and place an adhesive bandage or pressure dressing over the site. The patient may resume normal activities.

**Therapeutic Paracentesis**

A therapeutic paracentesis is similar to diagnostic paracentesis except that a larger bore needle (15- to 18-gauge) is used, and much greater amounts of fluid are removed. The removal of at least 5 L of fluid is considered a large volume paracentesis. Removal of all ascites (total paracentesis), even greater than 20 L, can be safely performed (5).

1.  Obtain the necessary equipment including a paracentesis tray with paracentesis catheter (7 in. long, with no. 14-gauge × 2-in. needle) and multiple 1-L vacuum bottles.

2.  Prepare the patient as for diagnostic paracentesis. Select the paracentesis site as described above. Clean and drape the selected site. Infiltrate the skin and subcutaneous tissue with local anesthetic.

3. Place an intravenous heparin lock if an albumin infusion of 5 g for each liter removed has been planned. Albumin has been recommended for removal of greater than 5 L to minimize increases in renin and aldosterone, and, therefore, to minimize volume depletion (5). However, no study has demonstrated a survival advantage for patients who have received albumin.

4. Using the paracentesis catheter attached to a 10-cc syringe, slowly advance the needle and catheter into the peritoneal cavity using the Z-tract technique. Intermittently aspirate fluid until a steady flow is achieved.

5. Attach tubing to the catheter and insert it into a 1-L vacuum bottle, or attach to a wall suction with a large canister.

6. Aspirate 4 to 6 L of ascitic fluid using this apparatus over 30 to 60 minutes.

7. Remove the catheter, and place a bandage or absorbable suture at the puncture site. A pressure bandage may be applied.

8. Send a sample of fluid from each paracentesis for white blood cell count and differential to detect the onset of unsuspected bacterial peritonitis.

## ANALYSIS OF FLUID

The analysis of the aspirated fluid will be determined by the individual patient and his or her presentation. If uncomplicated cirrhotic ascites is suspected, the initial laboratory investigation should include at least an ascitic fluid cell count and differential, total protein, and albumin (Table 10.1) (6). If the results of these tests are unexpectedly abnormal, further testing can be performed.

**Table 10.1.  Testing of ascitic fluid**

| Recommended |
| --- |
| Cell count and differential |
| Albumin |
| Culture |
| Gram stain |
| Glucose |
| Lactate dehydrogenase (LDH) |
| **Optional (depending on clinical setting and ascites appearance)** |
| Amylase |
| Triglycerides |
| Bilirubin |
| Tuberculosis staining |
| Cytology |

If ascitic fluid infection is suspected by the presence of fever, abdominal pain, or unexplained encephalopathy, bacterial culture in blood culture bottles should be performed at the bedside. Cell counts should be obtained. If there is concern for secondary bacterial peritonitis, total protein, lactate dehydrogenase, and glucose are obtained. Other studies, such as acid-fast bacilli (AFB) smear and culture, cytology, triglycerides, and bilirubin, can be ordered based on pretest probability of disease. Ascitic fluid profiles for various disease states appear in Table 10.2.

**Table 10.2. Ascitic fluid profiles**

| Type of ascites | Typical paracentesis findings |
| --- | --- |
| Portal hypertensive ascites | Clear, straw-colored fluid, with ascitic fluid neutrophil count of < 250 cells/mm$^3$; high serum-ascites albumin gradient (SAAG), i.e., serum albumin minus ascitic fluid albumin > 1.1 g/dL. |
| Spontaneous bacterial peritonitis | Ascitic fluid neutrophil count of > 250 cells/mm$^3$ (need to subtract 1 polymorphonuclear neutrophil (PMN) for every 250 red blood cells [RBCs] in hemorrhagic ascites); some variants may have as few as 100 cells/mm$^3$. Usually a single offending microbe. Glucose usually > 50 mg/dL. |
| Secondary bacterial peritonitis | Ascitic fluid neutrophil count of > 250 cells/mm$^3$ (need to subtract 1 PMN for every 250 RBCs in hemorrhagic ascites); surgically treatable intra-abdominal source of infection; often polymicrobial. Glucose usually < 50 mg/dL |
| Chylous ascites | Milky colored fluid, ascites triglycerides > 200 mg/dL, often accompanied by malignant cells, usually low SAAG. |
| Pancreatic ascites | Clear or straw-colored fluid, ascites amylase generally > 200 IU/L. Usually low SAAG. |
| Choleperitoneum (bile leak into ascites) | Brown-tinged fluid, ascites bilirubin > serum bilirubin and greater than 6 mg/dL. |
| Malignant | Often blood-tinged or chylous, may be clear. Usually low SAAG; malignant cells on cytology. |
| Tuberculous | May be clear, chylous, or blood-tinged. Low SAAG; positive smear for AFB. |
| Congestive heart failure | Clear. PMNs < 250 cells/mm$^3$. Usually high SAAG. |

## COMPLICATIONS

The incidence of serious complications from paracentesis is rare (2). Complications were reported in only about 1% of patients (abdominal wall hematomas), despite the fact that 71% of the patients had an abnormal prothrombin time. More serious complications, such as hemoperitoneum or bowel entry by the paracentesis needle, are rare (7). It is the practice of some physicians to give blood products such as fresh frozen plasma or platelets before paracentesis in cirrhotic patients with coagulopathy. This policy is not data-supported.

### CPT Codes

**49080** – Peritoneocentesis, abdominal paracentesis, or peritoneal lavage (diagnostic or therapeutic); initial.

**49081** – Peritoneocentesis, abdominal paracentesis, or peritoneal lavage (diagnostic or therapeutic); subsequent.

### REFERENCES

1. Runyon BA. Management of adult patients with ascites due to cirrhosis. *Hepatology* 2004;39(3):841–856.
2. Runyon BA. Paracentesis of ascitic fluid. A safe procedure. *Arch Intern Med* 1986;146(11):2259–2261.
3. McVay PA, Toy PT. Lack of increased bleeding after paracentesis and thoracentesis in patients with mild coagulation abnormalities. *Transfusion* 1991;13(2):164–171.
4. Sakai H, Mendler MH, Runyon BA. The left lower quadrant is the best site for paracentesis: an ultrasound evaluation. *Hepatology* 2002;36:525a.
5. Tito L, Gines P, Arroyo P. Total paracentesis associated with intravenous albumin management of patients with cirrhosis and ascites. *Gastroenterology* 1990;98(1):146–151.
6. Sartori M, Andorno S, Gambaro M, et al. Diagnostic paracentesis: a two-step approach. *Ital J Gastroenterol* 1996;28(2):81–85.
7. Webster ST, Brown KL, Lucey MR, Nostrantt TT. Hemorrhagic complications of large volume abdominal paracentesis. *Am J Gastroenterol* 1996;91(2):366–368.

# Percutaneous Liver Biopsy

Kimberly L. Beavers

Liver biopsy has a central role in the evaluation of patients with suspected liver disease. Percutaneous biopsy frequently provides important information on the exact nature of a liver disorder and the extent of hepatocellular damage. In addition, it may have prognostic and therapeutic implications. Although percutaneous liver biopsy is safe and is routinely performed, a transjugular approach should be considered when standard liver biopsy is contraindicated. Controversy continues to surround all of the technical aspects of liver biopsy, particularly the choice of needle and the use of ultrasound to mark or guide the biopsy site.

## INDICATIONS

1. Evaluation for liver pathology related to abnormal liver biochemical tests in association with a serologic workup that is inconclusive
2. Diagnosis of suspected primary liver disease
3. Assessment of the grade and stage of chronic liver disease
4. Evaluation of the efficacy and/or side effects of treatment regimens
5. Diagnosis of a liver mass
6. Evaluation of the transplanted liver
7. Evaluation of fever of unknown origin
8. Diagnosis of metabolic disease or multisystem disease
9. Monitoring of the effect of hepatotoxic drugs

## CONTRAINDICATIONS

Several absolute and relative contraindications to standard percutaneous liver biopsy have been generally agreed upon. Acceptable clotting parameters have been defined somewhat arbitrarily. However, some of these contraindications can be corrected by transfusion of platelets or fresh-frozen plasma and are therefore not absolute contraindications. An alternative approach such as transjugular biopsy should be considered in these situations.

Some controversy surrounds the utility of ultrasound-guided liver biopsy to avoid complications and improve diagnostic yield (1,2). In addition, cost-effectiveness has been questioned. To avoid possible complications, ultrasound marking is often used to confirm the biopsy site.

### Absolute Contraindications

1. Uncooperative patient
2. Bleeding tendency

a. Prothrombin time (PT) $\geq$ 3 seconds more than control
b. Partial thromboplastin time (PTT) $\geq$ 20 more than control
c. Platelet count < 50,000/mm$^3$
d. Prolonged bleeding time ($\geq$10 minutes)
e. Nonsteroidal antiinflammatory drug (NSAID) use within 7 days

3. Suspected hemangioma or vascular lesion

4. Inability to identify an adequate biopsy site by percussion and/or ultrasound

5. Massive ascites

6. Suspected echinococcal disease

**Relative Contraindications**
1. Morbid obesity

2. Infection in right pleural cavity

3. Infection below the right hemidiaphragm

**PREPARATION**
1. Complete a history and physical examination, assessing for personal or family history of excessive bleeding.

2. Review medications, particularly those known to affect bleeding parameters.

3. Evaluate coagulation status with prothrombin time, platelet count, and a complete blood count prior to the biopsy. Bleeding time may be considered (3), particularly in patients with renal failure or a history of excessive bleeding.

4. Obtain informed consent.

5. Some centers recommend NPO status prior to biopsy. In patients with an intact gallbladder, some centers recommend a light breakfast containing a small amount of fat to empty the gallbladder to minimize its risk of injury during the biopsy.

6. Conscious sedation is not routinely required. However, premedication with a benzodiazepine +/− a narcotic analgesia has been advocated (4).

7. Review computed tomography (CT) or magnetic resonance imaging (MRI) scans of the liver; this may aid in selection of a biopsy site.

8. Instruct the patient on what to expect and on the need to follow commands regarding respiration.

**SPECIAL SITUATIONS**
1. Chronic renal failure. Biopsy should be performed the day after dialysis. Prebiopsy deamino arginine vasopressin (DDAVP) has been recommended by some, even when traditional clotting studies are normal (5).

2.  Hemophilia. Biopsy can be safely performed after adequate replacement of clotting factors (6).

## EQUIPMENT

There are three different categories of liver biopsy needles.

1.  Aspiration needles (Jamshidi, Klatskin, Menghini)

2.  Cutting needles (Tru-cut, Vim-Silverman)

3.  Spring-loaded cutting needles that have triggering mechanisms

If cirrhosis is suspected, a cutting needle is preferred over an aspiration-type needle to minimize fragmentation of fibrotic tissue. The intrahepatic phase of the biopsy is shorter when using aspiration needles, potentially decreasing the risks of the procedure.

The following supplies will be needed at the bedside for the biopsy:

1.  Liver biopsy tray including biopsy needle, scalpel, gauze, saline, 10-cc syringe, and Betadine

2.  Sterile towels

3.  Gloves

4.  Lidocaine (5 cc of a 1% solution)

5.  Sterile containers for serology and culture specimens

6.  Adhesive bandage

## PROCEDURE

1.  Position the patient supine near the edge of the bed, with his or her right hand under the head and left arm by the left side.

2.  Percuss the area of maximum liver dullness in both inspiratory and expiratory phases over the right hemithorax in the mid-axillary line (usually between the eighth or ninth intercostal spaces), and mark the spot (Fig. 11.1).

3.  Confirm the selected biopsy site with bedside ultrasound. This is not mandatory unless the point of maximum dullness is uncertain.

4.  Disinfect the biopsy site using providone-iodine (Betadine)-soaked gauze pads.

5.  Infiltrate the site with local anesthetic, inserting the needle along the superior margin of the rib in order to avoid the intercostal artery.

6.  Prepare the biopsy needle. If a suction needle is used, attach it to a 10-cc syringe filled with sterile saline.

7.  Make a small skin incision so the needle can be passed easily through the skin.

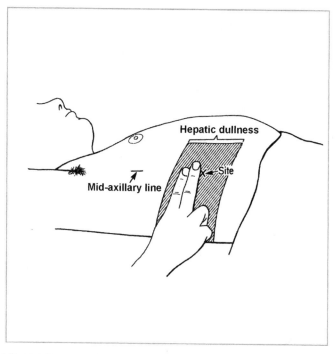

**Fig. 11.1. Percutaneous liver biopsy.**

8.  Insert the biopsy needle through the incision with the tip directed toward the xiphoid process, creating a tract that is parallel to the floor. Guide the needle with the left hand.

9.  After the needle passes through the subcutaneous tissue and the intercostal muscles, flush a small amount of saline into the peritoneal cavity to clear the needle. Place the left hand on the biopsy needle 3 cm from the skin.

10.  While the patient holds his or her breath in expiration phase, apply negative pressure on the syringe plunger, quickly advance the biopsy needle 3 cm within the liver, and come out quickly. Maintain suction at all times.

11.  If at least a 2-cm core of tissue is obtained, transfer the specimen to the appropriate container. Perform a second or third biopsy if more tissue is necessary. Clean the biopsy site and apply a bandage.

12.  Position the patient in the right lateral decubitus position to maintain constant body pressure on the biopsy site for about 2 hours. The patient then remains on bedrest for an

additional 2 to 4 hours, while his or her vital signs are monitored every 15 minutes.

13. Discuss detailed and clearly written postprocedure instructions with the patient before discharge.

## COMPLICATIONS

Sixty percent of complications occur within 2 hours of the procedure and 96% within 24 hours (7).

1. Pain over the liver and right shoulder occurs in 10% to 25% of patients but rarely requires analgesia. Approximately 2% to 3% of patients require hospital admission for management of complications, predominantly pain or hypotension (8).

2. Significant intraperitoneal hemorrhage occurs in 0.08% to 0.32% of biopsies (7,9).

3. Bile peritonitis occurs in approximately 0.09% of biopsies.

4. Pneumothorax and hemothorax are rare, with approximate incidences of 0.0078% and 0.063%, respectively, and seldom require therapeutic intervention.

5. The mortality rate following percutaneous liver biopsy is approximately 1 in 10,000 to 12,000 (9,10).

## CPT Codes

**47000** – Biopsy of liver, needle; percutaneous.
**47001** – Biopsy of liver, needle, percutaneous when done for indicated purpose at time of other major procedure (List separately in addition to code for primary procedure).

## REFERENCES

1. Caturelli E, Giacobbe A, Facciorusso D, et al. Percutaneous biopsy in diffuse liver disease: Increasing diagnostic yield and decreasing complication rate by routine ultrasound assessment of puncture site. *Am J Gastroenterol* 1996;91(7):1318–1321.
2. Friedman LS. Controversies in liver biopsy: who, where, when, how, why? *Curr Gastroenterol Rep* 2004;6(1):30–36.
3. Boberg KM, Brosstad F, Egeland T, et al. Is a prolonged bleeding time associated with an increased risk of hemorrhage after liver biopsy? *Thromb Haemost* 1999;81(3):378–381.
4. Alexander JA, Smith BJ. Midazolam sedation for percutaneous liver biopsy. *Dig Dis Sci* 1993;38(12):2209–2211.
5. Reddy KR, Schiff ER. Complications of liver biopsy. In: Taylor, Gollan, Steer, Wole, eds. *Gastrointestinal Emergencies*, 2nd ed. Baltimore: Williams & Wilkins, 1997:959–960.
6. McMahon C, Pilkington R, Shea EO, et al. Liver biopsy in Irish hepatitis C-infected patients with inherited bleeding disorders. *Br J Haematol* 2000;109(2):354–359.
7. Piccinino F, Sagnelli E, Pasquale G, Giusti G. Complications following percutaneous liver biopsy. A multicentre retrospective study on 68,276 biopsies. *J Hepatol* 1986;2(2):165–173.
8. Janes CH, Lindor KD. Outcome of patients hospitalized for complications after outpatient liver biopsy. *Ann Intern Med* 1993;118(2):96–98.

9. Van Thiel DH, Gavaler JS, Wright H, et al. Liver biopsy: its safety and complications as seen at a liver transplant center. *Transplantation* 1993;55(5):1087–1090.
10. McGill DB, Rakela J, Zinsmeister AR, et al. A 21-year experience with major hemorrhage after percutaneous liver biopsy. *Gastroenterology* 1990;99(5):1396–1400.

# III

# Advanced and/or Secondary Techniques

# Injection Therapy for Hemostasis and Anal Fissures

Lisa M. Gangarosa

Injection therapy in the field of gastroenterology is the directed delivery of a liquid agent into the wall of the gastrointestinal tract or adjacent structures. This is utilized for a variety of indications including but not limited to the following: to treat active GI bleeding from lesions such as esophageal varices, ulcers, arteriovenous malformations, diverticula, and iatrogenic lesions; to deliver botulinum toxin to the lower esophageal sphincter to treat achalasia or to the internal anal sphincter to treat anal fissures; to inject tattooing agents such as India ink submucosally to mark an area; to inject saline submucosally to lift a lesion prior to endoscopic removal; and to inject corticosteroids into refractory strictures prior to dilation.

This chapter will focus on the use of injection therapy for nonvariceal hemorrhage (section 1) and the treatment of anal fissures (section 2).

## HEMOSTASIS

### Indications
1. To achieve, or aid in achieving, the cessation of active bleeding

### Contraindications
1. See contraindications to upper (Chapter 5) and lower endoscopy (Chapters 8 and 9)
2. Known hypersensitivity to hemostatic agent

### Preparation
1. See upper endoscopy (Chapter 5) or lower endoscopy (Chapters 8 and 9)
2. Correct coagulopathy or thrombocytopenia. Goal international normalized ratio (INR) < 1.5, platelet count > 50,000.

### Equipment
1. Appropriate endoscope, lubricant, personal protective equipment (gown, gloves, mask with visor), working intravenous (IV) equipment, sedation medications.
2. Disposable injection needle within sheath (21- to 25-g, 4- to 6-mm needle, various sheath lengths available). These are supplied by a variety of manufacturers. There are no published studies comparing different injection needles (1).
3. A variety of agents are available (Table 12.1) including normal saline, epinephrine (1:10,000), ethanol, ethanolamine, morrhuate sodium, tetradecyl sulfate, polidocanol, and cyanoacrylate ( the last two are not commercially available

**Table 12.1. Strength and dosages of hemostatic agents for gastrointestinal bleeding**

| Hemostatic agent | Strength | Standard dose/site | Maximal total dose |
|---|---|---|---|
| Epinephrine | 1 mg/mL diluted 1:10,000 in normal saline | 0.5 to 2 mL | Unknown, up to 20 mL safe |
| Ethanol | 98% | 0.1 to 0.5 mL | 2 mL |
| Ethanolamine oleate | 5% | 1 to 2 mL | 20 ml |
| Morrhuate sodium | 50 mg/mL | 1 to 5 mL | 20 mL |
| Sodium tetradecyl sulfate | 1% | 0.5 to 2 mL | 10 mL |
| Polidocanol | 1% | 0.5 to 1 mL | 5 mL |
| N-butyl cyanoacrylate | 1:1 with lopiodol | 1 mL | 6 mL |

in the United States). Epinephrine may be used in combination with another agent. The agent of choice is drawn up in 5- to 10-cc syringes (1–6).

**Procedure**

1. Perform diagnostic endoscopy to locate the source of bleeding.

2. Have the assistant attach the syringe with the hemostatic agent of choice to the end of the injection device, and prime the device with the hemostatic agent until a few drops of fluid are seen to exit the needle.

3. Pass the injection device through the working channel until the tip of the sheath comes into endoscopic view.

4. Select the site around the bleeding lesion for injection.

5. Have the assistant advance the tip of the needle beyond the sheath. The assistant, via appropriate mechanism (varies by brand) on the device handle, can adjust the length of the needle protruding from the sheath. The endoscopist then advances the sheath to place the needle tip into the submucosa at the site chosen for injection.

6. Have the assistant push the end of the syringe to deliver the hemostatic agent. If the needle tip is placed appropriately in the submucosa, elevation of the mucosa will be noted. If the needle is too deep, no change will be observed. If the needle is too shallow, liquid will run onto the mucosa. Adjust the needle tip location accordingly, and have the assistant push the desired volume (Table 12.1). If using cyanoacrylate, flush the injection device with 2 to 3 cc lopiodol to fully deliver the adhesive.

7.   Have the assistant retract the needle into the sheath.

8.   Repeat Steps 4 to 7 until either hemostasis is achieved or a maximum volume of hemostatic agent felt to be safe has been delivered (Table 12.1).

9.   Retract the needle into the sheath prior to removing the entire injection device from the endoscope to avoid damaging the working channel of the scope with the needle.

10.  At this point, further adjunctive endoscopic therapy may be used if necessary (see Chapters 13, 14, and 32).

**Postprocedure**
1.   Monitor vital signs.

2.   Follow hemoglobin and hematocrit every 6 to 12 hours for 24 to 48 hours to evaluate efficacy of treatment.

3.   If evidence of rebleeding is observed, the endoscopist may need to repeat the procedure or obtain intervention by a surgeon and/or an interventional radiologist.

**Complications**
   The following are potential complications:

1.   Allergic reaction

2.   Ulcerations

3.   Perforation

4.   Laceration

5.   Infection

6.   Rebleeding

   Complication rates are low and vary by agent and site of injection (1). Other uses for this technique include

1.   To tattoo lesion or site

2.   To lift lesion prior to polypectomy

3.   To inject botulinum toxin into lower esophageal sphincter in patients with achalasia

4.   To inject steroids into refractory strictures

5.   To treat varices

6.   To palliate bulky tumors (1)

**ANAL FISSURES**
**Indications**
1.   To administer botulinum toxin, resulting in temporary decreased anal sphincter pressure. This decreases pain from and promotes healing of anal fissures (7).

**Contraindications**
1.   Hypersensitivity to botulinum toxin

2. Complicated hemorrhoidal disease
3. Active perianal or rectal inflammatory bowel disease

**Preparation**

No preparation is required. However, one should consider conscious sedation if the patient has significant perianal discomfort.

**Equipment**
1. A 1-cc syringe with 27-gauge needle
2. Botulinum toxin A (Botox, Allergan, Irvine, CA; 50 U/mL)
3. Gloves

**Procedure**
1. Perform a digital rectal exam.
2. Palpate the internal anal sphincter on either side of the fissure.
3. Inject 0.2 to 0.25 mL botulinum toxin (50 U/mL) into the internal anal sphincter on either side of the fissure (a total volume of 0.4 to 0.5 mL given). See Fig. 12.1 for location of injection sites.

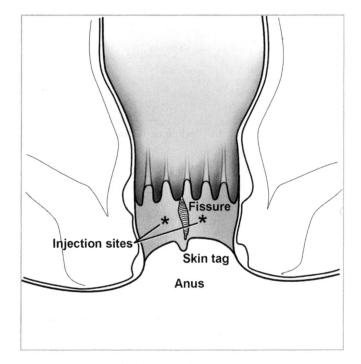

**Fig. 12.1. Schematic of injection sites for Botox treatment of anal fissures.**

**Note:** If the patient is too obese to easily palpate and visualize the fissure, the physician can perform flexible sigmoidoscopy (see Chapter 9).

4. Advance the injection needle through the endoscope. Then, retroflex the endoscope while in the rectum to visualize the anal canal. Inject 0.2 to 0.25 cc botulinum toxin on either side of the fissure.

5. If the anal fissure persists at 2 months, one can re-treat with an additional 25 U of botulinum toxin.

**Postprocedure**

1. Prescribe daily stool softeners and a high-fiber diet.

**Complications**

1. Transient incontinence of flatus (9%)

2. Transient incontinence of stool (5%)

3. Anal hematoma (5%)

4. Flu-like syndrome (3%)

5. Acute inflammation of external anal varices (2%)

6. Epididymitis (<1%)

7. Hemorrhoid prolapse (<1%) (8)

**CPT codes**

**43236** – Upper gastrointestinal endoscopy including esophagus, stomach, and either the duodenum and/or jejunum as appropriate; diagnostic, with submucosal injection.

**43255** – Upper gastrointestinal endoscopy including esophagus, stomach, and either the duodenum and/or jejunum as appropriate; with control of bleeding, any method.

**45334** – Sigmoidoscopy, flexible; with control of bleeding, any method.

**45335** – Sigmoidoscopy, flexible; with submucosal injection.

**45381** – Colonoscopy, flexible, proximal to splenic flexure; with submucosal injection.

**45382** – Colonoscopy, flexible, proximal to splenic flexure; with control of bleeding, any method.

**64640** – Destruction by neurolytic agent; other peripheral nerve or branch.

**REFERENCES**

1. Technology Committee of ASGE. Injection needles. *Gastrointest Endosc* 1999;50: 928–931.
2. Koyama T, Fujimoto K, Iwakiri R, et al. Prevention of recurrent bleeding from gastric ulcer with a nonbleeding visible vessel by endoscopic injection of absolute ethanol: a prospective, controlled trial. *Gastrointest Endosc* 1995;42:128–131.
3. Ethanolamine oleate. Drugdex Drug Evaluations, MICROMEDEX Healthcare Series Vol. 118, Thomson MICROMEDEX, 2003.
4. Sodium tetradecyl sulfate. Drugdex Drug Evaluations, MICRO-MEDEX Healthcare Series Vol. 118, Thomson MICROMEDEX, 2003.

5. Morrhuate sodium. Drugdex Drug Evaluations, MICROMEDEX Healthcare Series Vol. 118, Thomson MICROMEDEX, 2003.
6. Greenwald BD, Caldwell SH, Hespenheide EE, et al. N-2-butyl-cyanoacrylate for bleeding gastric varices: a United States pilot study and cost analysis. *Am J Gastroenterol* 2003;98:1982–1988.
7. Maria G, Cassetta E, Gui D, et al. A comparison of botulinum toxin and saline for the treatment of chronic anal fissure. *N Engl J Med* 1998;338:217–220.
8. Madalinski MH, Slawek J, Duzynski W, et al. Side effects of botulinum toxin injection for benign anal disorders. *Eur J Gastroenterol Hepatol* 2002;14:853–856.

# Bipolar Electrocautery and Heater Probe

## Lisa M. Gangarosa

When faced with an actively or potentially bleeding lesion, the therapeutic endoscopist now has a multitude of choices of endoscopic hemostatic devices. Contact thermal devices (heater probe and bipolar electrocautery) have been widely used since the 1980s. A heater probe consists of a Teflon-coated hollow aluminum cylinder with an inner heating coil and distal thermocouple, which maintains constant temperature. Tissue coagulation is the result of direct heat transfer (1). Bipolar (or multipolar) electrocautery probes generate heat indirectly by the passage of electrical current through tissue. Two electrodes in the tip of the probe complete a circuit through nondesiccated tissue (2). The heat generated by either type of device leads to swelling, protein coagulation (which requires temperature of at least 70° C), and vessel contraction. Both of these probes also allow for coaptive pressure on vessels. The resulting changes in the tissue and vessels usually lead to the desired effect of hemostasis (3).

### INDICATIONS
1. To treat actively bleeding lesions or lesions at high risk for bleeding including ulcers, arteriovenous malformations (AVMs) (naturally occurring, radiation-induced, and gastric antral vascular ectasias), Dielafoy lesions, Mallory-Weiss tears, and culprit lesions associated with diverticular hemorrhage

### CONTRAINDICATIONS
1. See contraindications to upper endoscopy (Chapter 5) or colonoscopy (Chapter 8).
2. Inability of patient to remain still during endoscopy
3. Uncorrectable coagulopathy

### PREPARATION
1. See preparation for upper endoscopy (Chapter 5) or colonoscopy (Chapter 8).
2. Correct coagulopathy or thrombocytopenia. Goal of international normalized ratio (INR) <1.5, platelet count >50,000.
3. Pretest all electrical equipment.

### EQUIPMENT
1. Appropriate endoscope (if 10-Fr probe to be used, then endoscope must have therapeutic-sized channel), lubricant, personal protective equipment (gown, gloves, mask with visor), working intravenous (IV) equipment, sedation medications

2. Device of choice: 7- or 10-Fr heater probe (Heat Probe, Olympus America, Melville, NY) or electrocautery probe (e.g., HEMArrest, Bard Interventional Products, Bellerica, MA; Gold Probe, Microvasive, Natick, MA; BICAP, Circon Acmi, Stamford, CT; or Quicksilver, Wilson-Cook Medical, Inc., Winston-Salem, NC) with integrated irrigation system

3. Appropriate electrosurgical generator with foot pedal control

4. Normal saline for irrigation

**PROCEDURE**

1. Perform diagnostic endoscopy to locate the source of bleeding or lesion to treat. The endoscopist may choose to use injection therapy (see Chapter 12) prior to thermal therapy.

2. Remove adherent blood clots.

**Bipolar Electrocautery**

1. Attach a bipolar probe to both the electrosurgical device and irrigation system filled with normal saline.

2. Turn on the electrosurgical device, and set the power to 15 to 20 W for a visible vessel, Mallory-Weiss tear, or Dielafoy lesion, and 10 to 15 W for AVMs or colonic diverticula vessels (4).

3. Advance the bipolar probe through the working channel of the endoscope.

4. The tip may be applied directly or tangentially to the lesion, but good apposition of the tip to tissue is necessary.

5. Depress the foot pedal to deliver current, and keep the tip in place for 2 to 10 seconds depending on the type, size, and depth of the lesion. Good therapy for visible vessels includes cauterization of the area previously housing the visible vessel.

6. Either directly remove the probe or use irrigation to remove the tip from the tissue if the coagulum from the tissue is adherent to the probe.

7. Repeat Steps 6 through 8 until coagulation/hemostasis is achieved.

**Heater Probe**

1. Attach both the heater probe and irrigation bottle to the generator.

2. Set the generator to deliver the appropriate amount of energy (20 to 30 J/pulse for visible vessels, 5 to 10 J/pulse for AVMs).

3. Advance the heater probe through the working channel of the endoscope.

4. The tip may be applied directly or tangentially to the lesion, but good apposition of the tip to tissue is necessary. Fig. 13.1 shows the method for coaptation of the vessel.

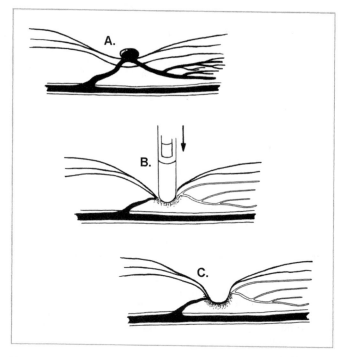

**Fig. 13.1. Heater probe treatment. A: Visible vessel seen above the surface of the ulcer crater. B: Heat applied by the probe that is tamponading the vessel. C: Postprocedure view showing the sealed vessel.**

5. Depress the foot pedal to deliver the heat pulse. Based on energy settings, the time of pulse is predetermined.

6. Either directly remove the probe or depress the irrigation pedal to irrigate the tip from the tissue.

7. Repeat Steps 7 through 9 until coagulation/hemostasis is achieved.

**POSTPROCEDURE**

1. Monitor vital signs.

2. For inpatients, if the lesion has been actively bleeding or remains at high risk for rebleeding, follow the hemoglobin and hematocrit every 6 to 12 hours for 24 to 48 hours to evaluate treatment efficacy.

3. If there is evidence of rebleeding, the procedure may need to be repeated or may require intervention by a surgeon and/or an interventional radiologist.

## COMPLICATIONS

1. Precipitation of bleeding: up to 5% with heater probe and 18% with bipolar electrocautery (3).

2. Perforation: 1.8 to 3% with heater probe; rarely in upper gastrointestinal lesions and up to 2.5% in right-colon AVMs with bipolar electrocautery (3).

### CPT codes

**43255** – Upper gastrointestinal endoscopy including esophagus, stomach, and either the duodenum and/or jejunum as appropriate; with control of bleeding, any method.

**43258** – Upper gastrointestinal endoscopy including esophagus, stomach, and either the duodenum and/or jejunum as appropriate; with ablation of tumor(s), polyp(s), or other lesion(s) not amenable to removal by hot biopsy forceps, bipolar cautery, or snare technique.

**45334** – Sigmoidoscopy, flexible; with control of bleeding, any method.

**45339** – Sigmoidoscopy, flexible; with ablation of tumor(s), polyp(s), or other lesion(s) not amenable to removal by hot biopsy forceps, bipolar cautery, or snare technique.

**45382** – Colonoscopy, flexible, proximal to splenic flexure; with control of bleeding, any method.

**45383** – Colonoscopy, flexible, proximal to splenic flexure; with ablation of tumor(s), polyp(s), or other lesion(s) not amenable to removal by hot biopsy forceps, bipolar cautery, or snare technique.

### REFERENCES

1. Fullarton GM, Birnie GG, MacDonald A, et al. Controlled trial of heater probe treatment in bleeding peptic ulcers. *Br J Surg* 1989;76:541–544.

2. Laine. L. Bipolar/multipolar electrocoagulation. *Gastrointest Endosc* 1990;36(Suppl):S38–41.

3. Nelson D, Barkon A, Block K, et al. Endoscopic hemostatic devices. *Gastrointest Endosc* 2001; 54:833–840.

4. Savides TJ, Jenson DM. Therapeutic endoscopy for nonvariceal gastrointestinal bleeding. In: Cappell MS, ed. High Risk Gastrointestinal Bleeding, Part II. *Gastoenterol Clin North Am* 2000;29:465–487.

# Clips and Loops

Emad M. Abu-Hamda and Todd H. Baron

Clips were initially developed for endoscopic use in 1971 for use in peptic ulcer hemostasis but now have many other applications (1). There are a number of designs available, which vary in terms of the length of the prongs and the angle of opening.

Loops were initially developed to help prevent postpolypectomy bleeding by their application to the stalks of large pedunculated polyps. Several other applications have been described including gastric and endoscopic variceal ligation (1,2). The loops are made of nylon that can be applied to the polyp stalk and released. Afterwards the polypectomy can be safely performed.

## INDICATIONS

### Endoclips

1. Treatment of actively bleeding vascular lesions such as a peptic ulcer or a Dielafoy's lesion

2. Treatment of lesions with high risk of rebleeding such as a peptic ulcer with a visible vessel

3. Treatment of medium-sized to large-sized arteries (2 to 3 mm) where other hemostasis methods such as contact thermal methods are suboptimal (3)

4. Treatment of actively bleeding or high-risk lesions in patients with coagulation disorders or who are on anticoagulants (e.g., warfarin) where contact thermal methods may be suboptimal

5. Treatment of postsphincterotomy bleeding

6. Treatment of postpolypectomy bleeding

7. Prevention of postpolypectomy bleeding with prophylactic placement of Endoclips to large pedunculated stalks (4,5)

8. Closure of small luminal perforations after endoscopic procedures

9. Temporary marking of colonic lesions preoperatively to assist surgical identification

10. Marking of proximal and distal edges of malignant tumors to facilitate endoscopic/fluoroscopic placement of endoluminal self-expandable metal stents

### Endoloops

1. Prevention of postpolypectomy bleeding by application to the polyp stalk prior to polypectomy

2. Esophageal and gastric variceal ligation by a modified Endocaps and Endoloop (mini Endoloop) (2)

3.  Hemostasis of bleeding lesions such as small ulcers with visible vessels or angiodysplasias by modified Endocaps

## CONTRAINDICATIONS

### Endoclips

1.  Ligation of esophageal or gastric varices

2.  Inability to get or obtain an enface view of the target lesion

3.  Inability to see the bleeding vessel

4.  Lesions that can only be seen in a retroflexed position

### Endoloops

1.  Contraindications similar to that of standard electrosurgical polypectomy (See Chapter 18)

## PREPARATION

1.  The patient should be *L. nil per os* (NPO) for 4 to 6 hours.

2.  Patients with gastrointestinal bleeding should be adequately resuscitated.

3.  The gastroenterology assistant should be well versed on the use, assembly, and deployment of Endoclips and Endoloops.

4.  If multiple clips are to be used, the gastrointestinal (GI) assistant should preassemble several devices (to alternate between two clip loading devices, hence very little time is spent loading clips while the endoscopist is waiting).

## EQUIPMENT

1.  An endoscope with at least a 2.8-mm accessory channel

2.  The appropriate-length loading device depending on whether a gastroscope or a colonoscope is used

3.  Reprocessed and disinfected single-shot, reusable loading device for Endoclips or Endoloops. After a clip or loop is deployed, a new clip or loop must be reloaded onto the loading device for further therapy.

4.  Onetime-only Endoclips and loading devices are available whereby the loading device is discarded after one use. This saves time between clip delivery and deployment, which is important when time is of the essence such as in emergent bleeders. However, disposable Endoclips are more expensive.

5.  Rotatable Endoclips are now available that allow the GI assistant to rotate the tip of the Endoclip, which allows for more accurate placement of the clip at the target lesion.

## PROCEDURE

### Endoclips

1.  Identify the lesion to be clipped. If a large amount of blood is obscuring visualization, hemostasis should be initially achieved with saline/epinephrine injection to allow identification of the bleeding vessel.

2. Position the target lesion enface.

3. Advance the preassembled clip-loading device with the attached clip through the accessory channel of the endoscope.

4. Bring the plastic sheath with the enclosed retracted clip into endoscopic view, and advance the endoscope toward the target lesion.

5. Ask the GI assistant to extend the clip from the tube sheath and lock it in place.

6. Have the GI assistant open the clip arms to their maximum width. This is identified endoscopically by disappearance of an 'X' at the base of the clip closest to the sheath.

7. Reposition the sheath and the endoscope as close as possible to the target lesion.

8. Advance the entire device to allow the fully extended clips to surround the target lesion, and firmly press against the surrounding tissue.

9. Ask the GI assistant to close and deploy the clip around the lesion.

10. Release the loading device from the clip by sliding the handle to its original position.

11. Evaluate the target lesion and the site of clip deployment, and repeat this sequence as needed. See Fig. 14.1 for sample placement of detached clips on vessels.

**Endoloops**

1. Identify the pedunculated polyp that will be snared, and place it at the 6 o'clock position in the endoscopic field.

2. Advance the preassembled loop-loading device with the attached loop through the accessory channel of the endoscope.

3. Once the sheath with retracted loop is in endoscopic view, advance the endoscope toward the target lesion.

4. Ask the GI assistant to extend the loop out of the sheath until it is fully opened.

5. Maneuver the nylon loop and the endoscope so that the loop fully surrounds the polyp. Carefully bring down the loop so it rests around the stalk of the polyp.

6. Ask the GI assistant to close the loop by pulling on the slider of the loading device until resistance is felt. It is important not to apply excessive force when ligating the polyp stalk, as this can inadvertently sever the polyp. Also, do not move the endoscope until the loop is released, as this can also sever the polyp and lead to bleeding.

7. Ask the GI assistant to push the slider until it touches the clamping ring. This will extend the hook from the sheath.

8. Ask the GI assistant to detach the loop from the hook in order to deploy the loop.

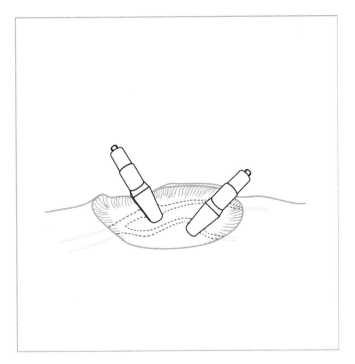

**Fig. 14.1. Sample clip placements on two exposed vessels in an ulcer crater.**

9.  After adequate ligation pressure is seen, as evidenced by bluish discoloration of the polyp, use a standard polypectomy snare to sever the polyp.

10. Place the polypectomy snare around the stalk a few millimeters above the previously placed Endoloop. The snare should not contact the Endoloop, as this can lead to their becoming fused. This may produce difficulty disengaging the snare or lead to premature cutting of the Endoloop with resultant bleeding.

**POSTPROCEDURE**

1.  Resuscitation and supportive care should continue in cases of GI bleeding.

2.  Patients with small postsphincterotomy, catheter-induced, or heater/bipolar electrocoagulation therapy (BICAP) probe-induced perforations in whom clipping was performed to close the perforation should be watched for signs of peritonitis or clinical deterioration. This would indicate failure of the clipping to seal the perforation and would

necessitate prompt surgical evaluation. Prophylactic antibiotics, nasogastric suction, and *L. nil per os* (NPO) should be instituted to assist in sealing the perforation.

3. Loops placed prophylactically on large polyps can prematurely dislodge; therefore, patients should be instructed to contact the endoscopist for any signs of lower GI bleeding.

4. Patients in whom loops are placed for obliteration of esophageal or gastric varices should have strong analgesics for postprocedural chest pain and consume clear liquids for 6 to 8 hours postvariceal ligation.

## COMPLICATIONS

1. Perforation
2. Bleeding
3. Chest pain (if esophageal varices ligated)

## OTHER USES FOR THIS TECHNIQUE

### Endoclips

1. Sealing of fistula from the GI tract to surrounding organs such as bronchioesophageal fistulas or colocutaneous fistulas (6)
2. Clipping of colonic manometry catheters to prevent premature migration of the manometry catheter tips distally due to normal colonic motility (7)
3. Clipping of jejunal extension of feeding tubes to prevent dislodgement
4. Endoscopic sealing of postsurgical anastomotic leaks such as in esophagogastric resections

### CPT Codes

There are no specific CPT codes for the use of the clips or loops.

### REFERENCES

1. Hepworth CC, Swain CP. Mechanical endoscopic methods of haemostasis for bleeding peptic ulcers: a review. *Baillieres Best Pract Res Clin Gastroenterol* 2000;14(3):467–476.
2. Hepworth CC, Burnham WR, Swain CP. Development and application of endoloops for the treatment of bleeding esophageal varices. *Gastrointest Endosc* 1999;50(5):677–684.
3. Hepworth CC, Kadirkamanathan SS, Gong F, Swain CP. A randomised controlled comparison of injection, thermal, and mechanical endoscopic methods of haemostasis on mesenteric vessels. *Gut* 1998;42(4):462–469.
4. Iida Y, Miura S, Munemoto Y, et al. Endoscopic resection of large colorectal polyps using a clipping method. *Dis Colon Rectum* 1994;37(2):179–180.
5. Cipolletta L, Bianco MA, Marmo R, et al. Endoclips versus heater probe in preventing early recurrent bleeding from peptic ulcer: a

prospective and randomized trial. *Gastrointest Endosc* 2001;53(2):147–151.

6. Familiari P, Macri A, Consolo P, et al. Endoscopic clipping of a colocutaneous fistula following necrotizing pancreatitis: case report. *Dig Liver Dis* 2003;35(12):907–910.

7. Fajardo N, Hussain K, Korsten MA. Prolonged ambulatory colonic manometric studies using endoclips. *Gastrointest Endosc* 2000;51(2):199–201.

# Injection Therapy of Esophageal and Gastric Varices: Sclerosis and Cyanoacrylate

Stephen H. Caldwell, Vanessa M. Shami, and Elizabeth E. Hespenheide

Variceal bleeding accounts for 10% to 30% of all upper gastrointestinal (GI) bleeding. Most, but not all, such patients have cirrhosis. The esophagus is the most common site for bleeding varices, but gastric varices are seen in about 10% to 20% of cases and may be particularly difficult to manage. Noncirrhotic patients account for about 10% of all gastric variceal bleeding. The presence of gastric varices necessitates imaging of the portal vascular bed to exclude splenic vein thrombosis, usually from pancreatitis or left upper quadrant neoplasm.

Currently, band ligation has largely supplanted sclerotherapy of esophageal varices. However, sclerotherapy is a viable option when visualization of the bleeding site is difficult due to active hemorrhage or occasionally when the banding device cannot be passed due to its relatively large size. Sclerosant agents cause marked local irritation to the veins producing acute occlusion from thrombus and eventually fibrosis of the vein. The most common agents in use are detergents which include ethanolamine oleate and sodium tetradecyl sulfate 1% to 2%; these work by forming a lipid bilayer which disrupts the cell surface membrane and removes essential cell surface proteins (protein theft denaturation) resulting in cell death.

In cirrhosis, esophageal varices usually represent collateral flow from the coronary vein which runs from the portal vein to the azygous system. Lesser curve gastric varices share this vascular anatomy, and these can usually be managed like more typical esophageal varices. However, gastric varices that lie in the fundus or fundic region of the gastric cardia are typically larger, often polypoid ("cluster of grapes"), and more difficult to manage. They represent collateral flow from the splenic vein to the left renal vein (spontaneous splenorenal shunting).

Due to their relatively large size, fundic-type gastric varices are not easily managed by either band ligation or conventional sclerotherapy, although occasionally use of both may temporize the problem. In the United States, many centers utilize transjugular intrahepatic portosystemic shunts (TIPS), but the optimal form of therapy for gastric varices widely practiced in Europe and Asia consists of varix "obturation" using cyanoacrylate. The greatest experience is with N-butyl 2-cyanoacrylate (Histoacryl, B. Braun, Melsungen, Germany), usually referred to as enbucrilate. Upon contact with blood, enbucrilate forms a glue polymer. Iodinated poppy seed oil (Ethiodol, also called

Lipiodol) is widely used and is radiopaque, which allows radio-logical visualization of the "plug." Eventually, the polymer is extruded through the mucosa, leaving a small mucosal defect and a vestigial, fibrotic vein.

Below is described first traditional sclerotherapy of esophageal varices and then enbucrilate therapy for gastric varices. In general these procedures are performed in the Intensive Care Unit although commonly more elective cases are handled in the Endoscopy Unit. Our experience with enbucrilate is based on an extended Federal Drug Administration (FDA)-approved pilot study.

## SCLEROTHERAPY OF ESOPHAGEAL VARICES

### Indications

1. Esophageal varices that are actively bleeding or that have evidence of prior bleeding

2. Eradication of some types of gastric varices which are in continuity with esophageal varices. These are typically small and usually extend in a linear configuration along the lesser curve (Type 1 gastroesophageal varices by the Sarin classification).

### Contraindications

1. A poorly sedated patient. The risk of perforation or bleeding by tearing the injected varix increases if the patient is unco-operative or agitated. In these circumstances, sedation and tracheal intubation is recommended.

2. Inability to achieve adequate visibility of the field

### Preparation

1. Place at least two large-bore intravenous (IV) tubes for administration of blood products and fluids.

2. Adequately sedate the patient to conduct the procedure as safely as possible. Intubation is often recommended to min-imize the chance of aspiration, especially in the setting of acute bleeding.

3. In the setting of an acute variceal bleed, give a bolus and subsequent continuous infusion of antiportal hypertensive medication (octreotide or vasopressin).

4. A balloon tamponade tube such as a Sengstaken-Blakemore tube should be readily available.

5. The need for correction of clotting indices is an unsettled issue. However, avoid use of plasma as this may worsen por-tal pressure and contribute to further bleeding.

6. Draw up the sclerosant agent into an injection needle before initiating endoscopy.

### Equipment

1. Upper endoscope. A therapeutic upper endoscope is pre-ferred because it has larger working channels for aspiration of blood.

2. Sclerosant drawn up in nondiluted form in a 10-mL syringe prior to endoscopy. The injection needle should be primed with the sclerosant.

3. Goggles

**Procedure**

1. Perform a complete examination of the upper gastrointestinal tract to exclude other nonvariceal sources of bleeding. If a site of active variceal bleeding is identified, complete the examination after control of the bleeding.

2. Administer prophylactic antibiotics with acute variceal bleeding. For patients with high-risk cardiac conditions (prosthetic heart valves, previous history of bacterial endocarditis, surgically constructed systemic pulmonary shunts or conduits, or complex cyanotic congenital heart disease) undergoing sclerotherapy, administer additional antibiotic prophylaxis (e.g., clindamycin 600 mg IV, cefazolin 1 g IV/intramuscularly (IM), or vancomycin 1 g IV) 30 minutes before the procedure.

3. Advance the upper endoscope to the gastroesophageal junction, and define the distal extent of the varices.

4. With the varix clearly in view, bring the needle out, and press it into the varix, next to the variceal lumen, or sequentially at both sites.

5. Inject between 0.5 mL and 2.0 mL of sclerosant at each site.

6. Withdraw the needle and cannula, and repeat the procedure as needed to eradicate all distended vessels.

7. Do not deliver more than 10 cc in a single session unless more is needed to achieve hemostasis.

8. For isolated esophageal varices, perform injections in a circumferential fashion at or just proximal to the gastroesophageal junction.

9. Pull the endoscope proximally 2 to 5 cm and repeat the injections.

10. With an actively bleeding varix, inject sclerosant immediately distal and proximal to the bleeding site. After bleeding has ceased, attend to all other varices.

**Postprocedure Care**

1. Observe for signs of blood loss, pulmonary complications, fever, and esophageal perforation. Pain medication may be needed.

2. With acute bleeding, keep NPO for at least 4 to 6 hours postprocedure as rebleeding may occur.

3. Consider using topical medications such as sucralfate and acid reducing agents.

4. If needed, place a nasogastric or soft feeding tube; these are usually tolerated for administration of medications. However, feeding tube perforation of the esophagus may occur if esophageal ulcers have formed prior to sclerotherapy.

**Complications**

Mild complications from the sclerosant or procedure are seen in up to 20% to 40%, with a mortality rate as high as 1% to 2% depending on the condition of the patient and the experience of the operator.

1.   Minor complications include transient chest pain, asymptomatic pleural effusions, transient difficulty swallowing, and fever. They will usually resolve within 48 hours.

2.   Allergic reactions to the solution

3.   Transient bacteremia

4.   Esophageal stricture may occur in 2 to 10%. This is usually managed by endoscopic dilation.

5.   Perforation may occur as a result of direct rupture with the needle or full-thickness esophageal wall necrosis secondary to the sclerosant.

6.   Bleeding may occur from the varix itself or, less frequently, from esophageal mucosal ulcerations.

7.   Aspiration pneumonia

8.   Mediastinitis

## ENBUCRILATE OBTURATION OF GASTRIC VARICES

**Indications**

Gastric varices usually of the type located in the fundus with active bleeding or stigmata of recent bleeding show red wale marking and/or the presence of a nipple or plug protruding from the surface of the varix.

**Contraindications**

1.   Increased risk of central nervous system (CNS) embolism. This may occur with hepatopulmonary syndrome or cardiac septal defects with right-to-left shunting.

2.   Bleeding to the extent that a clear field cannot be achieved. Consider first using a Blakemore tube or other hemostatic agents to gain control of bleeding prior to injecting the polymer.

**Preparation**

1.   Perform a diagnostic endoscopy to demonstrate large, high-risk gastric varices as the source of bleeding.

2.   Order octreotide, to be administered as a bolus if bleeding is active. A balloon tamponade tube (such as a Blakemore tube) should be available. Some recommend the use of recombinant activated factor VII in the setting of uncontrollable bleeding.

3.   Place the needle injector, cyanoacrylate, and oil on a clean pad.

4.   Have the assistant prepare the instruments while passing the endoscope.

5.   Cover the patient's eyes with a cloth.

6.   Have all personnel wear preventative plastic eye shields.

## Equipment and Additional Preparation

1. Because the procedure must be performed typically in the retroflexed position to visualize the fundus, short 60- to 70-cm (sigmoidoscope) endoscopes are preferred due to their much greater deflection. They also have larger working channels than typical diagnostic scopes and are less likely to have polymer become stuck within the channels.

2. Place a cup of nonsterile olive oil on the scope cart to irrigate the biopsy channel just before passing the injection needle. The oil prevents sticking of the injection needle and premature polymerization by preventing contact of the cannula tip with any blood or mucus which could be in the channel.

3. Add Simethicone (one dropper) to several hundred cc of water to provide additional irrigation fluid.

4. Keep the enbucrilate (Histoacryl) refrigerated (less than 5° C) until just before use. The small plastic vial contains 0.5 cc of polymer.

5. Use clean scissors to cut the tip off of the vial.

6. Squeeze the enbucrilate out of the plastic vial into a glass vial. Draw an equal amount of sterile iodinated poppy seed oil (Ethiodol) into a plastic syringe, and then add it to the enbucrilate thus making a final volume of 1 cc of enbucrilate-oil mixture.

7. Stir the mixture gently with the needle used to dispense the oil.

8. Draw 0.5 cc of the mixture into a 3-cc syringe.

9. Prime a 23-gauge Marcon-Haber (Wilson-Cooke Medical) cannula with sterile Ethiodol, and then load it with the enbucrilate-Ethiodol mixture.

10. "Push" the mixture to about 2 cm from the tip of the cannula. This leaves about 2 cm to 3 cm of oil between the needle tip and the enbucrilate-oil mixture and delivers about 0.25 cc of glue and about 0.25 cc of oil during the injection. The blue color of the enbucrilate makes this determination easier.

11. Fill a 10-cc syringe with sterile water, and then attach it to the hub of the needle cannula to be used as a pusher to express the column of enbucrilate-oil into the varix.

12. Other cannulas may be used but require testing to make sure that the hub is chemically compatible with the glue-oil mixture (dissolution of the hub with certain cannulas has been noted).

## Procedure

1. Pass the 70-cm scope, and bring the fundic varices into view, usually in the retroflexed position (Fig. 15.1).

2. Irrigate the field with the simethicone-water solution, and take several different views of the variceal complex to determine the best site for initial injection (usually to the patient's left as this is the likely "inflow" point).

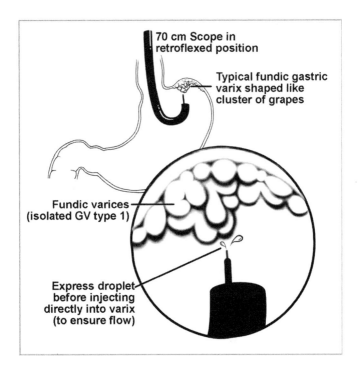

70 cm Scope in retroflexed position

Typical fundic gastric varix shaped like cluster of grapes

Fundic varices (isolated GV type 1)

Express droplet before injecting directly into varix (to ensure flow)

**Fig. 15.1. Enbucrilate obturation of gastric varices.**

3. Prime the biopsy channel with nonsterile olive oil before passing the injector needle.

4. Dip the needle cannula in the olive oil for additional protection, and then pass the cannula into the biopsy channel and visualize it through the scope.

5. With the varix in view, bring the needle into view, and express a small drop of the polymer mix to ensure liquidity and absence of premature hardening. Because the cyanoacrylate can polymerize in the cannula, it should not be passed through a pool of blood as this could cause premature polymerization.

6. Press the needle cannula into the varix at the chosen site, and instruct the assistant to squeeze the syringe filled with sterile water to cause the enbucrilate-oil mixture to pass into the lumen of the varix. The varix will swell and turn blue.

7. As the assistant presses the syringe, he or she should call out the volume delivered in cc increments.

8. As the volume reaches 2 cc, withdraw the needle while there is still flow from the tip (to avoid fixing the needle in the varix).

9. Quickly withdraw the needle cannula, and use the simethicone-water mixture to irrigate the freshly injected site. Some have advocated not suctioning after use of polymer out of concern for causing "glue" to stick inside of the scope. However, by waiting a few minutes for any excess polymer to harden and by using the simethicone-water mixture, there has not been a problem suctioning after injection.

10. Prepare a second needle cannula while cleaning up after the first injection.

11. Use the same steps to inject a second, third, and fourth site if needed. The average is about 2.5 injections per patient. However, if active bleeding develops, additional injections may be needed. Because each vial of enbucrilate produces two "loaded" needle cannulas, injections are usually performed in pairs.

12. Give a postprocedure intravenous dose of antibiotics if not previously administered.

**Postprocedure care**

1. Observe the patient for evidence of embolic problems.

2. Use sucralfate (Carafate) slurry po QID as a topical agent, oral antibiotics, and acid suppression routinely for at least 5 days postprocedure.

3. Perform follow-up endoscopy from 24 to 72 hours after the initial session. Perform subsequent endoscopies at regular intervals (usually 1 week, 1 month, and then every 3 months for the balance of a year). This schedule is based on FDA-approved protocol, but a more abbreviated schedule is probably suitable as repeat injections are required only in a minority of cases.

4. If esophageal varices are also present, these are typically managed by band ligation if they appear to be at high risk for bleeding (large with surface red marks).

**Complications**

1. Premature polymerization may occur, especially if precautions are not taken to avoid blood contact as noted above. Premature polymerization has also rarely been noted in the past with certain lots of iodinated poppy seed oil. This event results in piercing the varix but having no glue-oil mixture come out from the needle tip. It leaves a bleeding hole in the varix and requires urgent preparation of fresh injection material. This adverse event is best avoided in the steps noted above. The last step before the injection (expressing a drop of mixture from the needle tip under direct endoscopic visualization) ensures free flow of the mixture prior to piercing the varix.

2. Gluing the needle into the varix. This may occur if the needle is not withdrawn as the mixture is flowing. It may require clipping the cannula, removing the scope, and reinserting the scope with endoscopic scissors. Forceful removal

of an impacted needle should be avoided as it may "unroof'" the varix with severe bleeding.

3. Embolization of small pieces of glue. The risk of emboli varies with the degree of oil mixing, the type of cyanoacrylate, and probably with the coagulation status of the patient, although many of these variables have not been sufficiently studied. Minor emboli of radiopaque material to the lung fields have been observed in about 5% of cases. This is usually asymptomatic, and long-term sequelae have not been observed. However, if the patient has hepatopulmonary syndrome or any form of right-to-left shunting, the risk for severe arterial emboli becomes marked. Careful patient selection, as noted above, reduces this risk.

4. Local ulceration has rarely been noted. This is probably due to the relatively small volume of enbucrilate injected at each site.

5. Scope damage: As mentioned, some practitioners advocate avoidance of any suction. However, no problems have been noted with this, using the simethicone-water irrigation and waiting a few minutes before suctioning. Use of the larger channel 70-cm scopes probably also reduces this risk. Should enbucrilate adhere to the objective of the scope, it may be cleaned with acetone (fingernail polish remover).

6. Early rebleeding from persistent varix patency occurs in around 1% to 2% (within 72 hours) and can be retreated with additional injections. Localized ulcer bleeding (infrequent in our experience) or bleeding from another site should be excluded.

**OTHER USES**

1. Bleeding at other sites and enteric fistulae may respond to enbucrilate injection, but these have not been adequately tested

**CPT Codes**

**43243** – Upper gastrointestinal endoscopy including esophagus, stomach, and either the duodenum and/or jejunum as appropriate; with injection sclerosis of esophageal and/or gastric varices.

**Note:** Enbucrilate injection is not FDA approved.

**SUGGESTED READINGS**

Bernard B, Grange JD, Khac EN, et al. Antibiotic prophylaxis for the prevention of bacterial infections in cirrhotic patients with gastrointestinal bleeding: a meta-analysis. *Hepatology* 1999;29: 1655–1661.

Botoman VA, Surawicz CM. Bacteremia with gastrointestinal endoscopic procedures. *Gastrointest Endosc* 1986;32:342–346.

Greenwald BD, Caldwell SH, Hespenheide EE, et al. N-2-butyl-cyanoacrylate for bleeding gastric varices: a United States pilot study and cost analysis. *Am J Gastroenterol* 2003;98:1982–1988.

Huang Y-H, Yeh H-Z, Chen G-H, et al. Endoscopic treatment of bleeding gastric varices by N-butyl-2-cyanoacrylate (Histoacryl) injection: long term efficacy and safety. *GI Endoscopy* 2000;52:160–167.

Kim T, Shijo H, Kokawa H, et al. Risk factors for hemorrhage from gastric fundal varices. *Hepatology* 1997;25:307–312.

Laine L, Cook D. Endoscopic ligation compared with sclerotherapy for treatment of esophageal variceal bleeding: a meta-analysis. *Ann Int Med* 1995;123:280–287.

Lo G-H, Lai K-H, Cheng J-S, et al. A prospective, randomized trial of butyl cyanoacrylate injection versus band ligation in the management of bleeding gastric varices. *Hepatology* 2001;33:1060–1064.

Sarin SK, Jain AK, Jain M, Gupta R. A randomized controlled trial of cyanoacrylate versus alcohol injection in patients with isolated fundic varices. *Am J Gastroenterol* 2002;97:1010–1015.

Sarin SK, Lahoti D, Saxena SP, Murphy NS. Prevalence, classification and natural history of gastric varices: a long-term follow-up study in 568 portal hypertension patients. *Hepatology* 1992;16:1343–1349.

Suga T, Akamatsu T, Kawamura Y, et al. Actual behavior of N-butyl-2-cyanoacrylate (Histoacryl) in a blood vessel: a model of the varix. *Endoscopy* 2002;14:73–77.

# Endoscopic Variceal Ligation

Jason D. Conway and Roshan Shrestha

Chronic liver disease often leads to fibrosis and cirrhosis. Cirrhosis is the most common cause of elevated portal pressures and leads to dilation of portosystemic collaterals, including esophageal varices (1). Gastroesophageal varices are common in patients with cirrhosis, and up to one-third of patients with cirrhosis and varices will have a significant episode of upper gastrointestinal hemorrhage (2). The mortality rate for first variceal bleed is 30% to 50%, and in those who survive, the risk for rebleeding is about 60% to 70% within one year with a mortality of 20% at each episode (3,4).

Endoscopic variceal ligation was first described in humans in 1989 and was derived from band ligation of hemorrhoids (4). Since this time it has been shown to be superior to sclerotherapy and has become the endoscopic intervention of choice for acute esophageal variceal hemorrhage and subsequent variceal obliteration (5). A meta-analysis showed that variceal ligation has significantly lower rates of rebleeding, mortality, and complications when compared to sclerotherapy. Also, significantly fewer banding sessions were needed to obliterate varices compared to sclerotherapy (6).

**INDICATIONS**

1. Hemostasis of acutely or recently bleeding esophageal varices

2. Elective obliteration of esophageal varices to prevent recurrent hemorrhage

**CONTRAINDICATIONS**

1. Esophageal stricture, diverticula, or suspected esophageal perforation

2. Uncooperative patient

3. Patient hypersensitivity to latex (Speedband Superview Super 7 Multiple Band Ligator from Boston Scientific is a latex-free product)

**PREPARATION**

1. Obtain adequate intravenous (IV) access and start fluid resuscitation if indicated.

2. In the acute setting, start IV octreotide.

3. For patients who are acutely hemorrhaging or are very agitated, consider intubation for airway protection.

4. The patient's blood should be typed and crossed by the blood bank.

5. The patient should be NPO for 8 hours prior to the examination, if possible.

6. Obtain informed, written consent from the patient or a close relative.

7. Administer topical anesthetic for pharyngeal anesthesia.

8. Obtain medications for sedation (e.g., midazolam and fentanyl).

## EQUIPMENT

1. Upper endoscope. Make sure the ligator device is compatible with the outer diameter and accessory channel length of the endoscope.

2. Gloves, safety goggles, and gown

3. Lubricant

4. 50-cc syringe with Luer-lock tip and sterile saline or water for washing

5. 6- or 7-multi-band ligator (i.e., Saeed 6 Shooter Multi-Band Ligator from Wilson-Cook, Speedband Superview Super 7 Multiple Band Ligator from Microvasive, or UltraView Multiple Band Ligator from Bard)

## PROCEDURE

1. Perform diagnostic upper endoscopy to document esophageal varices and rule out other sources of bleeding.

2. Remove the endoscope, and attach the ligation device. *Refer to the specific device instructions for detailed setup instructions.* The UltraView Multiple Band Ligator from Bard is unique, features a retractable ligating unit, and mounts completely to the outside of the endoscope. In general, attachment and operation of the Saeed 6 Shooter Multi-Band Ligator from Wilson-Cook and Speedband Superview Super 7 Multiple Band Ligator from Microvasive are similar and are described below. Both ligator kits come with a ligating unit that is a clear plastic cylinder with preloaded bands and trigger string, a plastic or wire loader, a handle, and an irrigation adapter. Attach the handle to the accessory channel of the endoscope, and push the wire or plastic loader into the accessory channel of the endoscope until it exits the distal end of the endoscope. Affix the trigger string to the loader, and pull the string or wire until it is appropriately attached to the handle. Firmly press the ligating unit onto the distal end of the endoscope. When using Speedband Superview Super 7 Multiple Band Ligator, remove shrink-wrap from the ligating unit. Gently turn the handle to tighten the string, being careful to avoid deploying a band. Confirm that the trigger strings do not obstruct the view of the endoscope, and if they do, rotate the cap so that the strings are in the periphery of the viewing field. Finally, be sure the device handle is in the appropriate position to deploy a band.

3.  Lubricate the outside of the ligating unit, and insert it into the esophagus. Intubation may be more difficult than in normal upper endoscopy due to the added length and size of the ligation device.

4.  The first varix to be banded should be the largest or the one with stigmata of recent hemorrhage.

5.  Banding should start at the most caudal extent of the varix but above the Z-line. Bands should not be placed in gastric mucosa or on gastric varices.

6.  After the appropriate varix and site are chosen, the endoscope should be flexed so the varix is perpendicular (as much as possible) with the ligating unit (Fig. 16.1).

7.  Suction is applied, and the varix is sucked into the ligating unit (Fig. 16.2). When the varix is completely sucked into the ligating unit, "red out" will be seen. Misfire, or incomplete deployment of the band, may occur if the varix is not completely sucked into the ligating unit. Suction should be set to maximum to prevent this.

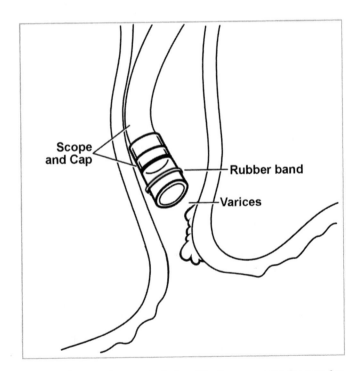

**Fig. 16.1. Correct placement of a band ligator on a varix. See text for details.**

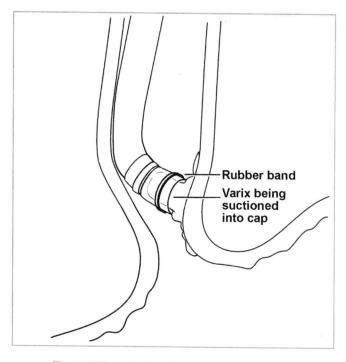

**Fig. 16.2. The varix is sucked into the ligating unit.**

8. The knob on the handle of the bander should be rotated approximately 180° clockwise. An increase in tension followed by immediate decrease in tension indicates the band has been deployed. On the Speedband Superview Super 7 Multiple Band Ligator, a "click" may be heard and an indent felt.

9. Continue suction for an additional 5 seconds to ensure complete ligation of the varix.

10. Apply air insufflation, and gently retract the endoscope. Inspect the varix for appropriate placement of the band, hemostasis, and decompression of the varix (Fig. 16.3).

11. Additional bands may be placed along the varix at 1- to 2-cm intervals cranially to the first band until it has been completely decompressed.

12. The procedure should be repeated until all varices are decompressed and hemostasis has been achieved.

13. Frequent irrigation using the 50-cc syringe, attached appropriately to the handle of the bander, with sterile water or saline should be used to maintain adequate visualization and to ensure hemostasis.

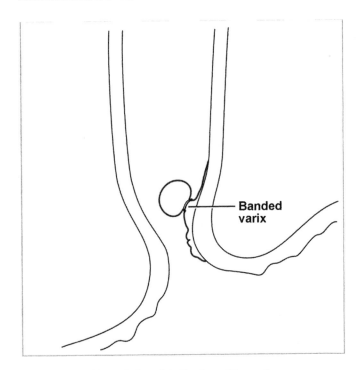

**Fig. 16.3. Complete ligation of the varix.**

14. Repeat band ligation of all varices at 10- to 14-day intervals until all varices are obliterated. An average of 3 to 4 banding sessions may be necessary to completely obliterate all varices (6).

**Note:** Band ligation may be ineffective for very small or Grade I varices. Sclerotherapy may be considered in the setting of small varices with acute or recurrent bleeding.

## POSTPROCEDURE

1. Monitor vital signs, and follow hemoglobin to make certain bleeding has stopped.

2. Elevate the head of the bed to reduce aspiration risk.

3. Give clear liquids for 24 hours, then advance the diet as tolerated.

4. Avoid nasogastric or feeding tube placement for 24 hours.

5. Short-term antibiotic prophylaxis (e.g., an oral quinolone for 5 to 7 days after procedure) has been shown to reduce

mortality and the incidence of bacterial infections in cirrhotic patients with variceal bleeding (7,8).

6. Acid suppression (e.g., proton pump inhibitor) for up to 4 weeks after all varices have been obliterated may reduce banding ulcer size and the risk of ulcer hemorrhage.

7. The patient should return for severe chest pain, fevers, shortness of breath, hematemesis, or blood per rectum.

## COMPLICATIONS

1. Continued variceal hemorrhage. This may necessitate placement of a balloon tamponade (i.e., Sengstaken-Blakemore or Minnesota tube), emergent transjugular intrahepatic portosystemic shunt (TIPSS), emergent surgery (portosystemic shunting or esophagogastric devascularization with gastroesophageal stapling, known as the modified Sugiura procedure), as well as continued medical management (i.e., IV octreotide, hemodynamic support, and correction of coagulopathy).

2. Superficial esophageal banding ulcers, which may bleed

3. Esophageal strictures

4. Esophageal perforation

5. Aspiration

6. Transient bacteremia

7. Esophageal obstruction

8. Dysphagia and/or odynophagia

9. Chest pain

## CPT Codes

**43244** – Upper gastrointestinal endoscopy including the esophagus, stomach, and either the duodenum and/or jejunum as appropriate; with band ligation of esophageal and/or gastric varices.

## REFERENCES

1. Sharara AI, Rockey DC. Gastroesophageal variceal hemorrhage. *N Engl J Med* 2001;345(9):669–681.
2. The North Italian Endoscopic Club for the Study and Treatment of Esophageal Varices. Prediction of the first variceal hemorrhage in patients with cirrhosis of the liver and esophageal varices; a prospective multicenter study. *N Engl J Med* 1988;319:983–989.
3. D'Amico G, Pagliaro L, Bosch J. The treatment of portal hypertension: a meta-analytic review. *Hepatology* 1995;22:332–354.
4. Stiegman GV, Goff JS, Sun J, Wilborn S. Endoscopic elastic band ligation for active variceal hemorrhage. *Am Surg* 1989;55(2): 124–128.
5. Stiegmann GV, Goff JS, Michaletz-Onody PA, et al. Endoscopic sclerotherapy as compared with endoscopic ligation for bleeding esophageal varices. *N Engl J Med* 1992;326(23):1527–1532.

6. Laine L, Cook D. Endoscopic ligation compared to sclerotherapy for treatment of esophageal variceal bleeding: a meta-analysis. *Ann Int Med* 1995;123(4):280–287.

7. Bernard B, Grange JD, Khac EN, et al. Antibiotic prophylaxis for the prevention of bacterial infections in cirrhotic patients with gastrointestinal bleeding: a meta-analysis. *Hepatology* 1999;29: 1655–1661.

8. Soares-Weiser K, Brezis M, Tur-Kaspa R, Leibovici L. Antibiotic prophylaxis for cirrhotic patients with gastrointestinal bleeding. *Cochrane Database Systematic Review* 2002;2:CD002907.

# Balloon Tamponade

Kim L. Isaacs

Esophageal varices occur as a consequence of portal hypertension and may develop in up to 50% of patients with cirrhosis. Approximately one-third of patients with varices will experience variceal bleeding (1). Acute endoscopic therapy, including band ligation and sclerotherapy, has been used as first line therapy in treating acute variceal bleeding. In patients whose bleeding cannot be controlled by endoscopic therapy, emergent transjugular intrahepatic portosystemic shunt (TIPS) may be performed (2). If TIPS is not available or the patient is exsanguinating, balloon tamponade plays a role in an attempt to control variceal bleeding while stabilizing the patient and setting up further intervention with TIPS or surgery.

The Minnesota four-lumen esophagogastric tamponade tube is used in the treatment of hemorrhage from varices in the esophagus and stomach (3) (Fig. 17.1). This tube is a modification of the widely used, three-lumen Sengstaken-Blakemore tube, which incorporates an internal separate esophageal suction port to the existing gastric suction port, gastric balloon, and esophageal balloon lumens (4). The Minnesota tube has been demonstrated to be fairly well tolerated by patients. Its design may help to prevent aspiration of esophageal contents (3).

The Minnesota tube is used for control of hemorrhage from esophageal varices, documented by endoscopy or, in rare cases, by angiography, which continue to bleed despite aggressive medical management including lavage, correction of blood-clotting abnormalities, intravenous octreotide or vasopressin infusion, and endoscopic therapy (band ligation and/or sclerotherapy) (5). An alternative approach is the use of a TIPS for uncontrollable bleeding (2).

## INDICATION

1. Acute bleeding from esophageal or gastric varices unresponsive to medical and endoscopic therapy, including band ligation and sclerotherapy

## CONTRAINDICATIONS

### Absolute

1. Cessation of variceal bleeding
2. Recent surgery involving the esophagogastric junction
3. Known esophageal stricture

### Relative

1. Poorly informed support staff (6)
2. Congestive heart failure
3. Respiratory failure

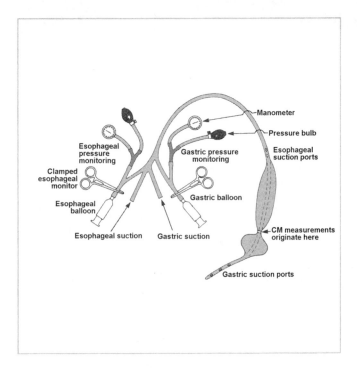

**Fig. 17.1. Minnesota four-lumen tube.**

4.  Cardiac arrhythmias

5.  Hiatal hernia

6.  Incomplete lavage

7.  Inability to demonstrate a variceal source of bleeding

8.  Esophageal ulceration (secondary to reflux esophagitis or previous endoscopic therapy—in these cases, the gastric balloon may be used but not the esophageal balloon)

**PREPARATION**

1.  Perform endoscopy to confirm the source of bleeding, and attempt band ligation or sclerotherapy as a primary mode of treating acute variceal bleeding.

2.  Start pharmacologic therapy with intravenous octreotide to reduce portal pressure (1).

3.  Protect the airway. In general, patients who require balloon tamponade for treatment of severe variceal bleeding should be intubated for airway protection.

4.  Transfuse as necessary for resuscitation and to improve coagulation abnormalities.

5. Anesthetize the oropharynx.

6. If endoscopy demonstrates large amounts of blood in the stomach, lavage the stomach with tap water using an adult gastric lavage or other large-bore tube.

7. Test the balloons by insufflating each with air and examining for leaks under water.

8. Connect a mercury manometer to the gastric balloon and inflate with 100-cc increments of air to 500 cc, recording manometric pressure at each point.

9. Instruct the staff caring for the patient in the use of the tube, complications that may arise, and measures for emergency removal.

## EQUIPMENT

A commercially available four-lumen tube with aspiration ports in the gastric and esophageal sections, a spherical gastric balloon capable of holding 500 cc of air, and a sausage-shaped esophageal balloon with reinforced rubber proximally attached to the gastric balloon (Blakemore Tube-4 Lumen Rubber, Rusch Inc., Duluth, GA). There are ports available for insufflation of esophageal and gastric balloons and for pressure monitoring of both of these balloons.

## OTHER EQUIPMENT

1. Topical anesthesia and tongue blades or swabs

2. Two wall-suction setups with plastic connectors to adapt gastric and esophageal ports to suction tubing

3. Hemostats to clamp closed the gastric and esophageal balloon ports

4. Two manometers with pressure bulbs attached by connector to one port of the gastric balloon lumen and one port of the esophageal balloon lumen

5. Water-soluble lubricant

6. Catheter-tipped syringes (60 cc)

7. An over-the-bed traction with a counterweight of 1 lb. Alternatively a football helmet or catcher's mask may be used, but can lead to pressure necrosis of the skin if severe edema occurs.

8. Adhesive tape

9. Scissors, which should be taped to the top of the bed

## PROCEDURE

1. Suction all air from the balloons, and insert plastic plugs.

2. Clamp hemostats on the two pressure-monitoring outlets.

3. Lubricate the tube, and pass it through the patient's mouth until the 45-cm mark is located at the dentate ridge. Do not pass the tube through the nares unless orogastric passage is impossible (due to increased risk of necrosis of the nasal

septum, sinusitis). The 45-cm mark is measured from the junction of the esophageal and gastric balloons. This should be taken into consideration in patients who have had esophageal or gastric surgery. If blind passage is not possible, endoscopically place a guide wire, then pass the Minnesota tube with the tip cut off over the guide wire (7). Confirm the position of the tube fluoroscopically so the tip is below the diaphragm.

4. Apply suction to the gastric and esophageal ports.

5. Remove the clamp and plastic plug from the gastric ports. Check the connection of the gastric pressure-monitoring outlet to the mercury manometer. Use the catheter-tip syringe to introduce 100-cc air increments through the gastric insufflation port. Check the manometer readings for correlation with pre-intubation readings. If the intragastric balloon pressure after intubation is more than 15 mm Hg greater than the pressure which was produced when the balloon was tested before insertion, then the balloon should be deflated as it may be located in the esophagus. Deflate the balloon immediately if the patient experiences chest pain.

6. When the gastric balloon is inflated with 450 to 500 cc of air, clamp the air inlet and pressure-monitoring outlets, and pull the tube back gently until resistance is felt against the gastroesophageal junction.

7. With a minimum of tension on the tube, fix the upper end of the tube to over-the-bed traction with a 1-lb weight or, alternatively, to the crossbar of a football helmet or a catcher's mask as it exits from the mouth (8).

8. Observe the nature of the drainage from the gastric and esophageal ports. If bleeding persists from either port, inflate the esophageal balloon. To do this, first check the connection between the esophageal pressure-monitoring port and the manometer, then inflate to a pressure of 25 to 45 mm Hg using the lowest pressure needed to stop bleeding through both the gastric and esophageal ports. Never inflate the esophageal balloon before the gastric balloon. Double clamp the tube. Check the esophageal balloon pressure with the mercury manometer every 3 hours, or keep the manometer attached for constant monitoring.

9. Elevate the head of the bed 6 to 10 in. Tape the scissors to the head of the bed for quick access in case the balloons need immediate deflation.

**POSTPROCEDURE**

1. Verify the tube position by stat portable x-ray.

2. Due to the risk of esophageal pressure necrosis, deflation of the esophageal balloon is performed for 5 minutes every 6 hours.

3. After bleeding has been controlled, reduce the pressure in the esophageal balloon 5 mm Hg every 3 hours until 25 mm Hg is reached without bleeding.

4. Manually check the tube tension at 3-hour intervals. Do not manipulate the tube unnecessarily.

5. Give nothing by mouth. Institute oral hygiene. If necessary, give medications through the gastric port.

6. Check both the gastric and esophageal return every 2 hours, and flush both lumens if there is any question of clogging. Barium should never be instilled through the tube, since impaction of balloons could occur, requiring removal of the tube

7. If respiratory distress occurs due to proximal migration of the esophageal balloon with occlusion of the airway, the tube must be removed immediately! *Grasp the tube at the mouth, transect with scissors above the grasping hand but below the entrance of the three channel inlets, and pull out the tube.*

8. If hemostasis persists for 24 hours, deflate the esophageal balloon. If there is no recurrence of bleeding over the next 6 to 12 hours, deflate the gastric balloon and release tension, but leave the Minnesota tube in place. If bleeding recurs, the gastric balloon and, if necessary, the esophageal balloon may be reinflated for an additional 24 hours (Fig. 17.2).

9. In the case of rebleeding, alternatives such as banding, sclerotherapy, TIPS, and surgery should be reconsidered as there is a high mortality rate among patients who rebleed (5).

10. If bleeding does not recur by 24 hours after deflation, remove the Minnesota tube, and transect it to ensure that it will not be reused. Removal is best done when there is adequate staff available to manage any rebleeding that might occur.

## COMPLICATIONS

### Major

1. Aspiration. In older series, this was a significant cause of death (9). The greatest risk for aspiration occurs during insertion. Airway protection with intubation should be strongly considered (10).

2. Airway occlusion secondary to proximal migration of the tube. This is usually secondary to deflation of the gastric balloon while the esophageal balloon remains inflated.

3. Pressure effects. Rupture of the esophagus, laceration or ulceration of the stomach, and pressure necrosis of the hypopharynx or alae nasi may occur with prolonged balloon inflation or excessive pressures. Rupture of the esophagus is a particular risk if sclerotherapy has been performed prior to tube placement.

4. Cardiac arrhythmias

5. Pulmonary edema

6. Bronchopneumonia

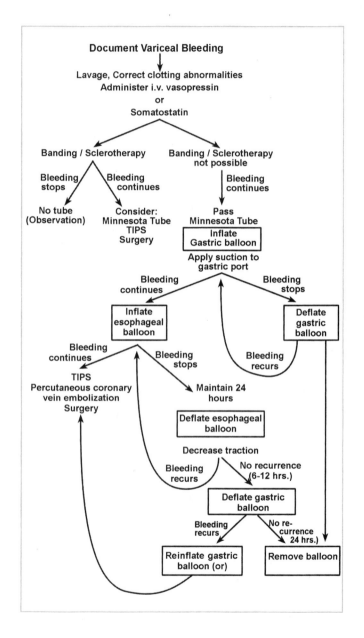

Fig. 17.2. Use of the Minnesota tube in a patient with variceal bleeding. TIPS, transjugular intrahepatic portosystemic shunt.

**Minor**

1. Unintentional deflation
2. Hiccoughs
3. Agitation

**EFFICACY**

The Minnesota tube has been demonstrated to be better tolerated than the older Sengstaken-Blakemore tube because of its softer rubber consistency. The Minnesota tube can be used safely in attaining initial hemostasis. The role of balloon tamponade is controversial. With the advent of improved endoscopic techniques and the availability of emergent TIPS procedure, balloon tamponade has a limited role in the primary treatment of bleeding varices. Its greatest role may be in temporarily stabilizing the actively bleeding patient in whom initial endoscopic therapy has failed while awaiting emergent TIPS procedure. The overall outcome of hemorrhage control by endoscopic techniques is dependent on the underlying condition of the patient (1).

The effectiveness of balloon tamponade has ranged from 50% to 92% in the published series. Permanent cessation of bleeding occurs in 40% to 50% of patients treated with balloon tamponade. In one study efficacy depended on the degree of hypovolemia at presentation, those who required less than 1,500 cc of fluid resuscitation had a higher rate of successful tamponade (10). Long-term efficacy in terms of rebleeding is dependent in part on the patient's underlying liver disease. Only 25% of patients with ascites, jaundice, and encephalopathy attain lasting hemostasis with balloon tamponade, whereas without these findings approximately 92% of patients will not rebleed (11).

**CPT Codes**

**43460** – Esophagogastric tamponade, with balloon.

**REFERENCES**

1. Sharara A, Rockey D. Gastroesophageal variceal hemorrhage. *N Eng J Med* 2001;345:669–681.
2. Chau T, Patch D, Chan Y, et al. "Salvage" transjugular intrahepatic portosystemic shunts: Gastric fundal compared with esophageal variceal bleeding. *Gastroenterology* 1998;114: 981–987.
3. Mitchell K, Silk D, Williams R. Prospective comparison of two Sengstaken tubes in the management of patients with variceal hemorrhage. *Gut* 1980;21:570–573.
4. Boyce H. Modification of the Sengstaken-Blakemore tube. *N Engl J Med* 1962;267:195–196.
5. Ferguson J, Tripathi D, Hayes P. Review article: the management of acute variceal bleeding. *Aliment Phamacol Ther* 2003;18:253–262.
6. Pitcher J. Safety and effectiveness of the modified Sengstaken Blakemore tube: a prospective study. *Gastroenterology* 1967;61:291–298.
7. Snow N, Almon M, Baillie J. Minnesota tube placement using a guide wire (Letter). *Gastrointest Endosc* 1990;36:420–421.

8. Kashiwagi H, Shikano S, Yamamoto O, et al. Technique for positioning the Sengstaken-Blakemore tube as comfortably as possible. *Surg Gynecol Obstet* 1991;172:63.

9. Conn H, Simpson J. Excessive mortality associated with balloon tamponade of bleeding varices; a critical appraisal. *JAMA* 1967;202:287–291.

10. Panes J, Teres J, Bosch J, Rodes J. Efficacy of balloon tamponade in treatment of bleeding gastric and esophageal varices: Results in 151 consecutive episodes. *Dig Dis Sci* 1988;33:454–459.

11. Novis B, Duys P, Barbezat G. Fiberoptic endoscopy and the use of the Sengstaken tube in acute gastroesophageal hemorrhage from esophageal varices. *Gut* 1976;17:258–263.

# Polypectomy, Endoscopic Mucosal Resection, and Tattooing

Gregory G. Ginsberg and Nina Phatak

Polyps are abnormal growths of tissue that protrude above the flat surface of the bowel wall. Many neoplastic lesions of the luminal digestive tract arise from the mucosal layer as polyps. Polyps may be pedunculated or sessile. Resection of cancer-containing and precancerous polyps prevents development of invasive cancer (1). Pedunculated polyps protrude on a stalk of nonneoplastic tissue and are resected via standard snare cautery polypectomy. Endoscopic mucosal resection (EMR) is the term applied to the addition of adjunctive techniques to achieve endoscopic resection of lesions otherwise not amenable to standard snare polypectomy. Endoscopic tattooing is performed to mark the location of a lesion, thereby facilitating future localization should further resection or confirmation of the completeness of prior resection be indicated.

## INDICATIONS

1.  Standard snare polypectomy

    a.  Resection of pedunculated luminal digestive tract polyps
    b.  Resection of moderate-sized (0.5- to 2.0-cm) sessile luminal digestive tract polyps

2.  EMR

    a.  Resection of large (> 2.0-cm) sessile luminal digestive tract polyps
    b.  Resection of early gastric cancer
    c.  Resection of esophageal focal high-grade dysplasia and intramucosal carcinoma associated with Barrett's esophagus or squamous dysplasia (2)

## RELATIVE CONTRAINDICATIONS

1.  Lesion has features suggestive of invasive carcinoma including ulceration, fixation, hard consistency

2.  Lesion is not readily accessible endoscopically

3.  Complete resection is not likely to be achieved even with multiple sessions; these are lesions greater than 5 cm in size, extending over two or more folds, and encompassing greater than one-third of the luminal circumference.

4.  Unaddressed bleeding or coagulation disorder

5.  Poor bowel preparation

6.  Poor general medical condition of the patient

7. No surgical backup for large lesions

8. "Nonlifting" sign after submucosal injection

9. Inability of the patient to physically tolerate or cooperate with the procedure

## PREPARATION

Endoscopic and colonoscopic polypectomy is routinely performed on an outpatient basis. However, overnight hospitalization should be considered on an individual basis, such as for those patients with coagulopathy, following resection of very large polyps, and when complications are suspected during or after the procedure. A complete colonoscopic or endoscopic evaluation is usually done prior to resection. Standard and simple saline-assisted polypectomy should be considered part of typical consent for endoscopy and colonoscopy. Lesions that are not amenable to standard polypectomy should have biopsies performed on them. The decision to undertake EMR should be considered with the patient in the context of the alternatives such as operative resection and endoscopic ablation. Lesion location determines the type of preparation needed for optimal results. For lesions in the upper gastrointestinal tract, patients should be kept NPO for 6 hours prior to the procedure. Per-rectal enemas suffice for rectal lesions. All other colonic lesions require a standard peroral bowel preparation.

Routine preprocedural laboratory testing is generally not recommended (3). Patients may be asked to discontinue aspirin, nonsteroidal antiinflammatory drugs (NSAIDs), and anticoagulants when polypectomy or EMR is anticipated.

## EQUIPMENT

### Polypectomy

1. Colonoscope

2. Monopolar electrosurgical generator

3. Grounding pad applied to the patient's thigh

4. Polypectomy snare (standard or specialty snare)

5. Retrieval apparatus (e.g., specimen container in circuit with suction line for small polyps aspirated through the accessory channel versus grasping devices and nets for larger lesions)

6. Hemostasis device for inadvertent postpolypectomy bleeding including contact or noncontact electrocautery, injection (epinephrine, sclerosant), mechanical (clips, loops, and/or bands)

### Adjuncts for EMR

7. Standard sclerotherapy injection needle

8. Submucosal injectant (e.g., normal saline, diluted epinephrine, 50% dextrose).

9. Spray catheter and chromoendoscopic agents. Indigo carmine is used as a topical contrast agent to discriminate

the margins of sessile lesions in the stomach and colon; Lugol's iodine is used as a vital stain to discriminate esophageal intestinal metaplasia and squamous dysplasia.

10. Transparent aspiration chamber for endoscopic mucosal resection with a cap (EMRC) method. This is commercially available in a dedicated EMR kit, or a similar device may be obtained from a variceal band ligation kit.

**Tattooing**

11. Injection needle

12. Tattooing agent: Spot (GI Supply, Camp Hill, PA), India ink

## PROCEDURE

### Standard Snare Polypectomy

Polyploid neoplasms are generally classified as pedunculated (protruding from the normal bowel wall attached to a stalk of nonneoplastic tissue) or sessile (flat or on a short, broad-based stalk). Repositioning the patient and/or manipulating the lesion with a device extended from the scope tip may better define its size and configuration (4).

*Techniques for Pedunculated Polyps*

1. Optimize the localization of the polyp to the 6 o'clock position, orienting it with the accessory channel of the endoscope by repositioning the scope or the patient.

2. Advance the closed snare in proximity to the lesion. Open the snare so that the wire loop is above the lesion. By manipulating the endoscope controls and shaft, negotiate the snare loop over the polyp head and down around the midsection of the stalk.

3. Gently push the base of the snare loop against the stalk. This will prevent the snare from riding up or down along the polyp stalk (Fig. 18.1).

4. Close the snare around the stalk until moderate resistance is encountered. While closing the snare, make sure no portion of the head of the polyp or any surrounding tissue is unintentionally caught. If the polyp is not well-positioned or surrounding tissue is caught in the snare, reopen the snare loop, and reposition it on the polyp. Ensure that the snare does not have other contact with the colon wall by gently pulling the polyp away from the wall.

5. Set the power level based on the manufacturer's recommendations and prior experience with your electrosurgical unit. Electrosurgical energy is applied using low-power pure coagulation or a blended cutting/coagulation current while the snare loop is tightened around the stalk. There should be a smooth but gradually resistive response. Look for visible swelling or whitening to indicate effective electrocautery. In 2 or 3 seconds, the snare will "snap" when the wire is pulled through the stalk.

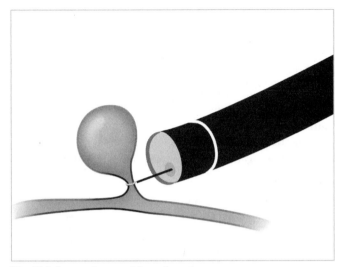

**Fig. 18.1. Snare placement for polypectomy.**

6. If a great deal of resistance is experienced, stop and reexamine for proper positioning of the snare and for blanching of the stalk. Do not pull through without coagulation! The snare catheter may be moved back and forth to help complete the transection. The rate of transection should be proportionate to the thickness of the polyp stalk.

7. Once transection is complete, retrieve the specimen with suction or a retrieval device. Examine the stalk for bleeding.

8. If active bleeding is observed to persist, endoscopic hemostasis should be undertaken with injection, thermal, and/or hemoclip therapies.

*Technique for Small Sessile Polyps (<1 cm)*

**SNARE TECHNIQUES**

1. The snare-cautery technique can be used to lasso small sessile polyps at their base. Gentle tightening produces a "pseudostalk" that can then be transected. "Tenting" the ensnared polyp, by deflecting the tip of the scope toward the lumen center, reduces thermal injury to the bowel wall.

2. Cold snare polypectomy may also be performed safely and effectively for polyps ≤ 0.5 cm without significant bleeding. Simply transect the ensnared polyp without applying electrosurgical current.

**BIOPSY TECHNIQUES.** Standard and large capacity cold biopsy forceps can be used to resect diminutive (< 5 mm) polyps as a single specimen or in piecemeal fashion. The "hot-biopsy" technique that employs the use of monopolar electrocautery directed to the tip of the forceps has fallen out of favor due to increased risk of thermal injury and delayed bleeding (5).

*Technique for Moderate-Sized Sessile Polyps (< 2 cm)*

A sessile polyp less than 2 cm in diameter can be removed with simple electrocautery snare resection similar to that described for pedunculated polyps.

1.  The opened snare is placed over the top of the lesion.

2.  The base of the open snare should be pushed snug up against the close edge of the polyp. Decompressing the lumen slightly by aspirating air while closing the snare will encourage the sessile polyp's margins into the snare loop.

3.  Close the snare about the base of the polyp until modest resistance is observed. Ideally, it is compressed to less than 1.5 cm in width.

4.  Proceed with the polypectomy as previously outlined.

### Endoscopic Mucosal Resection (EMR)

*Piecemeal Resection for Large Sessile Polyps (> 2 cm)*

This technique may be employed alone for rectal lesions (below the retroperitoneal reflection) and in conjunction with the "inject and cut" method for large sessile lesions elsewhere. A sessile polyp is removed in a piecemeal fashion by resecting portions of the polyp, in a manner similar to that described above for small sessile polyps, consecutively until complete resection is achieved (Fig. 18.2).

1.  The open snare engages the polyp obliquely at a lateral margin. The side of the snare loop abuts the edge of the lesion,

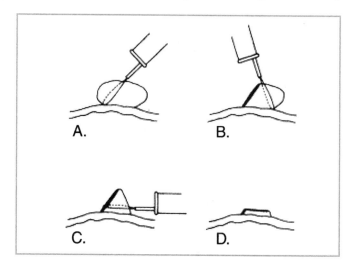

**Fig. 18.2. Removal of large sessile polyp. A: Piecemeal removal of polyp. B: Procedure repeated at other end of polyp. C, D: Top half of polyp is encircled and coagulated off (see text).**

and the open snare is leveled over a portion of the polyp. The loop is closed around the ensnared portion.

2.  Electrosurgical current is applied while the snare is closed, transecting the tissue.

3.  Repeat the procedure on the residual portions of the polyp.

4.  Retrieve all pieces for histopathologic evaluation.

*Inject and Cut Method*

Also known as "strip biopsy," "strip mucosectomy," and "saline-assisted polypectomy," the target mucosa is raised upon a cushion of fluid injected into the submucosal layer creating a "pseudostalk" more amenable to ensnarement (Fig. 18.3). The submucosal injectant also increases the distance from the serosa and decreases electrosurgical resistance. These features are thought to reduce the risk of perforation and transmural burn syndrome. This method can be used for removal of moderate-sized and large sessile adenomas.

1.  Normal saline solution (NSS) is the most commonly used injectant. Some enthusiasts use dilute epinephrine solution. More viscous solutions like hypertonic saline, 50% dextrose, and hyaluronate are investigational. Tinting the NSS with a

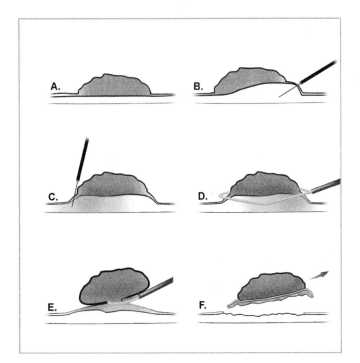

**Fig. 18.3A–F. Snare placement for polypectomy.**

drop of methylene blue creates a contrast agent that enhances discrimination of the lesion. Depending on the lesion size, one or more 10-cc syringes of sterile injectant should be prepared.

2. A standard injection needle should be primed with injectant. The exposed needle is preferentially plunged obliquely into the tissue at the edge of the lesion (insertion directly into the lesion proper is also allowed) and the solution injected at 1- to 2-cc increments. The injected solution should be seen to expand the submucosa and raise the lesion upon a bleb of injectant. Anywhere from 2 to 20 cc of injectant may be used depending on the extent of the lesion (6).

3. The lesion, now raised on a pseudostalk of submucosal injectant, is then ensnared and resected with standard electrocautery snare polypectomy technique. Resecting the lesion as a single specimen preserves the histopathological integrity of the cautery margins. However, large lesions may require piecemeal resection. Ideally, complete resection is accomplished in a single session.

*Endoscopic Mucosal Resection with a Cap*

Endoscopic mucosal resection with a cap is used to resect flat lesions primarily in the upper gastrointestinal (GI) tract, though it has been applied in the colorectum as well. The technique employs a specially designed transparent cap that is fitted to the tip of a diagnostic or therapeutic endoscope (7).

1. The cap is fit snugly over the tip of the endoscope and affixed with adhesive tape to reduce the risk of unintentional dislodgment.

2. Optionally, the periphery of the lesion may be predemarcated using vital staining or contact electrocautery.

3. Submucosal injection is then performed to elevate the target lesion as described above. Injection of up to 10 cc or more is commonplace.

4. A specially designed "crescent-shaped" snare is predeployed into the cap rim. To do this, the tip of the scope is directed away from the target tissue and directly opposed to a neighboring area of normal tissue. Gentle suction is applied, drawing tissue into the chamber and obscuring the open end. The snare is opened, and the wire loop slides neatly into the prefitting groove. The extent of snare opening is adjusted accordingly for a neat fit.

5. The scope tip is redirected to the target tissue and the suction button applied, drawing the lesion up into the cap chamber. The predeployed snare is closed, effectively strangulating the lesion, and suction is then released (Fig. 18.4). Gentle tugging on the ensnared lesion should demonstrate smooth movement over the fixed luminal wall. This "pseudopolyp" is then resected with electrosurgical current. If the wall is tugged along, it implies that the muscularis propria layer is ensnared, and the lesion should be released.

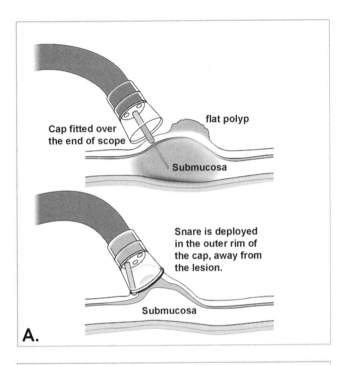

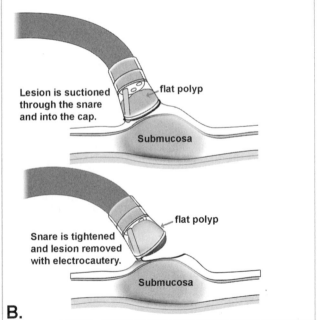

Fig. 18.4A–B. Endoscopic musocal resection with a cap.

*Endoscopic Mucosal Resection with Ligation*

This method for resection of flat lesions is a modification of the EMRC technique that employs commercially available variceal band ligation (VBL) devices.

1.   The target lesion is localized and submucosal injection is performed. Some enthusiasts forgo submucosal injection. The scope is removed.

2.   The VBL apparatus is assembled and the scope is reinserted. The target lesion is suctioned into the banding chamber, a band is deployed, and suction is released. The endoscope is again removed and the VBL apparatus is disassembled.

3.   The scope is again inserted, and the banded pseudopolyp is resected below the band using standard electrosurgical snare polypectomy technique.

*Endoscopic Tattooing*

This technique uses a staining agent to durably demarcate the location of a lesion or resection site for subsequent surveillance or resection (endoscopic or operative) (8).

1.   The tattooing agent (Spot or 1:100 dilution of sterile India ink in normal saline) is prepared in a 5- to 10-cc syringe. A standard injection needle is assembled and primed.

2.   The needle is inserted into the submucosa at a 45-degree angle. As the agent is injected, the depth of needle insertion should be adjusted so that a "bleb" of injectant is observed to form within the submucosa. Avoid injecting the tattooing agent through the bowel wall as this will discolor a broad outer surface and eliminate the intended benefit for preoperative marking.

3.   Inject 1 to 3 cc at one or more (up to four quadrants is recommended by some) points surrounding the lesion.

**POSTPROCEDURE**

1.   The resection site should be assessed as to the completeness of resection.

2.   Completion resection or thermal ablation (e.g., argon plasma coagulation) can be employed when residual neoplasia is observed.

3.   Postprocedure observation is as for any endoscopic procedure using sedation.

4.   Following colonic polypectomy and EMR, patients may resume their regular diet. After EMR of upper GI tract lesions, patients should be maintained on clear liquids for 12 hours, and a proton pump-inhibitor should be instituted to enhance resection site healing.

5.   Patients should be instructed to report symptoms of pain, bleeding, or fever.

6.   Endoscopic and colonoscopic surveillance intervals are lesion-dependent and pathology-dependent. When initial

resection is incomplete, repeat EMR should be scheduled at approximately 6 weeks to allow sufficient healing of the initial resection site.

**INTERPRETATION**

1. Endoscopic assessment of completeness of resection should be documented (9).

2. Adenomatous polyps and polyps containing carcinoma in situ are considered cured provided the polyp is completely excised.

3. Endoscopically resected pedunculated polyps containing invasive cancer are usually cured when favorable histological criteria exist such as when carcinoma is > 2 mm from the resected margin, the cancer is not poorly differentiated, and there is no lymphovascular invasion.

4. Endoscopically resected sessile polyps containing invasive cancer have a higher risk of metastasis, and further operative resection should be considered on an individual case basis.

**COMPLICATIONS**

The major risks of EMR and polypectomy include

1. Bleeding (immediate: 1.5%, delayed: 2%) is most often observed immediately, but can occur within the first 24 hours or rarely 5 to 7 days postprocedure. Most often these episodes are self-limited and do not require intervention. However, in some instances attention may be needed for brisk bleeding, especially immediately post-EMR. Low-concentration epinephrine saline solution is very effective in hemostasis when injected into the bleeding site, especially in the esophagus and colon. For more significant bleeding, hemodynamic stabilization of the patient must first be implemented. Other localized therapy such as heater probe therapy, electrocautery, argon plasma coagulation, laser, or endoscopic clips can be used to control bleeding and achieve hemostasis.

2. Perforation (0.04% to 2.1%) usually occurs when a transmural section, involving all layers from the mucosa to the serosa, is resected. Risk factors include inadequate submucosal saline injection, piecemeal resection without repeated submucosal saline injection, repeated attempts at resection at same site, and increased application of suction during EMR. Immediate surgical evaluation and possible exploratory laparotomy may be needed if clinical and radiographic suspicion is high.

3. Transmural burn syndrome (1%), also known as post-polypectomy syndrome, occurs when thermal energy during electrocoagulation extends to the muscularis propria and serosa, which produces peritoneal inflammation without perforation. The patient usually has localized peritoneal signs, abdominal pain, fever, and leukocytosis. These symptoms usually resolve with conservative management

including hospital observation for 1 to 2 days with bowel rest with intravenous fluids and antibiotics.

The most critical aspect of EMR is the proper placement of the submucosal bleb to ensure proper "lifting" of the lesion. This is important for two reasons. The first reason is to minimize transmural thermal injury to surrounding tissue, and the second is to recognize a nonlifting sign that is highly suspicious for a more advanced infiltrative process. The latter is more prone to perforation and will less likely be cured from an endoscopic approach.

## CPT Codes

**45385** – Colonoscopy, flexible, proximal to splenic flexure; with removal of tumor(s), polyp(s), or other lesion(s) by snare technique.

**45381** – With directed submucosal injection(s), any substance.

## REFERENCES

1. Muller AD, Sonnenber A. Prevention of colorectal cancer by flexible endoscopy and polypectomy. *Ann Int Med* 1995;123:904–910.
2. Ahmad N, Kochman ML, Long WL, Ginsberg GG. Efficacy, safety, and clinical outcomes of endoscopic mucosal resection: a study of 101 cases. *Gastrointest Endosc* 2002;55:390–396.
3. ASGE. Position statement on laboratory testing before ambulatory elective endoscopic procedures. *Gastrointest Endosc* 1999;50:906–909
4. ASGE Clinical Guideline. The role of colonoscopy in the management of patients with colonic polyps neoplasia. *Gastrointest Endosc* 1999;50:921–924
5. Gilbert DA, DiMarino AJ, Jensen DM, et al. Status evaluation: hot biopsy forceps. *Gastrointest Endosc* 1992;38:753–756.
6. Waye J. New methods of polypectomy. *Gastrointest Endosc Clin North Am* 1997;7(3):413–422.
7. Soetikno R, Gotoda R, Nakanishi Y, Soehendra N. Endoscopic mucosal resection. *Gastrointest Endosc* 2003;57(4):567–579.
8. Ginsberg GG, Barkun AN, Bosco JJ, et al. Endoscopic tattooing. *Gastrointest Endosc* 2002;55(7):811–814.
9. Cranley JP. Proper management of the patient with a malignant colorectal polyp. *Gastrointest Endosc Clin North Am* 1993;3(4): 661–671.

# Feeding Tubes (Nasoduodenal, Nasojejunal)

## William D. Heizer

Enteral feeding (tube feeding) is an effective way to provide nutrition to patients who cannot, should not, or will not eat. Although intravenous feeding is often favored because it can be more comfortable for patients and less time-consuming for nurses and doctors, enteral feeding is generally safer and more cost-effective. It is usually appropriate to feed into the stomach using either a large-bore nasogastric tube (14- to 18-Fr) which can also be used for suctioning or a small-bore tube (8- to 12-Fr). See Chapter 4 for nasogastric tube placement. Feeding distal to the pylorus, or preferably distal to the ligament of Treitz, is indicated when there is a high risk of gastroesophageal reflux and aspiration or markedly abnormal gastric emptying, or there are other compelling reasons to bypass the stomach or proximal duodenum. Among patients who can tolerate either gastric or postpyloric feeding there appears to be no advantage to postpyloric feeding (1) although some studies report fewer infections with postpyloric compared to gastric feeding (2). Small-bore tubes (8- to 12-Fr) should be used for nasoduodenal and nasojejunal feeding in adults.

### INDICATIONS

1. Acute pancreatitis
2. Gastric residual volume persistently >400 mL
3. Aspiration of gastric contents (likely to be catostrophic due to patient's compromised pulmonary status)
4. History of significant gastroesophageal reflux
5. History of severe gastroparesis
6. Severe trauma, burn, or other critical illness likely to cause significant gastric atony

### CONTRAINDICATIONS

1. Nasopharyngeal, esophageal, gastric, or pyloric obstruction
2. High-grade small bowel or colonic obstruction
3. Severe maxillofacial trauma and/or basilar skull fracture (can use orojejunal tube)
4. Severe uncontrolled coagulopathy
5. Bullous disorders of the esophageal mucosa
6. Severe mucositis
7. Intractable vomiting
8. Patient intolerance to tube

**PREPARATION**

1. Choose the method that will ensure that the small-bore tube will enter the esophagus and not the trachea. Inadvertent passage of small-bore tubes into the trachea is reported in 2% of attempts resulting in a major complication in 0.7% and death in 0.2% (3). If a tube that is stiffened with a stylet and has a tip less than 4 mm wide is passed into the trachea, it can perforate a small bronchus, pass into the lung tissue, and enter the pleural space with minimal if any detectable resistance. The risk that the tube will enter the trachea is significantly increased if the patient is unable to swallow on request, for any reason, or has an endotracheal tube (nasotracheal, orotracheal, or tracheostomy). For patients with either of these risk factors, special care must be taken to avoid bronchopulmonary injury. Several methods for achieving this goal have been published including a) fluoroscopic guidance; b) fiber-optic guidance (nasopharyngoscope or upper endoscope); c) two-step radiographic guidance—pass the tube to 30 cm from the nares, obtain a portable chest radiograph, advance the tube only if it is in the midline; and d) sampling for carbon dioxide through the feeding tube. Simpler methods including observing the patient for cough or hoarseness, placing the external end of the tube under water to observe for bubbles, and listening to the external end of the tube for air rushing over the feeding ports are all helpful but too insensitive to be reliable. Methods to detect when the tip of the tube has entered the stomach are ineffective for avoiding bronchopulmonary injury because if the tube enters the trachea and then is advanced far enough to be in the stomach (40 cm to 45 cm), lung injury is likely.

2. Choose the method that will be used to maneuver the tip of the tube from the stomach into the duodenum or jejunum. Several methods have been reported including a) spontaneous passage by natural peristalsis, b) peristalsis enhanced by a prokinetic agent, c) distention of the stomach with 350 mL to 1000 mL of air, d) bedside manipulation guided by auscultation, e) manipulation under fluoroscopy with or without a guidewire, f) endoscopic manipulation, g) passage over an endoscopically placed wire guide, h) use of a large external magnet to pull on a magnet imbedded in the tip of the tube (Gabriel Feeding Tube), and i) manual manipulation during laparotomy.

    Multiple techniques are reported for detecting when the feeding ports at the end of the tube have traversed the pylorus including a) auscultation, b) retrieval of infused air, c) checking aspirated fluid for pH and bile, d) plain radiography, e) endoscopy, f) fluoroscopy, g) pH probe on the tip of the tube, h) electrocardiographic tracing from the tube, and i) electromagnetic detection of the tip of the tube and the direction it is pointing.

3. Read the package insert for the feeding tube to be used, and retain the insert in the patient's chart.

4. Give nothing by mouth for at least 4 hours and preferably for 6 hours.

5.  If appropriate, have the patient sit upright, or raise the head of the bed. Alternatively, pass the tube with the patient in the left lateral position, which decreases the risk of aspiration compared to the supine position.

6.  Check for nasal obstruction. Use the most patent nostril.

## EQUIPMENT
### Bedside Nonendoscopic Placement

1.  Feeding tube 43 in. to 55 in. (109 cm to 140 cm) long, radiopaque, preferably polyurethane, preferably coated with hydromer water-activated lubricant in the lumen and on the tip, stylet that cannot exit the feeding ports of the tube, 8- to 12-Fr outer diameter (4). For adults, a 10-Fr outer diameter is the best compromise between patient comfort and likelihood of clogging. If the patient is unable to swallow on request or has an endotracheal tube, the feeding tube should have a tip that is equal to or greater than 5 mm wide (Fig. 19.1A).

    Contrary to expectations, data show that a tube without a weight at the tip is more likely to pass spontaneously from the stomach to the duodenum and is less likely to retract into the stomach after it is placed in the duodenum compared to a tube with a weighted tip.

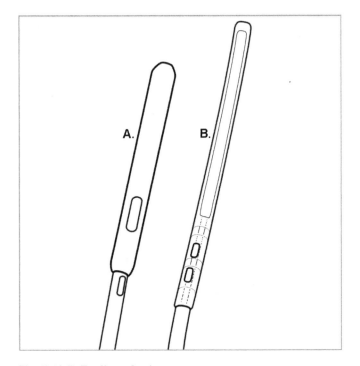

**Fig. 19.1A–B. Feeding tube tips.**

2. Sixty-mL syringe for aspirating through the tube

3. Water and 10-mL syringe to activate the hydromer lubricant coating the lumen and tip of the tube

4. Metoclopramide (10 mg) or erythromycin (250 mg) for intravenous (IV) injection. This is optional but recommended if the patient has diabetes.

5. Gloves

6. Lubricating jelly

## Placement with Fluoroscopic or Nasopharyngoscopic Guidance

Same as above except the tip of the tube can be the same diameter as the tube (Fig. 19.1B), because tracheal intubation will be avoided by visualizing passage of the tip of the tube into the esophagus.

## Placement Aided by Esophagogastroscopy

Same as above except tie suture material around the tube near the tip and 5, 10, and 15 cm proximal to the tip, leaving the ends of the suture material 2 cm long so they can be grasped with a forceps inserted through the endoscope channel.

## Placement Over a Guidewire Placed Endoscopically

1. Tube designed for insertion over a guidewire (e.g., Endo-Tube, Kendall HealthCare Products Co.)

2. Adult upper endoscope plus small plastic tube, scissors, and clamps suitable for transferring the external end of the guidewire from the mouth to the naris. Alternatively, use a neonatal or ultraslim upper endoscope (5- to 6-mm outer diameter) which can be passed through a nostril into the stomach and duodenum plus a topical anesthetic to anesthetize the nostril.

3. Ten-mL syringe containing 4 mL of spray cooking oil and 4 mL of water shaken to emulsify and injected into the tube. This emulsified oil, or liquid silicone if preferred, can be used to lubricate the tube lumen if the lumen is not coated with water-activated hydromer.

## PROCEDURE

### Bedside Nonendoscopic Placement

1. Give metoclopramide 10 mg IV by bolus or erythromycin 250 mg IV over 15 minutes before inserting the tube, especially if the patient is diabetic.

2. Identify marks on the tube that are 25, 45, 65, and 100 cm from the tip of the tube. When these marks are at the external nares the tip of the tube should be approximately at the upper esophagus, gastroesophageal junction, pylorus, and beyond the ligament of Treitz, respectively, assuming the patient is a normal-sized adult and that no significant loop of tube forms in the stomach.

3.  Examine the tube for defects. Fill the tube with water, and dip the tip of the tube in water to activate the hydromer lubricant. Insert the stylet into the tube if it is packaged separately. Bend the distal 5 to 10 cm of the tube slightly to give it a gentle 45-degree curve.

4.  With the patient in the appropriate position and the head flexed forward, gently advance the tip of the tube into the nostril, aiming the tip of the tube straight back toward the occiput. Using the curve placed in the tube, aim the tip down to conform to the nasopharynx.

5.  After the tip reaches the posterior pharyngeal wall, rotate the tube 180 degrees so that the curve placed in the tube will now cause the tip of the tube to hug the posterior pharyngeal wall near the opening to the esophagus and away from the opening to the trachea. Have the patient sip water through a straw, if possible. If the patient is unable to swallow on request, observe carefully for spontaneous swallows and advance the tube into the esophagus at the moment of a spontaneous swallow, if any. There should be minimal if any resistance to advancement of the tube in the patient who can swallow on request or swallows spontaneously. If spontaneous swallows are not observed, the tip of the tube must be gently forced through the potential opening into the esophagus. This is the most uncomfortable and potentially most dangerous part of the procedure because the tube may enter the trachea. A cuffed endotracheal tube increases the likelihood that the feeding tube will enter the trachea. Multiple indications that the tip of the tube has entered the trachea have been published and the person inserting the tube should pay attention to these indicators. They include observing the patient for coughing, hoarseness, or cyanosis; detecting air coming from the proximal end of the tube by placing the end of the tube under water; and detecting air rushing over the feeding ports by listening to the proximal end of the tube by ear or stethoscope. However, none of these are sensitive enough to reliably exclude tracheal intubation. If the tip of the tube is less than 5 mm in diameter, resistance is also not a reliable indicator that the tube has impacted in a bronchus. Once the tip of the tube reaches 25 to 30 cm from the external nares it is committed to either the esophagus or trachea unless it is coiled in the oropharynx.

6.  Once confident that the tip of the tube is in the esophagus (5-mm wide tip and no resistance, tube midline on plain chest radiograph, no air bubbling from the external end of the tube, or alert patient with no cough, cyanosis, or hoarseness), advance the tube to the 45- to 50-cm mark. At this point, it is appropriate to perform maneuvers to support the likelihood that the tip of the tube is in the stomach even though the methods are not completely reliable. Auscultation over the upper abdomen as air is insufflated into the tube is worthwhile but does not reliably distinguish between a tube in the stomach, a main stem bronchus, the pleura, or the peritoneum. Aspiration of fluid that is

unequivocally gastric (pH < 4) is good evidence that the tip of the tube is in the stomach. If results of auscultation and aspiration are not entirely reassuring, confirm tube placement radiologically before proceeding.

7. If feasible, turn the patient to the right lateral position, infuse 500 mL of air down the tube, and slowly advance the tube to the 75-cm mark. This encourages the tip of the tube to pass down the lesser curve to the pylorus. Tape the tube to the face with approximately 20 cm to 30 cm of slack so that the tube can advance by peristalsis to the 95- to 105-cm mark. Obtain a plain abdominal film immediately and at 12-hour intervals to check for progression of the tube into the jejunum. Advance the tube based on results of the radiographs. Bedside methods for more reliably and quickly advancing the tube into the duodenum have been published. They involve putting a substantial bend in the stylet near the tip of the tube (not approved by the manufacturers) and rotating the entire tube as it is advanced from 45 cm to 75 cm in the stomach. The bent tip of the tube follows a corkscrew pattern through the stomach, which increases the likelihood that it will advance to and through the pylorus (6).

Four bedside indicators have been used to predict that the feeding ports of the tube have passed from the stomach into the duodenum. The positive and negative predictive values of these signs are auscultation—progression of loudest sound locations from the left to the right abdomen—85% positive, 31% negative; vacuum effect—a change from $\geq$ 40 mL of aspirated air to $\leq$10 ml after 60 mL of air is instilled—86% positive, 45% negative; pH change of aspirate from $\leq$ 4.0 to $\geq$ 6.0—100% positive, 28% negative; and change of aspirate color to yellow—100% positive, 29% negative (7). These can be helpful at the bedside, but placement should be confirmed by a plain abdominal radiograph.

## Fluoroscopic or Nasopharyngoscopic Guidance

1. Consult radiology for assistance in passing the feeding tube safely into the upper esophagus and advancing it to the ligament of Treitz. For critically ill patients this is best done at the bedside using a portable fluoroscope and compatible bed, if other patients and staff can be adequately shielded from radiation.

2. Consult otolaryngology for bedside nasopharyngoscopic visualization to ensure that the tip of the feeding tube passes into the upper esophagus and not into the trachea.

## Placement Aided by Upper Endoscopy

1. Prepare the patient as usual for upper endoscopy.

2. Prepare the feeding tube with suture material as indicated in the *Equipment* section.

3. Insert the endoscope into the posterior pharynx, and observe as the feeding tube is passed through the naris in the pharynx. Observe to be sure the tip of the tube enters the esophagus, and then advance the endoscope into the stomach along with

the feeding tube. Use the endoscope to guide the tip of the feeding tube through the pylorus, using the forceps to grasp the suture material if necessary. Successively grasp the more proximal sutures, and push the feeding tube further into the duodenum until slight resistance is met or the 100- to 105-cm mark has reached the external naris.

4. Keep the stylet in place until the endoscope is removed. Remove the endoscope slowly with a rotating and jiggling motion while observing to be sure the feeding tube is not being dragged out due to friction between it and the endoscope.

5. Confirm appropriate tube placement radiographically.

**Placement Over an Endoscopically Placed Guidewire**

1. Perform upper endoscopy through the mouth with an adult upper endoscope or through the nose with an ultraslim or neonatal upper endoscope that is 5 mm to 6 mm wide (8). Advance the tip of the scope as far as possible into the duodenum by aspirating air from the stomach, using torque, and using external abdominal pressure to reduce the loop in the stomach.

2. Advance the wire packaged with the over-the-wire tube through the endoscope and beyond the tip of the scope until it begins to impact the wall of the small bowel.

3. Remove the endoscope slowly while feeding the guidewire through the channel to avoid moving the tip of the wire. Avoid creating a large loop in the stomach. Fluoroscopic guidance is helpful but not essential.

4. If the endoscope was passed orally, use the short cannula provided to transfer the guidewire from the oral to a nasal exit. Remove and discard the short cannula. Be careful to remove any slack in the wire from the posterior pharynx while at the same time avoiding any removal of the wire from the stomach or duodenum. Fluoroscopic guidance is useful but not essential.

5. Select the desired tube, which may be a single lumen nasoenteric feeding tube (e.g., Endo-Tube, Kendall HealthCare Products Co.) or a double-lumen gastric decompression and jejunal feeding tube (e.g., "StayPut," Novartis, or "Dobhoff feeding and decompression tube," Kendall HealthCare Products Co.). Flush the tube with 20 mL of water to activate the water-activated lubricant, if present. If the lumen of the tube is not coated with water-activated lubricant, instill 8 mL of oil emulsion consisting of 4 mL spray cooking oil and 4 mL water.

6. Now begins the most crucial step. With the help of at least two others, hold the wire at the patient's nose so that it is not inadvertently withdrawn, hold the distal end of the wire firmly at a point on a fixed object, and support the wire in a straight line from that point to the patient's nose. As the tube is passed over the wire, first the grasp on the wire at

the distal fixed point must be released and, subsequently, as the tip of the tube advances to the nose, the grasp of the wire at the nose must be released. However, at no time should both be released at the same time, and at no time should the wire and tube be allowed to sag or vary from a straight line between the nose and the fixed point. Keeping the above firmly in mind, insert the tube over the wire, and advance it into the patient to at least 105 cm and preferably 120 cm, which should be well beyond the ligament of Treitz. Fluoroscopic control is very helpful but not essential.

7. Remove the guidewire.

8. Confirm placement of the feeding tube radiographically.

## POSTPROCEDURE

1. Carefully tape the tube to the nose. Use a felt-tipped pen with permanent ink to mark the tube at the point where the tape stops so that if the tape around the tube loosens and the tube begins to slide out it will be easy to detect.

2. Because of the risk and expense of placing a nasoduodenal or nasojejunal tube, one should seriously consider placing a bridle to reduce the likelihood of inadvertent removal of the tube. This consists of a length of 5-Fr tubing looped around the nasal septum with an end extending a short distance from each nostril. These two ends are tied together close to, but not putting pressure on, the nasal septum and then tied to the feeding tube with three pieces of 3-0 silk (9).

## COMPLICATIONS

1. Regurgitation and aspiration of gastric contents. The presence of a feeding tube may increase the likelihood of gastroesophageal reflux. It may also increase the likelihood that the patient will aspirate oropharyngeal secretions.

2. Bronchopulmonary injuries during insertion of small-bore feeding tubes. The risk is greatest in patients who cannot swallow on request or have an endotracheal tube in place, if the tip of the tube is less than 5 mm wide or if the tube is passed without endoscopic or radiographic imaging. Instilling enteral formula into a tube inadvertently placed in the bronchial tree can cause severe pneumonia and death.

3. Perforation of the gastrointestinal tract

4. The tube can become clogged in several ways including instillation of a slurry of solid medication that is not ground finely enough; soluble medication precipitated in the tube by coming in contact with other, incompatible, fluids; hydrophilic materials such as psyllium gelling in the lumen of the tube; and inadequate irrigation.

5. Epistaxis, nasopharyngeal erosions, pharyngitis, otitis media, sinusitis, and vocal cord paralysis

6. Penetration of the brain by the tip of a small-bore tube

7. Tube rupture as a result of too much irrigation pressure is most likely to occur if a syringe smaller than 60 mL in size is used for irrigating or unclogging the tube.

8. Inadvertent withdrawal of the tube back into the stomach or completely out of the patient.

9. Necrotizing enteritis, if the patient is fed into the small bowel which has inadequate vascular perfusion or no motility.

10. Dumping symptoms are likely to occur if bolus feedings are given into a small bowel tube.

11. A small-bore tube can become tied into a knot in the stomach. The knot may cause damage to the esophagus or nasal passages during attempted removal and may require endoscopic removal.

## CPT Codes

**44500** – Nasoenteric tube placement.
**74340** – Nasoenteric tube placement with radiological supervision and interpretation.
**43241** – Upper GI endoscopy; diagnostic with transendoscopic intraluminal tube or catheter placement.

## REFERENCES

1. Marik PE, Zaloga GP. Gastric versus post-pyloric feeding: a systematic review. *Crit Care* 2003;7:R46–51.
2. Heyland DK, Dhaliwal R, Drover JW, et al. Canadian Critical Care Clinical Practice Guidelines Committee. Canadian clinical practice guidelines for nutrition support in mechanically ventilated, critically ill adult patients. *JPEN* 2003;27:355–373.
3. Rassias AJ, Ball PA. A prospective study of tracheopulmonary complications associated with placement of narrow-bore enteral feeding tubes. *Crit Care (Lond)* 1998;2:25–28.
4. Guenter P, Jones S, Sweed MR, Ericson M. Delivery systems and administration of enteral nutrition. In: Rombeau JL, Rolandelli RH, eds. *Clinical Nutrition. Enteral and Tube Feeding*, 3rd ed. Philadelphia: W.B. Saunders Company, 1997:240–267.
5. Lai CWY, Barlow R, Barnes M, Hawthorne B. Bedside placement of nasojejunal tubes: a randomized-controlled trial of spiral- vs straight-ended tubes. *Clin Nutr* 2003;22:267–270.
6. Zaloga GP. Bedside method for placing small bowel feeding tubes in critically ill patients. *Chest* 1991;100:1643–1646.
7. Welch SK, Hanlon MD, Waits M, Foulks CJ. Comparison of four bedside indicators used to predict duodenal feeding tube placement with radiography. *JPEN* 1994;18:525–530.
8. O'Keefe SJD, Foody W, Gill S. Transnasal endoscopic placement of feeding tubes in the intensive care unit. *JPEN* 2003; 27:349–354.
9. Popovich MJ, Lockrem JD, Zivot JB. Nasal bridle revisited: an improvement in the technique to prevent unintentional removal of small-bore nasoenteric feeding tubes. *Crit Care Med* 1996; 24:429–431.

# Percutaneous Endoscopic Gastrostomy (PEG) and Percutaneous Endoscopic Jejunostomy (PEJ)

Todd H. Baron

Percutaneous endoscopic gastrostomy (PEG) was introduced over 20 years ago and has supplanted surgical gastrostomy as a method of enteral access (1). There is now a wider range of indications for PEG placement since its original description. Endoscopic placement of jejunal feeding tubes (PEJ) can be achieved either indirectly, by passing a feeding tube through a PEG tube or existing PEG tract (PEG-J), or directly, by puncturing the small bowel (direct percutaneous jejunostomy [DPEJ]) (2). This chapter will discuss the indications and technique of endoscopic placement of PEG and PEJ tubes.

## PERCUTANEOUS ENDOSCOPIC GASTROSTOMY

### Indications

1. Enteral feeding in patients with any permanent or anticipated long-term inability to effectively swallow that prevents adequate maintenance of hydration or nutrition. Common causes are dysphagia secondary to cerebrovascular accident (CVA), neuromuscular disorders (multiple sclerosis [MS], amyotrophic lateral sclerosis [ALS]) dysphagia, esophageal obstruction, and dementia.

2. During preoperative radiation/chemotherapy for esophageal cancer

3. Underlying diseases with profound anorexia

4. Gastric decompression

### Contraindications

1. Large volume ascites

2. Uncorrected coagulopathy

3. Inability to obtain informed consent

4. Intraabdominal perforation

### Ethical issues

Most patients who receive PEG tubes have a limited life span. Additionally, some patients with severe dementia would otherwise die if enteral nutrition were not provided. These decisions are often made by family members rather than by the patient. The needs of the family as well as the patient must be addressed prior to PEG placement (3).

**Preparation**

1.  The patient should be NPO for at least 4 hours.

2.  Antibiotic prophylaxis: Antibiotics administered within several hours of the procedure reduce the risk of postprocedural infection at the PEG site. A first-generation cephalosporin is appropriate coverage in a non-PCN allergic patient. Patients who may already be receiving broad-spectrum antibiotics do not need additional prophylactic antibiotics (4).

3.  Adequate platelets and clotting parameters are necessary for safe PEG placement. Patients who have had normal labs within a recent period of time, have not had clinical changes, and have no history of bleeding do not necessarily need lab work done specifically for PEG placement. The international normalized ratio (INR) should be < 1.5 and the platelet count should be > 80,000.

4.  Correct coagulopathy.

5.  Place the patient in the supine position on the endoscopy table

**Equipment**

1.  Upper endoscope. Any endoscope that accepts a snare is adequate for performing PEG placement.

2.  Standard commercially available PEG tray. A variety of PEG feeding tube kits are available. All are designed to be removed by traction method (nonendoscopically). The diameters range from 16 Fr to 24 Fr in size.

3.  Abdominal binder for patients who are anticipated to inadvertently pull out their PEG tubes

**Procedure**

*The "Pull" Technique*

1.  Place the patient in the supine position.

2.  Pass the endoscope into the stomach.

3.  Dim the room lights. This will allow transillumination of the endoscope light, which is to be observed externally as bright red/orange. Generous air insufflation should be used to distend the stomach during this phase and throughout the procedure.

4.  At the maximum intensity of transillumination, apply a finger indentation externally and it should be noted endoscopically as a specific (not generalized), focal indentation of the anterior gastric wall. This area should be away from the xiphoid process or ribs by several centimeters to avoid damage to nerves and vasculature beneath the ribs and to avoid pain if the tube abuts bony tissue.

5.  Avoid previous abdominal surgical sites because adhered loops of bowel may be present at these sites, and subsequent injury to them may occur during PEG placement.

6.  Avoid the distal gastric antrum, if possible, since a PEG placed in this area may interfere with gastric peristalsis producing nausea and vomiting.

7.  At the chosen area, cleanse the skin with povidone-iodine (Betadine).

8.  Place a sterile drape over the site.

9.  Anesthetize the area of interest with lidocaine.

10.  Use a "finder needle" (enclosed in the kit), usually 19 g, to confirm the area of interest is suitable for gastrostomy. The needle is passed through the abdominal wall toward the maximum light intensity and should be confirmed endoscopically to have entered the gastric lumen.

11.  Make a superficial 1-cm skin incision at the anticipated site of entry to facilitate passage of the PEG tube using the scalpel enclosed on the PEG tray.

12.  Use a catheter with an indwelling trocar to puncture the site percutaneously in a thrusting motion while the endoscopist awaits the entry into the stomach with an open snare. The trocar and catheter are grasped with the snare, and the trocar is removed, leaving the catheter in place.

13.  Through the catheter, pass a vinyl "string" and readjust the snare to grasp only the string (Fig. 20.1A). Withdraw the endoscope and string together (Fig. 20.1B). At this point, the string enters the skin, passes through the anterior gastric wall, and exits the mouth.

14.  Attach the loop of the PEG tube to the end of the string exiting the mouth. Use the portion of the string on the abdominal side to pull the PEG through the mouth, esophagus, and gastric wall (Fig. 20.1C). Pull the PEG so it is snug against the anterior gastric wall (Fig. 20.1D). Reintroduction of the endoscope to assess the site may be performed but is not necessary (5). Some kits operate by having the PEG slide over the string, such that the inner bumper of the PEG enters the mouth last and is drawn into position by traction of the tubes.

15.  Shorten the external portion of the PEG tube appropriately using scissors. The external bumper (enclosed in the kit) is applied prior to shortening to prevent inward migration of the PEG tube (Fig. 20.1E). It is important to realize that excessive tension on the external bumper is not necessary and may lead to complications such as necrosis of the skin beneath it. The tube should be loose enough to allow free rotation of the PEG tube in the tract.

16.  Attach an adaptor onto the end of the PEG tube that allows a syringe to be connected to the tube for introduction of feeding.

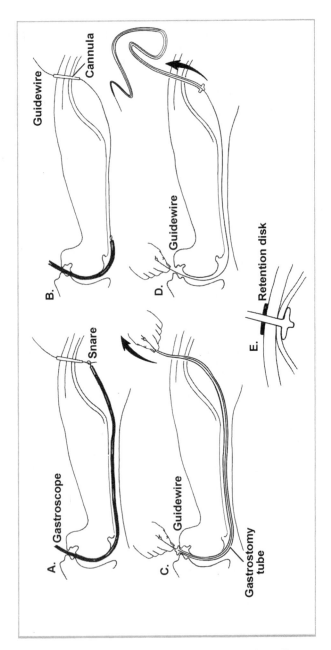

Fig. 20.1A–E. Correct placement of a PEG tube using the pull technique. See text for details.

*The "Push" Technique*

1. Perform Steps 1 through 12 for the pull technique as described.

2. Pass a guidewire through the catheter externally rather than a string, and grasp it with the snare. Withdraw the snare and endoscope, leaving the wire exiting the mouth.

3. Advance a push-PEG tube over the guidewire. It is important to keep tension on both ends of the guidewire as the PEG is advanced and pushed through the abdominal wall.

4. After the PEG exits the gastric wall, pull it snugly against the gastric wall.

5. Follow Steps 15 and 16 for the push technique as described.

**Postprocedure**

1. Feeding can be safely administered 3 hours after an uncomplicated procedure.

2. The external bolster should be placed 1 cm to 2 cm from the abdominal wall with no underlying dressing to avoid wound compression, infection, and tract breakdown.

3. In the first few days following placement, the PEG site should be examined at least once per day for erythema, drainage, induration, and other skin problems. Expect to see a small amount of clear drainage in the first few weeks following insertion.

4. Rotate the external bumper or other retaining device 90 degrees once a day to prevent irritation and pressure ulcers beneath it. Ensure that the site remains dry by changing dressings (over the external bumper) once or twice a day as needed.

5. Meticulous daily skin care is essential. Clean the area with a mild, pH-balanced soap or commercial cleanser or 0.9% sodium chloride. Use a cotton-tipped applicator to clean close to the tube to remove crusts or drainage. Be sure to rinse the exit site well and dry the skin completely.

6. After complete healing (usually by 2 weeks) the dressing can be eliminated.

**Complications (6)**

1. Those associated with upper endoscopy (see Chapter 5)

2. Oversedation

3. Aspiration

4. Bleeding

5. PEG site infection

6. Piercing of the colon or small bowel with fistula formation

7. Inadvertent removal with perforation

8. Buried bumper syndrome (In this situation, inner bumper of PEG is epithelialized over by the gastric wall, sometimes requiring surgical removal)

9. Migration with gastric outlet obstruction

10. Gastric ulcer

## Other Uses for This Technique

1. Percutaneous endoscopic cecostomy

2. Sigmoidopexy to prevent recurrent sigmoid volvulus

3. Correction of gastric volvulus

4. Reintroduction of bile from high-output external biliary drains

## JEJUNAL FEEDING

### Indications

1. Patients whose stomachs are obstructed or nonfunctional (diabetic gastroparesis)

2. Patients who have had documented aspiration of gastric feedings or a high risk for same

3. Patients with previous gastric resection or gastric bypass in whom PEG placement is not feasible

4. Intrathoracic stomach in those patients requiring enteral access

### Contraindications

The contraindications for jejunal feeding are the same as those outlined for PEG placement.

### Preparation

If a direct PEJ (DPEJ) is planned, the preparation is as outlined for patients with PEG. If a PEG-J or transgastric PEJ is planned with a prior PEG or PEG tract, then antibiotics and correction of coagulopathy are not necessary.

### Equipment

*For PEG Placement with J Extension*

1. Standard endoscope

2. Jejunal extension tube

3. Rat-tooth forceps

4. PEG tray if PEG not already in place

*For Transgastric PEJ*

1. Ultrathin endoscope

2. Single piece transgastric jejunal feeding tube

3. 0.035-in guidewire

4. Fluoroscopy

*For DPEJ*
1. Colonoscope (adult or pediatric) or small bowel push entero-scope
2. Standard "pull" PEG tray
3. Colon polypectomy snare
4. Glucagon

**Procedure**

*PEG placement with J extension*
1. Keep the patient in the supine position.
2. If an initial PEG tube has not been placed, it should be placed as described above.
3. The cap from the PEG tube is not put in place, or if previously placed it should be removed, to allow introduction of the jejunal (J) extension tube.
4. Further shorten the length of the external portion of the PEG tube to allow the J extension to pass distally.
5. Loosen the external bumper of the PEG.
6. Insert the endoscope orally into the stomach; grasp the internal PEG bumper with a rat-tooth forceps and advance to the pylorus (7).
7. With the stylet in the J extension tube, advance the J extension tube through the PEG tube beyond the pylorus and into the duodenum and jejunum. Fluoroscopy can be used to confirm that the distal end is beyond the ligament of Treitz. At this point the J tube, which has ports for jejunal feeding and gastric decompression, should be completely locked inside the PEG tube.
8. Bring the internal bumper back to its appropriate position against the anterior gastric wall by withdrawing the PEG tube externally away from the abdominal wall while monitoring the internal bumper position endoscopically.
9. Withdraw the endoscope.
10. Readjust the external bumper.

*Transgastric PEJ*
1. Place the patient in the supine position.
2. Once the gastrostomy tube tract has matured, the PEG may be safely removed by traction method.
3. Pass an ultrathin endoscope (5.8 mm) through the mature gastrostomy tract into the stomach and duodenum (8).
4. Advance the guidewire through the endoscope beyond the ligament of Treitz.
5. Withdraw the endoscope while advancing the guidewire so that it remains in position.

6. Pass a single piece of transgastric jejunal tube over the guidewire and beyond the ligament of Treitz using fluoroscopic guidance.

*Direct Percutaneous Endoscopic Jejunostomy (DPEJ)*

1. Place the patient in the supine position.

2. Pass a colonoscope or small bowel push enteroscope beyond the ligament of Treitz. Fluoroscopy may be used to assist in identifying the endoscope position and confirming it is beyond the ligament of Treitz.

3. Administer glucagon in 0.25-mg increments as needed to control motility.

4. Identify an area of transillumination and indentation as described for PEG tube placement, recognizing that the small bowel is not as easy to transilluminate and that the area may not be in the left upper quadrant.

5. Advance the 19-g "finder needle" in the PEG tray through the abdominal wall and into the jejunum.

6. Advance a standard polypectomy snare through the endoscope channel, and grasp the finder needle as tightly as possible. This keeps the small bowel in close apposition to the anterior abdominal wall (9).

7. Leaving the finder needle in place, advance the trocar and needle alongside the finder needle and into the jejunum.

8. Release the snare from the finder needle and place it around the trocar.

9. Remove the finder needle.

10. Withdraw the trocar needle, advance the plastic "string" through the trocar, and grasp it with the snare.

11. Remove the endoscope and string together, leaving the string exiting the mouth.

12. Make a small skin incision to facilitate entry of the tube through the abdominal wall.

13. Loop a standard pull-type PEG tube to the string and pull it through the abdominal wall.

14. Perform the remainder of the procedure as described for PEG placement.

**Postprocedure**

The care of the patient after PEG-J and DPEJ is the same as that described for PEG placement.

**Complications**

Complications are the same as those listed for PEG placement.

**Other Uses for This Technique**

This technique can also be used for endoscopic transgastric irrigation of necrotic pancreatic fluid collections.

## CPT Codes

**43246** – Upper gastrointestinal endoscopy including esophagus, stomach, and either the duodenum and/or jejunum as appropriate; with directed placement of percutaneous gastrostomy tube.

**44372** – Small intestinal endoscopy, enteroscopy beyond second portion of duodenum, not including ileum; with placement of percutaneous jejunostomy tube.

**44373** – Small intestinal endoscopy, enteroscopy beyond second portion of duodenum, not including ileum; with conversion of percutaneous gastrostomy tube to percutaneous jejunostomy tube.

## REFERENCES

1. Gauderer M. Twenty years of percutaneous endoscopic gastrostomy: origin and evolution of a concept and its expanded applications. *Gastrointest Endosc* 1999;50:879–883.
2. DiSario JA, Baskin WN, Brown RD, et al. Endoscopic approaches to enteral nutritional support. *Gastrointest Endosc* 2002;55:901–908.
3. Angus F, Burakoff R. The percutaneous endoscopic gastrostomy tube. Medical and ethical issues in placement. *Am J Gastroenterol* 2003;98:272–277.
4. Sharma VK, Howden CW. Meta-analysis of randomized, controlled trials of antibiotic prophylaxis before percutaneous endoscopic gastrostomy. *Am J Gastroenterol* 2000;95:3133–3136.
5. Sartori S, Trevisani L, Nielsen I, et al. Percutaneous endoscopic gastrostomy placement using the pull-through or push-through techniques: is the second pass of the gastroscope necessary? *Endoscopy* 1996;28:686–688.
6. McClave SA, Chang WK. Complications of enteral access. *Gastrointest Endosc* 2003;58:739–751.
7. Sibille A, Glorieux D, Fauville JP, Warzee P. An easier method for percutaneous endoscopic gastrojejunostomy tube placement. *Gastrointest Endosc* 1998;48:514–517.
8. Adler DG, Gostout CJ, Baron TH. Percutaneous transgastric placement of jejunal feeding tubes with an ultrathin endoscope. *Gastrointest Endosc* 2002;55:106–110.
9. Varadarajulu S, Delegge MH. Use of a 19-gauge injection needle as a guide for direct percutaneous endoscopic jejunostomy tube placement. *Gastrointest Endosc* 2003;57:942–945.

# Colonic Decompression

## Jeffrey T. Wei and Nicholas J. Shaheen

Colonic decompression involves removal of gas and fluid from the colon during colonoscopy. This procedure is most commonly performed for pathologic dilation of the colon secondary to mechanical or non-mechanical causes. Conservative management is usually attempted initially for incomplete colonic obstruction for a 24- to 48-hour period. This may include keeping the patient NPO, correcting metabolic and electrolyte disturbances, and providing intravenous (IV) fluids, nasogastric suction, and/or rectal tube decompression, if indicated. Medical therapy such as neostigmine may be beneficial in selected patients with colonic pseudo-obstruction, if complete obstruction has been ruled out. A contrast enema study may be helpful in some patients to evaluate for complete obstruction and to diagnose volvulus. There have been some reports of therapeutic benefit with enemas, particularly in the setting of sigmoid volvulus. If conservative management does not result in improvement, colonic decompression may then be performed with or without placement of a decompression tube. Use of a decompression tube may reduce the risk of recurrence of the dilation. In the setting of malignant obstruction of the colon, a metallic stent may also be placed as a bridge to surgery or for palliation. Alternatives to colonic decompression include endoscopic cecostomy/colostomy or surgery. There are no randomized controlled trials supporting the use of colonic decompression. Observational studies and anecdotal reports have suggested that there may be benefit in terms of symptom relief and a decreased need for subsequent surgical intervention.

## INDICATIONS

To decrease colonic dilation, provide symptomatic relief, and decrease need for surgical intervention from the following:

1. Colonic pseudoobstruction (Ogilvie's syndrome)

2. Sigmoid volvulus (success rate is much lower for cecal volvulus, with a higher risk of perforation)

3. Near-obstructing colorectal cancer

4. Dilation > 12 cm is a common standard diameter for decompression. However this threshold will vary depending on the clinical situation.

## CONTRAINDICATIONS

1. Colonic ischemia (relative contraindication)

2. Colonic perforation

3. Peritonitis

4. Fully obstructing lesion

## PREPARATION

1. Patients should be NPO.
2. Obtain written consent.
3. Do not give usual precolonoscopic bowel preparation.
4. Water enemas can be administered prior to procedure, although the cleansing effect on bowel may be minimal.
5. Start an intravenous line for the administration of systemic conscious sedation.

## EQUIPMENT

1. Colonoscope (sigmoidoscope may be adequate for distal dilation)
2. Decompression tube, if desired
3. Metallic stent for malignant obstruction
4. Fluoroscopy, if a stent is to be deployed
5. Lubricant
6. Gloves

## PROCEDURE

1. Perform colonoscopy with minimal insufflation of air.
2. In the case of colonic volvulus, apply gentle pressure, and advance the scope using minimal insufflation of air to allow straightening of the colon. Suction intermittently to decompress the colon and to avoid further colonic distension.
3. Suction excess gas and fluid when the scope reaches the area of colonic dilation at the time of withdrawal of the scope. A "whoosh" of air may be obtained with relief of a volvulus.
4. Inspect the mucosa for evidence of bowel ischemia.
5. If indicated, place the decompression tube over the guidewire just prior to the time the scope is being withdrawn (see instruction below).
6. To minimize air insufflation, detailed examination of the unaffected colonic mucosa is not recommended.

To place a decompression tube (fluoroscopy is recommended but is not essential):

1. Locate the colonoscope tip.
2. Insert the guidewire into the biopsy channel of the colonoscope until it exits the tip, and advance the guidewire as far as can be visualized by the scope.
3. Carefully withdraw the colonoscope, ensuring the guidewire remains stationary through periodic withdrawal of the scope.
4. If fluoroscopy is used, withdraw any excess wire to reduce loops.
5. Disassemble the decompression tube and preloaded guiding catheter.

6.  Flush the tube and guiding catheter with sterile water, or lubricate with water-soluble lubricant or a vegetable oil such as Pam.

7.  Reassemble the decompression tube and advance it into the colon over the guidewire, using fluoroscopic control when possible to avoid migration of the guidewire.

8.  Once the tube is advanced to the end of the guidewire, withdraw both the guiding catheter and the guidewire, leaving the decompression tube in place.

9.  Secure the external portion of the tube to the sacral crease by taping a gauze sponge to pad the area.

**POSTPROCEDURE**

1.  Monitor vital signs.

2.  Elevate the head of the bed to reduce aspiration risk.

3.  Connect the decompression tube to a vented Foley bag for drainage, and flush with 20 to 30 mL of normal saline or water every 2 to 4 hours to maintain patency.

4.  Obtain an abdominal radiograph to assess adequacy of decompression and to confirm position of the tube.

5.  Due to the high risk of recurrence, advancement of the patient's diet should be reserved for when symptoms and colonic dilation have definitively improved.

6.  Symptoms or signs of perforation (fever, abdominal pain/dilation, peritoneal signs) require immediate evaluation.

**COMPLICATIONS**

1.  Perforation has been described in up to 3% of patients undergoing colonic decompression.

2.  Mortality associated with colonic decompression in colonic pseudo-obstruction has been reported as 1%. Mortality associated with this procedure, however, is highly variable depending on underlying etiology of colon dilation and comorbidities.

3.  Recurrence of dilation is common, up to 33%, although the risk may be substantially reduced with placement of a decompression tube.

4.  In addition to perforation, complications specific to colonic stent placement include stent migration, malpositioning, occlusion, and bleeding.

**CPT Codes:**
**45337** – Flexible sigmoidoscopy; with decompression of volvulus.
**45321** – Proctosigmoidoscopy, rigid with decompression of volvulus.
**Note:** No additional code is available if decompression tube is deployed.
**45378** – Colonoscopy; with or without decompression.

## SUGGESTED READINGS

Baron TH. Expandable metal stents for the treatment of cancerous obstruction of the gastrointestinal tract. *N Engl J Med* 2001; 344(22): 1681–1687.

Bender GN, Do-Dai DD, Briggs LM. Colonic pseudo-obstruction: decompression with a tricomponent coaxial system under fluoroscopic guidance. *Radiology* 1993;188:395–398.

Dulger M, Canturk NZ, Utkan NZ, et al. Management of sigmoid colon volvulus. *Hepatogastroenterology* 2000;47(35):1280–1283.

Eisen GM, Baron TH, Dominitz JA, et al for the American Society for Gastrointestinal Endoscopy, Standards of Practice Committee. Acute colonic pseudo-obstruction. *Gastrointest Endosc* 2002;56(6): 789–792.

Geller A, Peterson BT, Gostout CJ. Endoscopic decompression for acute colonic pseudo-obstruction. *Gastrointest Endosc* 1996;44(2): 144–150.

Harig JM, Fumo DE, Loo FD, et al. Treatment of acute nontoxic megacolon during colonoscopy: tube placement versus simple decompression. *Gastrointest Endosc* 1988;34:23–27.

Jetmore AB, Timmcke AE, Gathright JB, et al. Ogilvie's syndrome: colonoscopic decompression and analysis of predisposing factors. *Dis Colon Rectum* 1992;35:1135–1142.

Lee JG, Vigil H, Leung JW. A randomized controlled trial of total colonic decompression after colonoscopy to improve patient comfort. *Am J Gastroenterol* 2001;96:95–100.

Ponec RJ, Saunders MD, Kimmey MB. Neostigmine for the treatment of acute colonic pseudo-obstruction. *N Engl J Med* 1999;341(3):137–141.

# Dilation of the Esophagus: Mercury-Filled Bougies (Hurst and Maloney)

Douglas Morgan

Dilation of the esophagus is most frequently required for the management of peptic strictures related to gastroesophageal reflux disease (GERD). Luminal narrowings of the esophagus requiring dilation also result from other fibrosing etiologies (radiation, caustic, anastomotic), benign stenoses (Schaztki's ring, web), and esophageal carcinoma. One of the original, least expensive, and still regularly used dilation methods utilizes mercury-filled bougies of graded sizes. The two main types available are the blunt, rounded Hurst dilators and the tapered Maloney dilators (Fig. 22.1).

## INDICATIONS

1. Esophageal fibrotic strictures

    - GERD-related peptic stricture
    - Caustic stricture
    - Radiation-induced strictures
    - Anastomotic strictures

2. Benign esophageal luminal stenoses

    - Schatzki's ring
    - Esophageal webs

3. Esophageal carcinoma, for palliation

4. Empiric dilation for dysphagia

## CONTRAINDICATIONS

1. Bleeding diatheses (international normalized ratio [INR] < 1.5; platelets > 50,000 to 100,000). For patients on anticoagulants, peridilation anticoagulation management should follow American Society for Gastrointestinal Endoscopy (ASGE) guidelines.

2. Recent esophageal biopsies—within 14 days—are a relative contraindication.

3. Active food impaction, with impacted bolus or mucosal maceration

4. Neck immobility (e.g., severe cervical arthritis)

5. Lack of patient cooperation

6. Esophageal diverticulum

## PREPARATION

1. Obtain prior radiologic and/or endoscopic evaluation of the esophagus. A barium swallow is recommended for tortuous or long strictures.

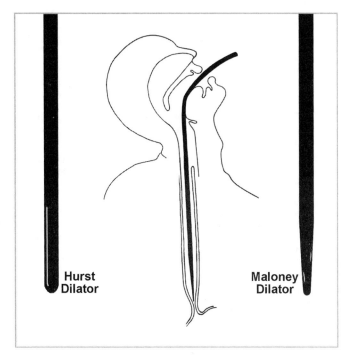

**Fig. 22.1. Dilator types and Hurst dilator being passed through esophageal stricture.**

2. Nothing by mouth for 8 hours. For severe luminal narrowing, a liquid diet is recommended 1 to 3 days prior to the procedure.

3. Obtain informed, written consent.

4. Anesthetize the pharynx with a topical agent.

5. Conscious sedation is not required but may be appropriate for certain patients.

6. If the patient has a prosthetic valve, antibiotic administration should follow the ASGE guidelines (see Chapter 1).

**EQUIPMENT**
1. Hurst or Maloney dilators
2. Dilator lubricant
3. Fluoroscopic equipment (desirable, but not essential) to allow confirmation of dilator position

**PROCEDURE**
1. Either the Hurst or Maloney dilator may be used initially. The Hurst dilator with its blunt end is the appropriate

bougie for mild to moderate luminal narrowings. Maloney dilators with their tapered ends may be used for tight or long strictures because the tapered end serves as a lumen finder.

2. Start with the size most appropriate, based on the previous endoscopic examination or a prior dilation. For example, if the stricture was judged to be 6 mm in transverse diameter on endoscopic exam, an 18-Fr Hurst bougie should be used as the initial dilator (1 mm is roughly equivalent to 3 Fr). If the patient was dilated to 30 Fr a week earlier, it would be appropriate to start the subsequent dilation with the same size bougie.

3. The patient may be placed either in the seated position or the left lateral decubitus position. The patient's neck should be gently extended.

4. Holding the dilator in the dominant hand like a pencil, slide the dilator over the bite block and into the posterior pharynx, resting it on the cricopharyngeus. Ask the patient to swallow. Pass the tube while the nurse assists by keeping the weighted column of mercury above the patient's head.

5. If stricture passage is difficult, it may help to place the volar surface of the index and middle fingers of the nondominant hand against the hard palate to anchor the bougie in place while exerting mild pressure with the right hand on the bougie. Most often a "give" can be felt as the stricture is passed. Greater resistance is noted when pulling the dilator back through the stricture.

6. Dilations are usually carried out with a series of three sequential dilators, depending on the ease of the procedure and patient tolerance. Stop the dilation at the point where blood is noted on the dilator or if the patient complains of pain. In general, dysphagia should be significantly improved with a luminal diameter of 14 to 16 mm (43 to 50 Fr). The goal of dilation is relief of dysphagia, rather than a specific luminal diameter.

7. Narrow peptic strictures may require repeat dilation in 14 days, starting with size of the last dilator from the previous dilation. If passage is difficult, it may be necessary to decrease 1 to 2 bougie sizes.

8. Fluoroscopic confirmation is necessary when there is a question as to whether the bougie is passing through the stricture. At times, the bougie may simply curl in or stretch the esophagus.

9. Endoscopic biopsy specimens to exclude a neoplasm may be obtained immediately after the dilation or 14 days prior. It is controversial whether either predilation or recent biopsies (1 to 7 days) increase the risk of perforation. Dilation should not be delayed if nutrition intake cannot be maintained. Brush cytology specimens may be obtained prior to the procedure.

10. For dilation of a lower esophageal ring (Schatzki's ring), two methods have been recommended. One approach is to use graded Hurst or Maloney dilators with progressive dilation. This allows one to stretch as well as rupture the mucosal ring. The other approach is a single dilation with one large (44- to 50-Fr) bougie.

## POSTPROCEDURE

1. The procedures described in this chapter are usually performed in an outpatient setting. The physician and nursing staff must advise the patient to notify them immediately if there is chest or back pain, hematemesis, regurgitation, or fever.

2. For significant esophageal strictures or difficult dilations, the patient should take nothing by mouth for 6 to 8 hours after the procedure.

3. Consider administration of a short course (5 days) of either sucralfate slurry and/or a proton pump inhibitor dependent upon the specific clinical situation.

## COMPLICATIONS

1. Esophageal perforation (0.1%)

2. Hemorrhage (0.1%)

3. Aspiration

4. Bacteremia

## CPT Codes

**43450** – Dilation of esophagus, by unguided sound or bougie, single or multiple passes.
**43456** – Dilation of esophagus, by balloon or dilator, retrograde.

## SUGGESTED READINGS

Rosenow EC. Techniques of esophageal dilation. In: Payne WS, Olsen AM, eds. *The Esophagus*. Philadelphia: Lea Febiger, 1974:55–64.

Patterson DJ, Graham DY, Smith JL, et al. Natural history of benign esophageal stricture treated by dilation. *Gastroenterology* 1983; 85:346–350.

Welsh JD, Griffiths WJ, McKee J, et al. Bacteremia associated with esophageal dilation. *J Clin Gastroenterol* 1983;5:109–112.

Tulman AB, Boyce HW Jr. Complications of esophageal dilation and guidelines for their prevention. *Gastrointest Endosc* 1981;27: 299–334.

# Dilatation of the Esophagus: Wire-Guided Bougies (Savary and American Endoscopy)

Nicholas J. Shaheen

Wire-guided dilatation offers the ability to dilate difficult and convoluted strictures with some control over the path of the bougie. Although these systems were initially developed for use by fluoroscopic guidance, multiple groups have now reported their use in subjects not receiving fluoroscopy, with good results (1,2). Both of the two available systems, the Savary-Gilliard and the American endoscopy systems, offer a wire with a spring tip for insertion into the stomach. Neither system has been demonstrated to be superior to the other with respect to safety of quality of the dilatation.

Although confirmatory studies are not available, many authorities feel that wire guidance decreases the possibility of perforation with bougienage when compared to traditional, unguided methods such as use of Hurst and Maloney dilators. Previous entries in the field of wire-guided dilatation, such as Eder-Puestow olives, are now largely obsolete.

## INDICATIONS

1. To provide relief of dysphagia in subjects with esophageal strictures secondary to acid-peptic disease, lye ingestion, or other causes
2. To dilate esophageal webs or rings
3. As short-term palliation in esophageal malignancy

## CONTRAINDICATIONS

1. Cardiac instability, respiratory insufficiency, or other life-threatening cardiopulmonary conditions
2. Significant bleeding diathesis
3. Warfarin or heparin use
4. Lack of patient cooperation
5. An impacted food bolus (dilatation may be performed after disimpaction, however)
6. Severe cervical spinal arthritis

## PREPARATION

1. Subjects should be NPO for 6 hours prior to the examination.
2. Obtain written consent.
3. Administer a topical anesthetic for pharyngeal anesthesia.
4. Start an intravenous line for the administration of systemic conscious sedation

**EQUIPMENT**

1. Upper endoscope
2. Spring-tipped wire
3. Appropriate range of available dilator sizes, generally from 5 mm up to at least 17 mm
4. Lubricant
5. Gloves
6. Available fluoroscopy, for complex or tight strictures

**PROCEDURE**

1. Perform diagnostic upper endoscopy. If the esophageal stricture is too tight to allow passage of the adult upper endoscope, a pediatric or neonatal scope may be necessary to traverse the stricture. Special note should be made of any tortuosity, diverticula, or angulation, as these conditions may increase the risk of complication or ineffective bougienage. The approximate minimal diameter of the stricture should be noted by comparing it to the scope tip or to an open forceps.

2. Under direct endoscopic observation, place the spring-tipped guidewire into the gastric antrum, spring tip first. In situations when the stricture is not traversable even by a small caliber endoscope, the guidewire may be placed on the greater curve with fluoroscopic guidance. In situations when fluoroscopy is not available and the stricture is short, the wire may be passed through the stricture as long as it does not meet resistance. For longer strictures, blind passage of the guidewire is inadvisable, and the best course would be to postpone the procedure until fluoroscopic guidance is available. With such strictures, a barium study can provide valuable information regarding stricture morphology.

3. After the guidewire is placed in the antrum, withdraw the scope slowly, and advance the guidewire 5 cm through the scope for every 5 cm of scope withdrawn. In this fashion, the wire tip will remain in the antrum even after complete withdrawal of the endoscope.

4. After the endoscope has been removed from the patient, have an assistant hold the wire position firmly at the patient's mouth, then slide the scope completely off of the wire and remove the endoscope.

5. Note the wire position at the incisors. Approximately 60 cm of wire should be inside of the patient. If this is not the case, the endoscope may need to be reinserted and the wire repositioned. The wire often has markings every 20 cm. If so, assess the wire marking at the mouth to ensure that there is no migration of the wire for the remainder of the procedure (3).

6. Pass a dilator approximately 1 mm to 2 mm larger than the smallest diameter of the stricture onto the wire.

7. When the dilator is just outside the patient's mouth, ask the assistant to fix the wire in space, so that proximal

migration of the wire into the patient does not occur with passage of the dilator.

8. Slightly hyperextend the patient's neck to allow for smoother passage of the dilator.

9. With the wire fixed by the assistant, pass the dilator, holding it in the dominant hand like a pencil, so that the resistance to the dilator is easily appreciable.

10. Pass the dilator into the patient, until all but 3 in to 4 in is in, or until anything greater than mild-moderate resistance is encountered (Fig. 23.1). If greater resistance is encountered, consider withdrawal of the dilator and initiation of a smaller caliber dilator.

11. After passage of the dilator, slowly withdraw the dilator over the guidewire. After complete withdrawal, assess the wire placement at the mouth to confirm that the wire has not migrated.

12. Repeat Steps 6 through 11 with the next largest dilator.

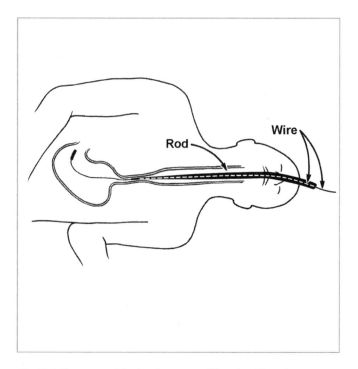

**Fig. 23.1. Correct positioning for savary dilatation. Note the extension of the patient's neck, as well as the position of the wire in the antrum.**

13. Although few data support it, most endoscopists use the "rule of threes" for dilatation: Pass no more than three dilators to resistance at any given sitting. Any more than small amounts of blood on the dilator should also prompt termination of the procedure.

14. After three dilations, remove the last dilator and the wire together as one unit.

## POSTPROCEDURE

1. Monitor vital signs.

2. Elevate the head of the bed to reduce aspiration risk.

3. Give clear liquids for the rest of the day.

4. Continue an acid suppressive regimen with proton pump inhibitors for acid peptic strictures to reduce the rate of recurrence (4).

5. Instruct the patient to return for chest pain, fevers, shortness of breath, hematemesis, or blood per rectum.

## COMPLICATIONS

1. The most dreaded complication of dilatation is esophageal perforation. In large series, this appears to occur about 0.3% of the time.

2. Esophageal hemorrhage, less than 0.1% of cases

3. Aspiration causing respiratory distress, >0.1% of cases

4. Transient bacteremia, probably occurring commonly. Resulting sepsis is very rare (>0.1%), as is infection of prosthetic heart valves (>0.1%) (2,5).

## CPT Codes

**43248** – Upper gastrointestinal endoscopy including esophagus, stomach, and either the duodenum and/or jejunum as appropriate; with insertion of guidewire followed by dilation of esophagus over guidewire.

## REFERENCES

1. Marshall JB, Afridi SA, King PD, et al. Esophageal dilation with polyvinyl (American) dilators over a marked guidewire: practice and safety at one center over a 5-yr period. *Am J Gastroenterol* 1996;91(8):1503–1506.
2. Chan MF. Complications of upper gastrointestinal endoscopy. *Gastrointest Endosc Clin North Am* 1996;6(2):287–303.
3. Fleischer DE, Benjamin SB, Cattau EL Jr, et al. A marked guide wire facilitates esophageal dilatation. *Am J Gastroenterol* 1989; 84(4):359–361.
4. Swarbrick ET, Gough AL, Foster CS, et al. Prevention of recurrence of esophageal stricture, a comparison of lansoprazole and high-dose ranitidine. *Eur J Gastroenterol Hepatol* 1996; 8(5):431–438.
5. Zubarik R, Eisen G, Mastropietro C, et al. Prospective analysis of complications 30 days after outpatient upper endoscopy. *Am J Gastroenterol* 1999;94(6):1539–1545.

# Pneumatic Dilation for Achalasia

## Joel E. Richter

Achalasia is a primary disorder of esophageal motility of unknown etiology. Patients present with dysphagia for both solids and liquids, bland regurgitation of food and saliva, and sometimes chest pain and weight loss. Achalasia is characterized by abnormal lower esophageal sphincter (LES) relaxation and aperistalsis in the distal smooth muscle portion of the esophagus. The goal of treatment is to disrupt the hypercontracting LES muscle, thereby facilitating esophageal emptying by gravity and the hydrostatic pressures generated by swallowing and retaining food and liquid in the esophagus. This is best accomplished by either pneumatic dilation or Heller myotomy, usually performed laparoscopically. Although losing favor in some centers, pneumatic dilation often is considered the preferred treatment for many patients with achalasia because it is easy to perform as an outpatient procedure and has a low rate of troubling gastroesophageal reflux when compared to esophageal myotomy. Long-term studies generally show similar efficacies between pneumatic dilation and Heller myotomy (1).

### INDICATIONS
1. Achalasia. It is important to confirm the diagnosis of achalasia by appropriate testing prior to performing pneumatic dilation.

### CONTRAINDICATIONS
The major contraindication for pneumatic dilation is

1. Older age or comorbid illnesses (especially cardiac and pulmonary) that do not make the patient fit for surgery. Age alone should not be a contraindication as, our clinic has performed pneumatic dilation in healthy adults up to 84 years of age after a thorough discussion of the risks and a failure to respond to less invasive treatments.

Other contraindications include

1. Lack of patient cooperation
2. Significant bleeding diathesis
3. Warfarin or heparin use

In the latter setting, pneumatic dilation can be safely done during a "heparin window," restarting anticoagulation 6 to 8 hours after pneumatic dilation. Other relative contraindications reported in the literature include vigorous achalasia, large hiatal hernia, and associated epiphrenic diverticulum. Finally, a prior Heller myotomy is not a contraindication for pneumatic dilation. Because of the associated scarring, these patients often are done initially with a larger balloon, and dilations are not as effective as in untreated cases.

## PREPARATION

1. Barium esophagram. Characteristic features of the barium esophagram include dilation of the esophagus with retained secretions, loss of peristalsis, and a smooth narrowing at the gastroesophageal junction (bird's beak appearance). Early in the course, the esophagus may be minimally dilated, sometimes causing confusion with a peptic stricture. Routinely, it is also important to assess esophageal emptying in the upright position using a simple "timed barium esophagram" technique (2). In the upright position, the patient ingests 100 mL to 200 mL of low-density barium over 30 or 45 seconds. Three-on-one-spot films are obtained 1, 2, and 5 minutes after ingestion. The degree of esophageal emptying may be estimated by measuring the percent change in the height and width of the barium column over 5 minutes.

2. Esophageal manometry. Esophageal manometry findings characteristic of achalasia include aperistalsis in the smooth muscle portion of the esophagus with waves that are usually not true contractions and are mirror images of each other (common cavity phenomena). The LES is elevated in about half of the cases, but relaxation of the sphincter is always abnormal, with approximately 75% of patients demonstrating absent or incomplete relaxation and 20% to 30% showing relaxation that is very short (< 6 seconds, but complete).

3. Upper endoscopy. Endoscopy is important to confirm the absence of structural abnormalities such as a stricture and, more importantly, to rule out tumor at the gastroesophageal junction. This is particularly important in elderly patients with short duration of symptoms and profound weight loss. However, since the suspicion of pseudoachalasia is low in most patients, endoscopy is advisable at the time of pneumatic dilation and not as a separate procedure. Patients with recurrent dysphagia after Heller myotomy may be problematic. In these patients, an initial endoscopy should be done to assess for esophagitis, exclude a peptic stricture, and define the presence or absence of a fundoplication.

4. Informed consent. All symptomatic patients with achalasia in good health are presented with a complete discussion about the pros and cons of the more definitive treatments of achalasia—either pneumatic dilation or laparoscopic Heller myotomy—We do not consider botulinum toxin injection an alternative therapy in otherwise healthy subjects. All patients being considered for pneumatic dilatation must be fit for surgery in case this need arises because of an esophageal perforation. In patients who are poor risks for surgery, alternative treatments including botulinum toxin injection or drug therapy (calcium channel blockers or nitrates) are discussed.

5. Preprocedural fast. Pneumatic dilation is an outpatient procedure. Minimizing the amount of retained food and

secretions in the esophagus is critical for a careful evaluation of the esophageal mucosa and for decreasing the risk of aspiration during the procedure. A 12-hour fast is usually sufficient in patients with mild to moderately dilated esophagi up to 6 cm to 7 cm. In patients with megaesophagus, some may require several days of clear liquids and lavage through a wide-bore Ewald tube before the procedure. Rarely, a patient will need hospitalization, esophageal lavage via an Ewald tube, and overnight low-pressure nasogastric tube suction.

## EQUIPMENT

1. Pneumatic balloon. In the United States, the most commonly used balloon is the Rigiflex System (Boston Scientific Corp, Boston, MA). This is a graded, polyethylene balloon system mounted on a flexible catheter similar in design to the through-the-scope balloons. The Rigiflex balloon is 10 cm long and comes in three diameters including 3.0, 3.5, and 4.0 cm. This balloon is not visible under fluoroscopy but has several radiopaque markers on the shaft that define the upper, middle, and distal borders of the balloon. The Rigiflex balloon is noncompliant, meaning that it inflates maximally to a designated diameter only. Further inflation pressures increase the pounds per square inch (psi) within the lumen but not the balloon diameter. Once the maximum psi for any balloon is exceeded, it simply ruptures without ever increasing the diameter.

    The other pneumatic dilator is the Witzel dilator (U.S. Endoscopy, Mentor, OH), which is made of a 20-cm–long polyvinyl tube surrounded by a 15-cm–long polyurethane balloon which is passed in a retrograde fashion over the endoscope. The Witzel dilator has the advantage of direct endoscopic visualization of the balloon position during dilation. However, its utility is limited because it comes in only one size, a 4.0-cm balloon diameter, and has a two to three times higher perforation rate than the Rigiflex balloons (1).

2. Other supplies for upper endoscopy (see Chapter 5)

## PROCEDURE

1. Perform pneumatic dilation in a room with fluoroscopy the morning after an overnight fast. Administer antibiotics if the patient has significant valvular heart disease or an artificial valve. Obtain written consent, and remind the patient about the risk of perforation the day of the procedure.

2. Prior to beginning the procedure, choose the appropriate dilator size, inflate the balloon to check for leaks, and confirm the sphygmomanometer is correctly functioning. Use the smallest balloon diameter (3.0 cm) at the first procedure. If there is no response, use a 3.5-cm balloon after 4 weeks or longer and then a 4.0-cm balloon if necessary. In patients with a prior pneumatic dilation or Heller myotomy who are still symptomatic, begin with a 3.5-cm balloon.

3. Prior to beginning the procedure, give standard topical anesthetic for pharyngeal anesthesia and intravenous (IV) conscious sedation using meperidine and midazolam. Titrate as necessary to keep the patient comfortable and often amnesic for the procedure. Supplemental nasal oxygen ($O_2$) may be required.

4. Perform a complete endoscopy in the left lateral position with special attention to the cardia to exclude a tumor and assess for the presence of a hiatal hernia. Remove residual fluid in the esophagus by suction. Sometimes further Ewald lavage is required.

5. After a careful endoscopy is completed, place a Savary guidewire in the stomach, and remove the endoscope. It is important to deflate the stomach after placing the guidewire, which allows the air in the balloon to be seen easily by fluoroscopy during the dilation. Regardless of the degree of esophageal tortuosity, pass a stiff Savary wire, although a softer, more pliable wire can also be used if the esophagus is relatively straight. Using this technique, dilation is successful as long as the stomach is entered with the Rigiflex system.

6. Still in the left lateral position, use a 50-cc syringe attached to the balloon port to pass the selected Rigiflex balloon, which is covered with lubricant (e.g., K-Y jelly) and completely deflated, into the esophagus and stomach. This is done with the bite block in place and the head tilted slightly backward, which straightens the posterior pharynx, allowing for a smoother intubation of the esophagus.

7. The key to a successful dilation is accurate placement of the balloon. With the patient in the supine position, the balloon is centered across the gastroesophageal junction by fluoroscopy. This may be difficult, especially if a good waist caused by the surrounding hypercontracting LES is not easily seen. Partial inflation and repositioning may be required to get the balloon in proper position, i.e., with half of the partially inflated balloon above the waist and half below the waist (Fig. 24.1A).

8. Then gradually inflate the balloon under fluoroscopic guidance until the waist disappears (Fig. 24.1B). This usually requires 7 psi to 12 psi of air, with this pressure being maintained for 60 seconds. Although not scientifically studied, abrupt effacement of a persistent waist is very suspicious of a perforation. As the balloon is inflated, there is a tendency for the dilator to be pulled down into the stomach, especially with the larger balloons. This can be counteracted by maintaining a constant upward traction at the mouthpiece during the procedure (Fig. 24.2). The duration of balloon inflation does not appear to be as important as making sure the waist is obliterated. This was recently confirmed in a study comparing the efficacy of 6- or 60-second balloon inflation times (3). Some authors suggest repeat inflation for up to 3 minutes, but none of these variables has been prospectively studied.

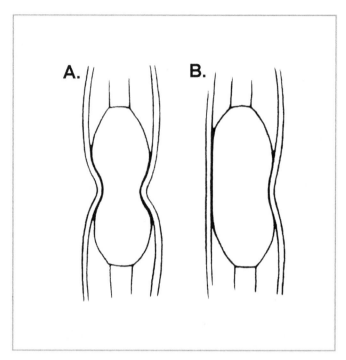

**Fig. 24.1. Appearance of the pneumatic balloon before (A) and after (B) sphincter disruption.**

9. Reposition the patient in the left lateral position, and remove the balloon and guidewire after deflation. The amount of blood on the balloon is noted but is not a prognostic indicator of success or perforation.

**POSTPROCEDURE**
1. Take the patient to the recovery room for 30 to 60 minutes or until awake, with the head of the bed elevated to reduce aspiration risk.
2. Perform a Gastrografin swallow with x-rays taken in the area postrema (AP) and lateral views. If no perforation is seen, thin barium is administered to provide better anatomic detail. The x-rays are obtained solely to identify early esophageal perforations and not to assess esophageal emptying, which may be poor secondary to edema or LES spasm.
3. Upon return to the endoscopy suite, give the patient water to drink.
4. On rare occasions in which severe postdilation pain occurs, give sublingual nitroglycerin or nifedipine.

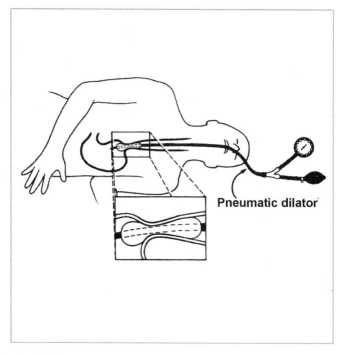

**Fig. 24.2. Correct position of balloon in patient.**

5.  Once the patient is stable and tolerating fluids, discharge him or her after 3 to 4 hours of observation. Before 1994, nearly all achalasia patients were observed overnight in the hospital after dilation, but since the report by Barkin et al. (4), nearly all patients go home after outpatient observation.

6.  All patients are followed up in clinic in one month to assess symptoms and esophageal emptying with the timed barium esophagram, using the same volume as the initial study. If symptoms and/or barium esophageal emptying are not markedly improved, then repeat dilation is scheduled with the next-larger-size balloon. This "aggressive" technique is used because patients have longer remission rates with pneumatic dilation in those having concurrent improvement in symptoms and esophageal emptying (2).

## COMPLICATIONS

Complications after pneumatic dilation are reported in up to 33% of patients, with most complications being mild (5).

1.  The most serious complication is esophageal perforation. Although the perforation rate varies in the literature from 0% to 16% (1), the overall perforation rate of 2.3% with the new

Rigiflex balloon dilators is very acceptable. Efforts to use the 3.5-cm balloon, comparable in diameter to the older Browne-McHardy dilator, showed perforation rates unacceptably high at 10.6% (6). Now, beginning with the 3.0-cm balloon results in perforation rates of 2% in 200 patients. This observation confirms the safety of a graded approach to pneumatic dilation (7). As previously discussed, after pneumatic dilation, patients undergo a Gastrografin swallow to exclude obvious and subtle perforations. Others suggest a more selective approach, performing x-rays only if patients have prolonged chest pain, tachycardia, shortness of breath, or fever (8). Patients with free perforation to the mediastinum, pleural, or peritoneal space should undergo surgery to close the perforation, preferably through an open posterior thoracotomy. If performed within the first 8 to 12 hours, a myotomy on the contralateral esophageal wall also can be done. Perforations that seem contained within the muscle wall can be treated medically with nasogastric suction, parenteral alimentation, and intravenous antibiotics for 10 to 14 days (9). If the perforation is recognized early, Schwartz et al. (10) found no difference in the duration of the operation, intensive care stay, hospitalization days, or the long-term outcome in seven patients who had surgical repair for pneumatic perforation as compared to five patients undergoing elective myotomy during the same period. However, it must be emphasized that the surgical myotomy in these patients was an open rather than laparoscopic myotomy, which has become the routine in recent years.

2. Postdilation chest pain

3. Aspiration pneumonia

4. Hematemesis

5. Fever that resolves spontaneously

6. Esophageal mucosal tear without perforation

7. Esophageal hematoma

**CPT Codes**

**43458** – Dilation of esophagus with balloon (30-mm diameter or larger) for achalasia.

**REFERENCES**

1. Vaezi MF, Richter JE. Diagnosis and management of achalasia. American College of Gastroenterology guidelines. *Am J Gastroenterol* 1999;94:3406–3412.
2. Vaezi MF, Baker ME, Achkar E, Richter JE. Timed barium oesophagram: better predictor of long term success after pneumatic dilation in achalasia than symptom assessment. *Gut* 2002; 50:765–770.
3. Khan AA, Shah SWH, Alam A, et al. Pneumatic balloon dilation in achalasia: a prospective comparison of balloon distention time. *Am J Gastroenterol* 1998;93:1064–1067.

4. Barkin JS, Guelrad M, Reiner DK, et al. Forceful balloon dilation. An outpatient procedure for achalasia. *Gastrointest Endosc* 1990;36:123–125.
5. Eckhardt VF, Kanzler G, Westermeir T. Complications and their impact after pneumatic dilation for achalasia: a prospective long-term follow-up study. *Gastrointest Endosc* 1997;45: 349–353.
6. Stark GA, Castell DO, Richter JE, et al. Prospective randomized comparison of Browne-McHardy and Microvasive balloon dilator in the treatment of achalasia. *Am J Gastroenterol* 1990;85: 1322–1326.
8. Kadakia SC, Wong RKH. Graded pneumatic dilation using Rigiflex achalasia dilators in patients with primary achalasia. *Am J Gastroenterol* 1993;88:34–38.
9. Ciarolla DA, Traube M. Achalasia. Short term clinical monitoring after pneumatic dilation. *Dig Dis Sci* 1993;38:1905–1908.
10. Michel L, Grillo HC, Malt RA. Operative and non-operative management of esophageal perforation. *Ann Surg* 1981;194: 57–63.
11. Swartz AM, Cahou CE, Traube M. Outcome after perforation sustained during pneumatic dilation for achalasia. *Dig Dis Sci* 1993;38:1409–1413.

# Through-the-Scope Balloon Dilation

Elena I. Sidorenko and Prateek Sharma

Through-the-scope (TTS) balloon dilation is a common method of dilation of complex esophageal strictures and, less commonly, of gastrojejunostomy and other accessible surgical strictures, and rectal and colonic strictures. Data comparing the efficacy and safety of different dilating systems are lacking. Standardization of the procedure technique is also lacking. In this review, we discuss the advantages and disadvantages of TTS balloons, the technical aspects of the procedure and comment on mistakes often made during the procedure. Complications related to the technique are also addressed.

Hydrostatic balloons for TTS dilation became available in the mid-1980s. They have since become widely used among endoscopists. Data comparing the efficacy and side effects of different dilating systems are conflicting. Some initial data had suggested that TTS dilation is safer than push-type dilators because only radial forces are applied, causing circumferential stretching, but with a reduction of shear stress. However, most studies agree that both rigid and balloon dilators are equally safe in the treatment of benign lower esophageal strictures (1,2). Studies have shown no significant differences in the immediate relief of dysphagia and the need for repeat dilation at one year between rigid- and balloon-treated patients with benign distal esophageal strictures (2). Physician experience and the characteristics of the stricture eventually determine whether balloon dilation will be effective, as well as the size and type of balloon used. The advantages of TTS balloons are the ease of passage, elimination of repeated esophageal intubations, and direct endoscopic visualization of stricture with improved placement control. The disadvantages of the TTS balloons include difficult judgment of the resistance at the stricture level, limited life span of the balloons, and their cost. A learning curve is required to be comfortable with TTS use.

## INDICATIONS

The primary clinical goal of esophageal balloon dilation is the long-term symptomatic relief of dysphagia. On occasion this dilation is used to treat strictures of the gastrointestinal tract accessible to the endoscope. Specific indications include (1,3)

1. Dilation of severe, lengthy, irregular, and complex strictures (such as in multiple, closely placed strictures in the cervical esophagus); and/or strictures associated with large hiatal hernia, esophageal diverticula, tracheoesophageal fistulas; and/or when another method of dilation has failed

2. Occasionally, dilation of esophageal rings and webs, when they are narrow and of firmer consistency

3. Dilation of surgical anastomoses in patients with previous gastrectomy or gastric bypass surgery

4. Dilation with intent to minimize oropharyngeal shearing stress in certain conditions (e.g., epidermolysis bullosa)

5. Occasionally, dilation of colonic or small bowel strictures (e.g., Crohn's disease)

## CONTRAINDICATIONS (4)

### Absolute

1. Acute abdomen

2. Acute or incompletely healed esophageal or other gastrointestinal perforation

3. Lack of informed consent

### Relative

1. Bleeding disorders

2. Use of anticoagulants (American Society for Gastrointestinal Endoscopy [ASGE] guidelines should be followed for stopping anticoagulation before dilation)

3. Severe pulmonary disease

4. Recent myocardial infarction

5. Recent perforation or surgery at area of stricture

6. Pharyngeal or cervical deformity

7. Recent laparotomy

8. Large thoracic aneurysm

## PREPARATION

1. The patient should have been fasting for 12 hours prior to the procedure.

2. Obtain written consent.

3. The procedure is performed under conscious sedation.

4. Fluoroscopy should be available for complicated cases.

## EQUIPMENT

1. TTS balloons of various length and diameter

2. Dilating gun or inflation device to maintain pressure

3. Stopcocks to ensure a constant pressure during inflation

The size of the dilator is expressed either in metric system (mm) or French (Fr) units. The diameter, expressed in French units, equals the diameter in millimeters multiplied by *pi* (3.14, or approximately by 3). The size of TTS balloons varies, ranging from 18 Fr to 60 Fr, and they are 3 cm to 8 cm long, with a polyethylene shaft of 60 cm to 200 cm. Short balloons frequently suffer displacement during dilation, and balloons that are 8 cm long usually are used for esophageal dilation. Wilson-Cook (Wilson-Cook Medical, Inc., Winston-Salem, NC), Bard (C.R. Bard, Inc.,

Tewksbury, MA), and Microvasive (Boston Scientific Corporation, Watertown, MA) are the manufacturers of balloon dilators. Microvasive makes Rigiflex balloons, available in balloon diameter sizes of 6, 8, 10, 12, 15, and 18 mm, as well as a new multi-diameter controlled radial expansion (CRE) balloon dilator. The CRE balloons can be inflated to three progressively larger sizes by increasing pressure up to the maximum inflation pressure, but unfortunately they are single-use balloons. Balloons can be inflated with air, water, or contrast material.

## PROCEDURE

Fluoroscopic guidance is not required in most cases for TTS balloon advancement, even when the endoscope cannot be passed beyond the stricture.

1. Endoscopy and the first dilation are frequently performed at the same session.

2. Pass the endoscope through the stricture if possible.

3. Use a balloon 1 mm to 2 mm (3 Fr to 6 Fr) larger than the stricture diameter. Some endoscopists rarely use balloons larger than 15 mm at the initial dilation.

4. Test the balloon for leaks by attaching the balloon to the manometer and the inflator. Fill the entire system with water or contrast. Inflate the balloon to the maximum range of pressure, and then deflate it.

5. Apply silicone to the tip of the balloon catheter.

6. Pass the balloon through the biopsy channel of the endoscope until the tip of the TTS balloon is seen in the lumen.

7. Withdraw the scope to the midportion of the stricture, and then place the balloon in the tightest area of the stricture (Fig. 25.1A). Inflate the balloon slowly.

8. If the endoscope is unable to be passed through the stricture, the balloon or guidewire can be carefully advanced through the stricture. The passage should be stopped if resistance is encountered, and an alternative method for dilation or fluoroscopic guidance should be used (3). For fluoroscopy, the balloon should be filled with 1:3 dilution of water-soluble contrast. Obliteration of the balloon waist seen under fluoroscopy corresponds to the stricture stretching or splitting (Fig. 25.1B).

9. Inflate the balloon gradually using a 10- to 20-mL syringe or the inflation gun. The manometer attached to the balloon measures the pressure in the balloon. Pressures should not be higher than those recommended by the manufacturer.

10. Pressures are kept constant, during which period the stricture wall is observed through the transparent balloon wall.

11. Duration of balloon inflation has not been standardized and varies from institution to institution. Usually it varies

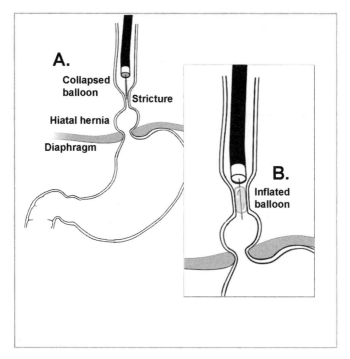

**Fig. 25.1. Dilatation of a peptic stricture in a subject with a hiatal hernia using a TTS balloon. A: Collapsed balloon. B: Inflated baloon.**

between 30 seconds to 2 minutes in one session. Some have suggested 30 seconds of dilation followed by redilation a second or third time after repositioning of the balloon. It is not clear how fast the balloon should be distended and how many times dilation needs to be performed with the same size balloon.

12. The distended balloon should be able to slide easily through the strictured area to confirm dilation.

13. Deflate the balloon by applying negative pressure to the syringe.

14. Examine the mucosa of the stricture for mucosal breaks.

15. Straighten the tip of the endoscope prior to removing the balloon from the channel.

16. Dilation can be repeated using balloons of larger diameter during the same session if the patient remains comfortable and vital signs are stable.

17. Keep in mind the "rule of threes:" Never dilate more than three consecutive dilator sizes during one session, to minimize

the risk of perforation. This rule is usually applied to bougie dilators but has little data support. A single large (e.g., 50-Fr) dilator can be used for rings or webs.

18. Several sessions could be required for successful dilation. On each subsequent dilation it is usually wise to use a dilator at least one size smaller than the largest dilator passed during the previous session.

## POSTPROCEDURE

1. Observe the patient according to the standard post-endoscopy protocol.

2. Discharge the patient with the following instructions:

   a. Follow standard antireflux measures.
   b. For esophageal dilation, start medical therapy with proton pump inhibitors to delay restricturing process and to reduce the need of redilations in case of peptic stricture.
   c. Advise the patient to return if chest/abdominal pain, hematemesis, blood per rectum, shortness of breath, or fever occur.
   d. Schedule a follow-up visit to assess for recurrent dysphagia.

## INTERPRETATION

The overall success rate of balloon dilation is 80% to 90%. Symptomatic relief is often more obvious than objective evidence of improvement. Both subjective and objective measures (e.g., a passage of a 12-mm barium tablet) can be used as an end point for dilation (5). Initial dilation usually should be limited to a diameter of no more than 45 Fr. With dilation to 45 Fr, patients should be able to eat a modified regular diet; dilation to 54 Fr allows intake of regular food. Patients who have an esophageal lumen less than 39 Fr will continue to experience solid food dysphagia.

## COMPLICATIONS

### Procedure-Related Complications

1. Perforation is reported as 0.3% for balloon dilation of all types of esophageal strictures (6). Studies have not shown an increased perforation rate with the use of TTS balloons compared to other types of dilators (7). The risk increases when larger balloons are used; however, no prospective data are available.

2. Bleeding is usually minor, and transfusions are rarely required.

3. Bacteremia is common after esophageal dilation, with a frequency as high as 22.8% (8). Bacteremia usually does not result in severe infectious complications. Antibiotic prophylaxis guidelines are reflected in ASGE recommendations (9).

### Common Mistakes During Dilation

1. Use of small biopsy channel endoscopes for the larger balloons (3)

2.  Use of inflation pressures above the one recommended by the manufacturer

3.  Attempts to remove the balloon before it is completely deflated

4.  Excessive angulation of the endoscopic tip

5.  Dilation of the narrow stricture to normal esophageal diameter in one endoscopic session

## OTHER USES FOR THIS TECHNIQUE

Balloon dilation is an alternative to surgical treatment of selected patients with gastric outlet obstruction, including pyloric stenosis caused by peptic ulcer disease, postoperative strictures, and Crohn's disease. Although relief of symptoms has been reported in 77% of patients (10) following TTS dilation, data regarding long-term relief of obstructive symptoms are lacking. Duration of the balloon insufflations, the frequency and adequacy of the dilation, and the size of the balloon have not been standardized.

## CPT Codes

**43220** – Esophagoscopy; with balloon dilation (less than 30-mm diameter).

**43245** – Upper gastrointestinal endoscopy; with dilation of gastric outlet obstruction (balloon, guidewire, bougie).

**43249** – Upper gastrointestinal endoscopy; with balloon dilation of the esophagus (less than 30 mm in diameter).

## REFERENCES

1.  Shemesh E, Czerniak A. Comparison between Savary-Gilliard and balloon dilation of benign esophageal strictures. *World J Surg* 1990;14:518–522.

2.  Scolapio JS, Pasha TM, Gostout CJ, et al. A randomized prospective study comparing rigid to balloon dilators for benign esophageal strictures and rings. *Gastrointest Endosc* 1999; 50(1):13–17.

3.  Shailesh C, Kadakia SC, Wong RKH. Transendoscopic balloon therapy: what is its role for esophageal strictures and with which balloon? In: Barkin JS, O'Phelan CA, eds. *Advanced Therapeutic Endoscopy*, 2nd ed. New York: Raven Press, Ltd., 1994:85–93.

4.  American Society for Gatsrointestinal Endoscopy Guidelines. Esophageal dilation. *Gastrointest Endosc* 1998;48(6):702–704.

5.  Saeed ZA, Ramirez FC, Hepps KS, et al. An objective end point for dilation improves outcome of peptic esophageal strictures: a prospective randomized trial. *Gastrointest Endosc* 1997;45(5): 354–359.

6.  Kozarek RA. Hydrostatic balloon dilation of gastrointestinal stenosis: a national survey. *Gastrointest Endosc* 1986;32:15–19.

7.  Hernandez LJ, Jacobson JW, Harris MS. Comparison among the perforation rates of Maloney, balloon, and Savary dilation of esophageal strictures. *Gastrointest Endosc* 2000; 51(4):460–462.

8.  Nelson DB. Infection control during gastrointestinal endoscopy. *J Lab Clin Med* 2003;141(3):159–167.

9. American Society for Gastrointestinal Endoscopy Guidelines. Infection control during gastrointestinal endoscopy. *Gastrointest Endosc* 1999;49(6):836–841.

10. Hewitt PM, Krige JEJ, Funnell IC, et al. Endoscopic balloon dilation of peptic pyloroduodenal strictures. *J Clin Gastroenterol* 1999;28(1):33–35.

# Stenting of Esophageal Cancers: Placement of Expandable Stents

Kenneth K. Wang

Esophageal stents are the most common method to palliate esophageal carcinomas. Although nonexpandable plastic stents had been used in the past, the need to dilate the esophageal cancer to large diameters (17 mm to 18 mm) led to frequent and devastating complications such as esophageal perforation. The expandable stents that have been created by multiple manufacturers including Wilson-Cook, Boston Scientific, Polyflex, and Bard all allow the endoscopist to place a stent through an esophageal tumor with only minimal diameters required for dilation. Studies have shown that these expandable stents can be placed with fewer complications than plastic stents (1,2). None of these systems are superior to the others in all tumor types, and all can relieve dysphagia in over 90% of patients (3). Some stents have some theoretical advantages in supplying greater radial force in tumors that have large bulky extramural components.

## INDICATIONS

1. To relieve dysphagia produced by neoplastic strictures of the esophagus

2. To relieve dysphagia in chronic nonneoplastic strictures that have not responded to routine dilation (Polyflex only)

3. To seal fistulas between the trachea and esophagus due to neoplastic causes (covered stents)

## CONTRAINDICATIONS

1. Those associated with upper endoscopy (see Chapter 5)

2. Compression of the trachea by esophageal cancer. This may require bronchoscopy to assess.

3. Anticipated chemotherapy or radiotherapy. These methods have reasonable success in decreasing tumor and allowing palliation of dysphagia so a stent may not be necessary. There is considerable debate over whether stent placement followed by radiation or chemotherapy increases complications (4–6).

4. Poor patient functional status with anticipated survival less than a month

5. Complete loss of appetite in patients who are able to tolerate their oral secretions

6. Severe cardiac and/or respiratory disorder

7. Food impaction in the esophagus (removal is necessary prior to stent therapy)

8. Lack of patient cooperation

9. Bleeding diathesis

10. Anticipated need for chronic anticoagulation

11. Severe cervical spinal arthritis or spinal instability

**PREPARATION**

1. Fast the patient for at least 8 hours prior to the procedure.

2. Obtain informed consent from the patient that outlines the possible complications of the procedure as well as alternative methods of treatment.

3. Assess the patient's airway by bronchoscopy if the tumor involves the tracheal bifurcation by radiographical imaging or the patient is exhibiting signs of pulmonary compromise.

4. Administer a topical anesthetic for pharyngeal anesthesia.

5. Start an intravenous line for administration of systemic sedation.

6. Obtain oral suction in the case of retained fluid or inability to clear secretions during the procedure.

**EQUIPMENT**

1. Upper endoscope

2. Spring-tipped wire (at least 180 cm in length)

3. Fluoroscopy (stents can be placed safely without fluoroscopy by experienced endoscopists) (7,8)

4. A variety of expandable stent lengths (8 cm to 15 cm in length). Stent types also vary between coated and noncoated stents. Most expandable stents are coated to prevent tumor ingrowth. In addition, antireflux valves have been placed in some stents to prevent gastroesophageal reflux, although these have been associated with increased obstruction (9).

5. A variety of dilators, both through-the-endoscope and over-the-wire

6. Radiopaque markers, either hemoclips or contrast solution for injection through a sclerotherapy needle

7. Leaded aprons for radiation safety

8. Radiation dosage badges for personnel

9. Lubricant

10. Gloves

11. Intravenous sedatives

**PROCEDURE**

1. Assessment of the tumor. Perform a diagnostic upper endoscopy to assess tumor location and dimensions and to

determine the need for dilation. If the tumor does not allow the passage of a standard adult endoscope, dilation will be required. As the endoscopist traverses the tumor, the degree of stenosis will need to be determined. The expandable stents have different degrees of radial force. (Radial force is generally thought to be greatest with the Wallstent followed by the Z-stent and then the Ultraflex.)

2. Dilation of the tumor. Perform dilation as needed to ensure easy passage of the stent delivery system. This will vary according to the type of stent chosen but generally will be to a diameter of 5 mm to 14 mm. Most commonly this is done with through-the-endoscope balloons to allow visualization of the results and to ensure dilation of the entire tumor area. However, if the tumor is very stenotic (does not allow passage of the endoscope or dilating balloon), over-the-wire dilators may need to be employed using fluoroscopic guidance.

3. Marking tumor dimensions. Since the stents are placed under fluoroscopy, the tumor dimensions (proximal and distal extent) must be carefully assessed by both endoscopic determination of distance from the incisors and by radiopaque markers placed at the distal and proximal ends of the tumor. During these measurements, the correct length of the tumor should be determined. The correct stent length will be longer than the length of the tumor but will vary depending on the degree of contraction of the stent when it is deployed. Some stent types will deploy at precisely the length of the stent, but other expandable stents will actually contract while being deployed, and the endoscopist should be familiar with the characteristics of the stent type available. Generally the stent contraction is greatest with the Ultraflex followed by the Wallstent and then the Z-stent. Injection of the distal and proximal ends of the tumor is often done using hypaque, but this can diffuse into an unusable smear unless the stent is rapidly placed after injection. Oil-based radiopaque solutions more readily maintain a discrete formation after injection. Some endoscopists prefer using hemoclips to fluoroscopically identify normal mucosa proximal and distal to the tumor.

4. Placement of the stent delivery system. After marking the tumor, the endoscope is advanced into the stomach, and a flexible wire is left in place in the antrum of the stomach. The endoscope is then withdrawn from the esophagus, leaving the wire in the stomach (Fig. 26.1A). The radiopaque markers should be visualized on fluoroscopy with the tumor visualized in its entirety by the fluoroscopic image. The wire should not have slack in the esophagus in order to perform as a guide for the stent delivery system. There has to be sufficient wire outside of the mouth to allow the stent delivery system to be placed onto the extracorporeal wire. The endoscopist should then select the appropriate size stent for use and assemble the stent delivery system. Though there are individual differences, the delivery systems usually entail a folded wire mesh stent that is compressed over a semirigid

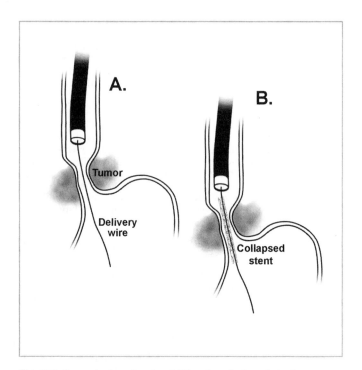

**Fig. 26.1. Correct wire placement (A) and undeployed stent placement through lesion (B).**

plastic catheter that can be introduced over a wire (Fig. 26.1B). The stent can be released from its compressed state by either withdrawing a plastic overtube that is placed over the stent or by withdrawing string that is wound around the compressed stent. The endoscopist should remember that most expandable stents expand from the distal end to the proximal end. The patient's neck should hyperextend to allow easy insertion of the stent delivery systems. The stent delivery system should then be inserted over the wire and placed into position in the tumor. The stent itself should be visible under fluoroscopy and should overlap both the proximal and distal markers of the tumor. This must be carefully confirmed before the stent is deployed.

5. Stent deployment. The patient should be well-sedated at this point, as patient motion during stent deployment could interfere with good stent positioning. The stent is then deployed distally to proximally, with the endoscopist continually monitoring deployment under fluoroscopy (Fig. 26.2A). The expansion of the distal end of the stent will cause the stent to migrate distally unless the endoscopist is vigilant. If the stent does not expand as anticipated, the endoscopist

must consider the possibility that the tumor is too stenotic or that the stent is in an incorrect position. If the distal portions of the stent are not expanding in normal tissue, the stent will not achieve its required hourglass-like shape, which anchors the stent in position. Adjustments can be made to the stent position until a specified portion of the stent is deployed (stent dependent), then the stent can no longer be recompressed by the stent delivery system. It is generally easier to reposition the stent proximally by gently pulling the delivery catheter than to move the stent more distally.

6. Withdrawal of the stent delivery system. Once the stent is fully deployed (Fig. 26.2B), it must be allowed to expand for several minutes. Premature withdrawal of the stent delivery system before adequate expansion of the stent can lead to the delivery system actually dislodging the stent position. It is often advantageous to torque the delivery system from side to side to prevent the delivery system from engaging the mesh wires of the stent and causing the stent to migrate. During the withdrawal of the stent delivery system, the wire can also be withdrawn. Fluoroscopic monitoring of the stent while removing the delivery system will minimize the risk of stent displacement.

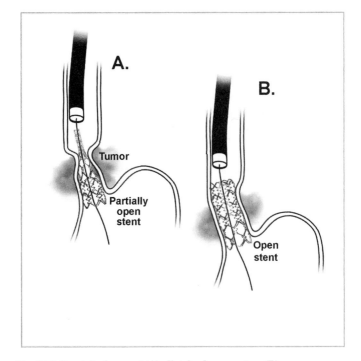

**Fig. 26.2. Stent deployment (A), distal release system (B).**

7. Stent placement without fluoroscopy. Endoscopists have reported placement of stents without the use of fluoroscopy by placing colored marks on the proximal portion of the stent delivery system and relying on the endoscopic measurements to determine the distal portion of the stent. In expert hands, this appears to be successful and does simplify the process. However, endoscopists who choose this method should recognize that this technique is not consistent with some manufacturers' suggested placement techniques (10).

8. Assessment of the stent after placement. The patency of the stent should be confirmed under fluoroscopy; if the stent has drifted distally, the stent can be withdrawn using the endoscope and a pair of grasping forceps. The positioning of the stent should be observed under fluoroscopy. Proximal migration of the stent cannot generally be corrected without removal of the misplaced stent. It is not necessary to confirm placement of the stent with endoscopy unless fluoroscopic images are unclear, and passing an endoscope through a freshly placed stent may actually cause stent displacement.

9. Second stent placement. Whereas a single esophageal stent is ideal therapy, occasionally a second or even third stent can be placed within the initial stent to increase the length of the stent or to seal a fistula. Even tracheoesophageal fistulas will seal with a single coated stent (11).

## POSTPROCEDURE

1. Vital signs should be monitored for at least an hour postprocedure.

2. The head of the bed should be elevated.

3. The patient should be instructed on care of the stent, avoidance of difficult-to-digest meats, avoidance of lying supine or bending over after eating, and sleeping with the head of the bed elevated.

4. Clear liquids should be given for at least 24 hours, and then full liquids should be given for another day to allow the stent to fully deploy.

5. The patient should return if there is rapid onset of dysphagia, hemetemesis, melena, dyspnea, or marked chest pain.

6. If the stent traverses the lower esophageal sphincter, the patient should be instructed as to the increased risk of reflux and aspiration.

## COMPLICATIONS

Stent-related complications are common (20% of patients) and include

1. Chest pain (5% with severe pain)

2. Perforation (5%)

3. Bleeding (3% to 5%)
4. Tumor ingrowth (4%)
5. Gastroesophageal reflux (1% severe reflux)
6. Compromise of the respiratory system (0.1%)
7. Aspiration (5%)
8. Stent migration (10%)

## CPT Codes

**43219** – Esophagoscopy, rigid or flexible; with insertion of plastic tube or stent.

**47511** – Introduction of percutaneous transhepatic stent for internal and external biliary drainage.

**47555** – Biliary endoscopy, percutaneous via T-tube or other tract; with dilation of biliary duct stricture(s) without stent.

**47556** – Biliary endoscopy, percutaneous via T-tube or other tract; with dilation of biliary duct stricture(s) with stent.

**43268** – Endoscopic retrograde cholangiopancreatography (ERCP); with endoscopic retrograde insertion of tube or stent into bile or pancreatic duct.

**43269** – Endoscopic retrograde cholangiopancreatography (ERCP); with endoscopic retrograde removal of foreign body and/or change of tube or stent.

## REFERENCES

1. Knyrim K, Wagner HJ, Bethge N, et al. A controlled trial of an expansile metal stent for palliation of esophageal obstruction due to inoperable cancer. *N Engl J Med* 1993;329:1302–1307.
2. Kozarek RA, Raltz S, Brugge WR, et al. Prospective multicenter trial of esophageal Z-stent placement for malignant dysphagia and tracheoesophageal fistula. Erratum appears in *Gastrointest Endosc* 1996;44(6):764.
3. Siersema PD, Hop WC, van BM, et al. A comparison of 3 types of covered metal stents for the palliation of patients with dysphagia caused by esophagogastric carcinoma: a prospective, randomized study. Comment. *Gastrointest Endosc* 2001;54:145–153.
4. Sumiyoshi T, Gotoda T, Muro K, et al. Morbidity and mortality after self-expandable metallic stent placement in patients with progressive or recurrent esophageal cancer after chemoradiotherapy. *Gastrointest Endosc* 2003;57:882–885.
5. Siersema PD, Schrauwen SL, van BM, et al. Self-expanding metal stents for complicated and recurrent esophagogastric cancer. *Gastrointest Endosc* 2001;54:579–586.
6. Raijman I, Siddique I, Lynch P. Does chemoradiation therapy increase the incidence of complications with self-expanding coated stents in the management of malignant esophageal strictures? *Am J Gastroenterol* 1997;92:2192–2196.
7. White RE, Mungatana C, Topazian M. Esophageal stent placement without fluoroscopy. *Gastrointest Endosc* 2001; 53:348-351.
8. Austin AS, Khan Z, Cole AT, Freeman JG. Placement of esophageal self-expanding metallic stents without fluoroscopy. *Gastrointest Endosc* 2001;54:357–359.

9. Dua KS. Antireflux stents in tumors of the cardia. *Am J Med* 2001;111:3.

10. White RE, Mungatana C, Topazian M. Esophageal stent placement without fluoroscopy. Comment. *Gastrointest Endosc* 2001; 53:348–351.

11. Raijman I, Siddique I, Ajani J, Lynch P. Palliation of malignant dysphagia and fistulae with coated expandable metal stents: experience with 101 patients. *Gastrointest Endosc* 1998;48: 172–179.

# Biliary Sludge Analysis

Jason D. Conway

Biliary sludge, or microlithiasis, can be defined as abnormal precipitates in gallbladder bile, predominantly cholesterol monohydrate crystals and calcium bilirubinate granules (1).

Microlithiasis is present asymptomatically in a large proportion of the population, and the clinical course varies widely from disappearance in 17.7% to formation of gallstones in 8.3% after an average follow-up of over two years (2). An estimated 10% of patients with microlithiasis may eventually develop biliary colic (3,4). In patients with idiopathic pancreatitis, up to 74% have been shown to have microlithiasis (5).

The sensitivity of transabdominal ultrasound for detecting microlithiasis is only 55%, while endoscopic ultrasound has a sensitivity of 96% and a specificity of 86% (6). However, direct microscopic examination of gallbladder bile sediment, as described below, is considered the gold standard for the diagnosis of microlithiasis (1).

## INDICATIONS

1. Idiopathic pancreatitis

2. Pain of suspected biliary origin with normal imaging and laboratory evaluation

## CONTRAINDICATIONS

1. Any contraindication to nasogastric (NG) or feeding tube placement under fluoroscopy.

2. Allergy to cholecystokinin

## EQUIPMENT

1. Centrifuge

2. Glass slides and cover slips

3. Polarizing microscope

4. Cholecystokinin for intravenous infusion

## PROCEDURE

1. Cholecystokinin (0.04 mcg per kg body weight) should be infused intravenously over 10 minutes just prior to collection of bile.

2. Bile should be collected by aspiration of duodenal secretions immediately after cholecystokinin infusion for 10 to 20 minutes. This can be accomplished during endoscopy or by placing an NG or feeding tube in the duodenum under fluoroscopic guidance and applying mild intermittent negative suction (–5 to –10 mm Hg). Five to 15 cc of duodenal fluid should be collected.

3.  Aspirated bile should be kept at room temperature and immediately centrifuged at 3000 *g* for 15 minutes. At this point the sediment may only be frozen for further analysis.

4.  The supernatant can be discarded, and the sediment resuspended in a drop of distilled water, placed on the slide, and examined under the microscope.

**INTERPRETATION**

1.  Generally, two or more crystals or clumps per ×100 power field is consistent with microlithiasis. More than four crystals in an entire sample is also consistent with microlithiasis. Normal bile is brown in color with no precipitates.

2.  Cholesterol monohydrate crystals are rhomboid in shape with a notched corner and are birefringent under cross-polarization (Fig. 27.1).

3.  Calcium bilirubinate granules are reddish brown in color and nonbirefringent, appearing much like grains of sand.

4.  Each sample should be examined in triplicate and compared to positive and negative controls.

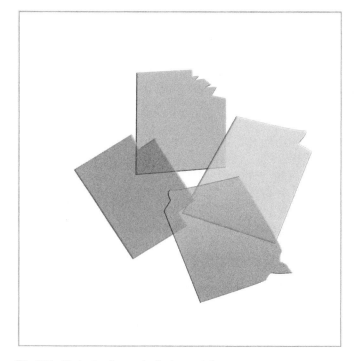

**Fig. 27.1. Cholesterol monohydrate crystals.**

5.  It should be noted that biliary sludge might form in situations of starvation, critical illness, long-term total parenteral nutrition (TPN), pregnancy, and in those who have bile stasis from obstructed large bile ducts.

## REFERENCES

1.  Ko CW, Sekijima JH, Lee SP. Biliary sludge. *Ann Intern Med* 1999;130:301–311.
2.  Lee SP, Maher K, Nicholls JF. Origin and fate of biliary sludge. *Gastroenterology* 1988;94:170–176.
3.  Moskovitz M, Min TC, Gavaler JS. The microscopic examination of bile in patients with biliary pain and negative imaging tests. *Am J Gastroenterol* 1986;81:329–333.
4.  Ohara N, Schaefer J. Clinical significance of biliary sludge. *J Clin Gastroenterol* 1990;12:291–294.
5.  Lee SP, Nicholls JF, Park HZ. Biliary sludge as a cause of acute pancreatitis. *N Engl J Med* 1992;326:589–593.
6.  Dahan P, Andant C, Levy P, et al. Prospective evaluation of endoscopic ultrasonography and microscopic examination of duodenal bile in the diagnosis of cholecystolithiasis in 45 patients with normal conventional ultrasonography. *Gut* 1996;38:277–281.

# Endoscopic Sphincterotomy (Including Precut)

John S. Goff

Endoscopic sphincterotomy (ES) has become a very important component of endoscopic retrograde cholangiopancreatography (ERCP). With the advent of many other methods for studying the biliary and pancreatic ductal system, such as magnetic resonance cholangiopancreatography (MRCP) and endoscopic ultrasonography (EUS), diagnostic ERCP is becoming less frequent than therapeutic ERCP. Endoscopic sphincterotomy is literally the opening of the door for the majority of the procedures performed during a therapeutic ERCP. It is therefore extremely important for any endoscopist who is doing ERCP to become proficient in ES so that the procedure can be used to its fullest. Endoscopic sphincterotomy is a task that requires moderate to high skill as it can produce serious complications. In order to perform ES one must be skilled at doing diagnostic ERCP and should be very familiar with the anatomy of the papilla. The bile duct and pancreatic ducts come together in the wall of the second part of the duodenum in several different configurations, which are not necessarily apparent by just observing the papilla. The bile duct is usually heading in an 11 o'clock direction from the orifice, and the pancreatic duct is usually straight inward. The ducts may enter the duodenum via a common channel of variable length or may have separate openings into the duodenal lumen. The papilla may be in or near a diverticulum, which can alter the ductal orientation. There are vessels in the lateral aspect of the papilla that can bleed excessively if inadvertently cut with the sphincterotome.

## INDICATIONS

Endoscopic sphincterotomy is the first step in most therapeutic procedures involving ERCP.

1. Removal of bile duct stones

2. To facilitate placement of biliary stents, especially multiple or large stents

3. To keep bile duct stents from compressing the pancreatic duct orifice, thus reducing the risk of pancreatitis

4. To facilitate choledochoscopy using the "mother-daughter" scope technique

5. To treat postsurgical or traumatic bile leaks by encouraging bile flow into the duodenum and facilitating bile duct leak closure; ES is frequently combined with stent placement to bridge the leak.

6. To temporarily relieve biliary obstruction from an adenoma or carcinoma at the papilla

7. To treat sphincter of Oddi dysfunction (SOD)

8. To treat the "sump syndrome" that may develop after a biliary enteric anastomosis

9. To treat some patients with a symptomatic choledochocele

10. To create better access to the pancreatic duct for therapeutic endeavors, or to treat SOD of the pancreatic portion of the sphincter of Oddi

## CONTRAINDICATIONS

### Absolute

1. A lack of informed consent

2. An inability to adequately sedate the patient (i.e., combativeness during diagnostic part of the ERCP)

3. Unfavorable anatomy (obstruction, surgical changes)

4. Coagulopathy and thrombocytopenia are also significant contraindications if they are not easily correctable or are associated with portal hypertension.

## PREPARATION

1. Obtain informed consent, which includes a detailed discussion with the patient and possibly the patient's family about the risks and benefits of the procedure. Effectively communicating the inherent risks (bleeding, perforation, infection, etc.) will avoid difficulties related to any adverse outcomes.

2. Do not allow food or fluid ingestion for 6 hours prior to the procedure.

3. If the patient has had contrast studies during the week prior to the ES, obtain abdominal radiography to check for retained contrast in the colon, which may interfere with adequate visualization during ES.

4. Obtain adequate intravenous access.

5. Monitor the patient's pulse, blood pressure, and oxygen saturation.

6. Give supplemental oxygen during the procedure.

7. Consider capnography, especially if using propofol for sedation.

8. Set up two suction sources, one for the endoscope and the other for removing oral secretions.

9. Insert the mouth guard.

10. Give antibiotic prophylaxis if indicated for appropriate cardiac or prosthesis indications (see Chapter 1). Some recommend giving antibiotics prior to ERCP in any patient with biliary obstruction to avoid colonizing areas that may not be adequately drained even after a successful ES. Antibiotic prophylaxis is appropriate when planning pancreatography on a patient with a pseudocyst to avoid infection. Antibiotics also need to be given to any patient with cholangitis.

**EQUIPMENT**

1.   Standard side-viewing or therapeutic side-viewing endoscope. The side-viewer is needed to adequately visualize and orient the papilla. With a Billroth II anastomosis, some endoscopists advocate using an end-viewing endoscope. However, most endoscopists feel that the advantage of having the elevator in the endoscope to increase catheter movement outweighs any angle advantage of the end-viewing scope.

2.   A cautery unit that has connecting wires matched to the type of sphincterotome(s) to be used and that generates the desired cutting force. Olympus and Valley Lab produce good units that will generate a powerful initial cutting force rather than just coagulating the tissue. However, the ERBE electrosurgical generator produces a controlled current output that is automatically adjusted to tissue resistance.

3.   Sphincterotome. Keep several sphincterotomes on hand in order to make selections that fit the clinical situation, which may not be known until the procedure is well under way. These may include (a) pull- and push-type sphincterotomes with and without separate channels for guidewires and contrast (some have a built-in balloon for extracting stones) and (b) specialized sphincterotomes for patients with Billroth II anatomy and for doing precut papillotomies.

4.   A fluoroscopy room

5.   Lead aprons, thyroid shields, and protective eyewear

6.   Water-soluble contrast agents suitable for intravenous use. If the patient has an iodine allergy, a contrast agent with no iodine (nonionic) needs to be used (e.g., iopamidol [Isovue]); determine if the patient needs to be premedicated with diphenhydramine (Benadryl) and/or steroids.

7.   Ancillary devices and equipment necessary for the therapeutic procedure planned after the ES (e.g., balloon catheters, baskets, stents, etc.)

**PROCEDURE**

1.   Place the patient in the standard position for ERCP. This is the left lateral decubitus position with the left arm behind the back, so the patient can be moved to the prone position once the endoscope is in the duodenum. This usually puts the papilla in the most favorable alignment for cannulation.

2.   Alternatively, ERCP can be done with the patient on his or her back; however, the nursing assistant will need to pay attention to the airway to avoid aspiration.

3.   Cannulate and inject the bile duct and pancreatic duct with contrast first in order to establish the patient's anatomy.

4.   Cannulate the bile duct with the sphincterotome. Perform a free, deep cannulation so that the sphincterotome can be positioned in the correct direction.

5.  Position the sphincterotome in the 11 o'clock-to-noon direction with no more than one half of the sphincterotome wire inside the duct. This will allow for easier cutting because there is less tissue in contact with the wire and thus less tissue to heat up before the cutting starts. If either low power is used initially or there is too much coagulation of the tissue, there may be a sudden rapid cutting when the cutting wire gets through this higher resistance area and enters tissue with low resistance ("zipper effect"). This can either result in too big a cut with a perforation or excessive bleeding. The ERBE device can limit excessive rapid cutting.

6.  Place the cautery device on a setting of two or three for the Olympus or Valley Lab unit and set at 200 for the ERBE device. The preferred setting is pure cutting with the first two cautery units (though some experts advise a blended current) and Endocut for the ERBE unit.

7.  Make the cut using the power pedal with short bursts while gently bowing the cutting wire, and use the elevator or the scope tip deflection dials to apply upward pressure with the cutting wire to the tissue. The ERBE unit will do the short bursts automatically with continuous activation of the footswitch.

8.  The sphincterotomy needs to be large enough for stone removal. However, the length of the sphincterotomy will be limited by the length of the intraduodenal portion of the duct and the overall size of the duct. Generally, the cut will be 1 cm to 1.5 cm and extend to the fold just above the papillary os. The sphincterotomy can rarely be made any larger than this. If the patient's stones are bigger than the sphincterotomy, they will need to be crushed/fractured before attempting to extract them.

9.  The sphincterotomy can be done over a guidewire (Fig. 28.1). The wire can be placed via the standard catheter after contrast injection, or it can be used to help cannulate the bile duct opening when there is difficulty using just the standard catheter. Use a coated guidewire to prevent current leakage. Several sphincterotomes are available that can be passed over the guidewire and then used to make the sphincterotomy. The advantage of the guidewire is that exchanges can be done with less chance of losing access to the duct since the wire always maintains its position in the bile duct.

10. Consider a precut sphincterotomy if one cannot enter the bile duct freely with deep cannulation or cannot enter it at all. This technique requires even more skill and a precise understanding of the biliary and pancreatic duct anatomy.

11. There are four different techniques for accomplishing a successful precut.

    a.  The first uses a sphincterotome with the wire that exits directly from the tip and then loops back up the catheter a few centimeters and reenters into the catheter. Cut into the bile duct by wedging this sphincterotome

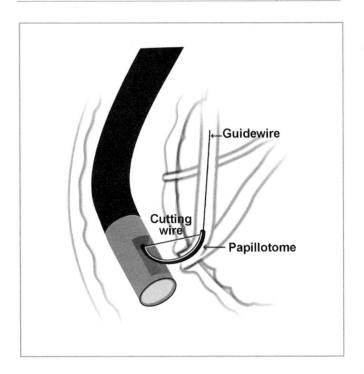

**Fig. 28.1 Biliary sphincterotomy over a guidewire.**

into the papillary os. Then apply current to make a small cut with a combination of bowing and directing the cutting wire toward the suspected direction of the bile duct. Probe the cut area with the catheter, especially after bile comes from the cut. This permits full bile duct cannulation, which is then followed by completing the ES.

b.  The next two methods for creating a precut involve the precut needle-knife sphincterotome (NKS). These sphincterotomes have a cutting wire that protrudes as a single straight retractable wire of 3 mm to 5 mm. The most common method is to place the NKS in the papillary os and make upward strokes to cut into the bile duct. The alternative is to make downward strokes with the NKS to enter the bile duct. However, the latter method is more likely to damage the pancreatic duct and is not widely recommended. Once it is suspected that the bile duct is opened, gently inject and inject a standard sphincterotome. If there is no extravasation of contrast and deep cannulation is achieved, then the ES can be completed in the usual fashion. It is advisable to make a few practice strokes with the NKS before applying current. Do not cut deep initially, but with successive passes, slowly cut deeper as needed to gain access.

c. Another method to gain access to the bile duct is to use the NKS to create a fistula into the duct above the papilla in the intraduodenal portion of the bile duct. Burrow the NKS directly into the bile duct through the supra-os tissue of the duodenum wall. This is easier if the duct is bulging due to a distal obstruction or from a choledochocele. Again, once access is achieved, pass a standard sphincterotome to complete the ES.

d. The final precut method for obtaining access to the bile duct uses the standard sphincterotome. Place the sphincterotome into the pancreatic duct, which is often the easier of the two ducts to cannulate. With only a couple of millimeters of wire within the duct, make a cut in the 11 o'clock direction. The final cut is usually no more than 5 mm. After making the cut, withdraw the sphincterotome, and probe the cut surface to gain access to the bile duct and to complete the ES. This method has the potential to cause pancreatitis since the cut starts in the pancreatic duct. This theoretical increased risk has not been borne out by most endoscopists who use this technique.

All of the precut techniques, which have high degrees of success in the hands of their developers, seem to be transferable to adequately trained community gastroenterologists. Occasionally, it may be necessary to perform a second ERCP a few days after the precut to finally gain access to the bile duct. This is because the anatomy is easier to work with once any swelling induced by the cutting or probing of the papilla has subsided.

12. Special Circumstances

a. It is a challenging task to perform a sphincterotomy in a patient with a previous Billroth II gastrojejunostomy. Use the side-viewing scope with an elevator to aid in cannula positioning. Since the papilla usually ends up in an upside-down position, it is generally best to use the special sphincterotome (e.g., Wilson-Cook) that works in a similarly upside-down fashion. Sometimes the papilla is too far away after a Billroth II to be reached. Occasionally, an end-viewing endoscope provides a better orientation.

b. Sphincterotomy can also be done on the pancreatic duct but with extreme caution. The intraduodenal wall portion of the duct is very short, and thus a cut that is too long can more easily lead to perforation. The sphincterotomy can be done with a standard sphincterotome or the NKS with or without a simultaneous ES of the bile duct. Many endoscopists feel that a small, short (3-cm, 5-Fr) stent should be placed after the ES on the pancreatic duct to decrease the occurrence of pancreatitis. A stent placed in the pancreatic duct prior to the ES can be used as a guide for the cutting of the sphincter with the NKS. This is the method of choice if a sphincterotomy is being attempted on the accessory papilla.

## POSTPROCEDURE

1. Monitor vital signs closely until the patient is alert. Usually this is about an hour after sedation.

2. Overnight monitoring in the hospital is recommended for many post-ES patients, especially if the patient is from out of town, lives alone, is elderly, has had extensive manipulation of the papilla during the ERCP/ES, or has other risk factors that might predispose the patient to post-ERCP/ES pancreatitis (e.g., pancreatic duct ES, sphincter of Oddi dysfunction, prior history of pancreatitis).

3. Keep the patient NPO until alert, and give clear liquids until the next day.

4. Advance the diet if there are no signs of pancreatitis or other complications.

5. Start antibiotics if signs of cholangitis are found during the procedure or if a perforation is suspected.

## COMPLICATIONS

Complications from ES range from 5% to 13% in various series, while the mortality rate ranges from 0% to 6.6%. The primary complications directly related to ES are pancreatitis, bleeding from the sphincterotomy, which can occur immediately or with up to a 2-week delay, and perforation. Complications after a precut ES are similar, but the frequency ranges up to 20%.

## CPT Codes

**43262** – Endoscopic retrograde cholangiopancreatography (ERCP); with sphincterotomy/papillotomy.

## SUGGESTED READINGS

1. Larkin CJ, Huibregtse K. Precut sphincterotomy: indications, pitfalls, and complications. *Curr Gastroenterol Rep* 2001;3:147–153.
2. Freeman ML. Complications of endoscopic sphincterotomy. *Endoscopy* 1998;30:A216–220.
3. Choudari CP, Fogel E, Gottlieb K, et al. Therapeutic biliary endoscopy. *Endoscopy* 1998;30:163–173.
4. Al-Kawas FH, Geller AJ. A new approach to sphincterotomy in patients with Billroth II gastrectomy. *Gastrointest Endosc Clin North Am* 1996;43:253–255.
5. Shields SJ, Carr-Locke DL. Sphincterotomy techniques and risks. *Gastrointest Endosc Clin North Am* 1996;6:17–42.
6. Sherman S, Uzer MF, Lehman GA. Wire-guided sphincterotomy. *Am J Gastroenterol* 1994;89:2125–2129.
7. Shakoor T, Geenen JE. Pre-cut papillotomy. *Gastrointest Endosc* 1992;38:623–627.
8. Muhldorfer SM, Kekos G, Hahn EG, et al. Complications of therapeutic gastrointestinal endoscopy. *Endoscopy* 1992;24:276–283.

# Management of Lithiasis: Balloon and Basket Extraction, Endoprosthesis, and Lithotripsy

David Horwhat and M. Stanley Branch

The management of patients with symptomatic cholelithiasis has greatly improved with the widespread availability of laparoscopic cholecystectomy, and most patients are successfully treated operatively. Despite improvements in laparoscopic surgical technique for cholelithiasis, choledocholithiasis remains a problem. Common bile duct (CBD) stones may be noted prior to cholecystectomy or may not become evident until afterward due to passage into the CBD perioperatively, a falsely negative intraoperative cholangiogram, or, less commonly, as a result of de novo formation of stones within the common bile duct. Because intraoperative cholangiography and laparoscopic CBD exploration are not universally practiced, there remains a role for the gastroenterologist in the evaluation and management of choledocholithiasis. Other scenarios that may require therapeutic biliary endoscopy for choledocholithiasis include selected patients with acute biliary pancreatitis, high-risk surgical patients, and patients who are not considered for surgery on the basis of advanced age or medical frailty. A review of the endoscopic management of choledocholithiasis reported that overall duct clearance could be expected in at least 90% of those undergoing successful sphincterotomy which translates to an overall success rate of 80% to 95% for complete endoscopic stone clearance (1). See Chapter 28 for sphincterotomy technique. This chapter will describe techniques for the successful endoscopic management and/or removal of choledocholithiasis.

## SOME GENERALIZATIONS

1. Some authors have suggested that stones smaller than 1 cm may pass spontaneously after sphincterotomy (1). The recommended approach has been to remove all CBD stones if possible with a basket or balloon as stones may not always pass if the sphincterotomy is small and/or the stone is not smooth.

2. Stones between 1 cm and 2 cm in size can generally be removed after endoscopic retrograde cholangiopancreatography (ERCP) and sphincterotomy with basket or balloon.

3. Stones larger than 2 cm will generally require lithotripsy for fragmentation into smaller pieces for successful removal.

The approach to patients with stones that cannot be removed with balloons, baskets, or mechanical lithotripsy depends on the extent of medical comorbidity, the presence or absence of the gall bladder (both of which impact the decision to pursue surgical options), and the availability of local endoscopic expertise.

## INDICATIONS FOR ENDOSCOPIC MANAGEMENT OF CHOLEDOCHOLITHIASIS

1. Choledocholithiasis documented by transabdominal ultrasound (US), endoscopic US (EUS), magnetic resonance cholangiopancreatography (MRCP), or ERCP

2. Signs and/or symptoms related to choledocholithiasis (e.g., right upper quadrant pain, cholangitis, biliary pancreatitis, elevations in serum alanine aminotransferase [ALT], and/or serum bilirubin in the appropriate setting)

## CONTRAINDICATIONS

1. Inability to safely undergo ERCP with biliary sphincterotomy (see Chapter 7 and Chapter 28)

2. Lack of interventional radiology and/or general surgery availability is a relative contraindication

   • These services should be available for establishing biliary drainage in the event that endoscopic therapy of choledocholithiasis is unsuccessful.
   • If not available, consider possible transfer of the patient to a facility with these capabilities.

## PREPARATION

See Chapter 7 and Chapter 28.

## EQUIPMENT

Basic equipment for ERCP with biliary sphincterotomy as outlined in Chapter 7 and Chapter 28 plus additional equipment as outlined in the sections below. The therapeutic duodenoscope (4.2-mm working channel) is necessary for most therapeutic endoscopy.

## COMPLICATIONS

Many of the possible complications are related to the performance of ERCP and sphincterotomy. These have been described in Chapter 7 and Chapter 28. Procedure-specific complications will be addressed in the pertinent sections below.

## STANDARD TECHNIQUES

### Basket Extraction

The Dormia-type basket is the preferred stone retrieval device for many endoscopists and is especially useful in the setting of a massively dilated duct wherein balloon extraction catheters are too small to be usefully employed. Baskets are available from various manufacturers in 4-, 5-, 6-, and 8-wire models. Some baskets are wire-guided, and some are compatible with the Soehendra mechanical lithotripter (see below). The basket may also function as a lithotripter to reduce the size of large soft calcium bilirubinate stones to smaller pieces that may then be removed by either balloon or basket. Care must be taken if using a basket to fracture large stones, since the wires can impale the stone, resulting in impaction of the instrument. Fracture of the wires may also occur when trying to break hard stones. Our approach is to change to a formal lithotripsy basket if fracture of stones is anticipated. We would also recommend using baskets compatible with the Soehendra lithotripsy device as this allows "escape" if the basket should become entrapped. Extraction baskets are available as single-use/disposable and reusable instruments.

*Procedure*

1.  Endoscopic retrograde cholangiopancreatography and biliary sphincterotomy will have already been performed prior to basket extraction to ensure the greatest chance for complete duct clearance.

2.  With the basket wires fully withdrawn into the sheath, introduce the basket into the instrument port of the duodenoscope, and recannulate the bile duct (with or without guidewire assistance as needed).

3.  Using fluoroscopic guidance, advance the basket sheath to just above the level of the most distal stone (Fig. 29.1). Removing the most distal stone first reduces the risk of entrapping the basket above a conglomerate of multiple stones. Contrast can be injected via most baskets but may require opening the basket slightly. This will allow identification of the stone under fluoroscopy.

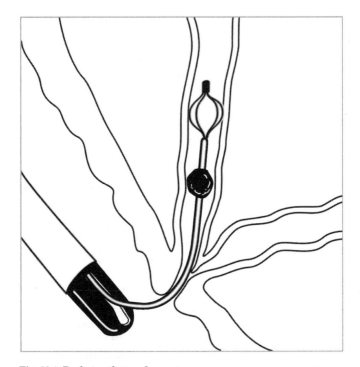

**Fig. 29.1. Basket catheter above stone.**

4. Open the basket by pushing in the handle, and maneuver the basket under fluoroscopy until the stone is seen to be within the wires of the basket. A "jiggling" motion is often helpful to capture the stone.

5. Gently close the basket to avoid impaling the wires in the stone, realizing the basket does not need to be completely closed to remove the stone. In fact, in most cases the partially closed basket can be used almost as a "net" to sweep the duct. Avoiding tight closure of the basket upon the stone decreases the risk of basket entrapment.

6. Withdraw the basket under fluoroscopy into the duodenum and release the stone. Repeat Steps 2 through 4 as needed for additional stones. Remember to remove the most distal stone first, and progressively clear the biliary tree.

7. Exercise care when withdrawing the basket in the long scope position as the tip of the basket could potentially impale the duodenal wall with enough force to cause mucosal injury or even perforation.

**Balloon Extraction**

Balloon extraction catheters are available in balloon diameters ranging from 8 mm to as large as 18 mm and are useful for the clearance of multiple small stones as well as sludge and microlithiasis. Balloons are advantageous in the setting of smaller-caliber common bile ducts where a basket cannot be fully deployed. Further advantages include the ability to use differing amounts of air to vary the balloon size (though the optimal shape is with full inflation), ability to test the adequacy of sphincterotomy prior to stone extraction, ability to perform occlusion cholangiography (with dual-lumen and triple-lumen balloon catheters), and the absence of risk for impaction of the device. Disadvantages include the fact that the inflated balloon must fill the entire lumen to effectively sweep the duct. Therefore, they cannot be used as effectively in massively dilated ducts. Another relative disadvantage is that balloons are more fragile compared to wire baskets and may break on a pointed edge of a stone. Finally, there can be mechanical disadvantages compared to baskets with attempts at balloon extraction whereupon the stone may slip past the balloon. Balloons are single-use, disposable instruments.

*Procedure*

1. Endoscopic retrograde cholangiopancreatography and biliary sphincterotomy will have already been performed prior to balloon extraction to ensure the greatest chance for complete duct clearance.

2. After passing the balloon catheter through the instrument port, down the duodenoscope, across the elevator, and into the duodenum, test the integrity of the balloon by inflating it in the duodenal lumen. This ensures the balloon has not inadvertently been perforated on a lifted elevator.

3. While in the short scope position, recannulate the biliary orifice with the balloon catheter (with or without guidewire assistance as needed), and advance the balloon proximally into the bile

duct under fluoroscopic guidance. Position the balloon above a single stone. Again, the technique should be to remove the most distal stones first (go for the "low hanging fruit").

4. Again using fluoroscopic guidance, slowly inflate the balloon with air, ensuring the stone remains below the balloon. If needed, many balloon catheters, especially double-lumen or triple-lumen models (when using a guidewire), can be used to inject contrast to help localize the stone for extraction.

5. Withdraw the balloon catheter distally to bring the stone out of the duct and into the duodenal lumen. Deflate the balloon, and repeat Steps 2 through 4 as necessary, retrieving one stone at a time until the duct is clear.

6. If resistance is felt when trying to bring the stone through the sphincterotomy site, repositioning the endoscope may be helpful. Initially the duodenoscope should be tipped up against the sphincterotomy site and the balloon catheter pulled down, bringing the stone into the very distal bile duct. Then the duodenoscope may need to be brought slightly into the long position by advancing the duodenoscope, turning the small wheel to the right, bringing the endoscope tip down (big wheel away) and turning the endoscopist's body to the right. This will create the mechanical force down in line with the bile duct to remove the stone (This technique can also be used with a basket). Alternatively, the sphincterotomy may not be large enough. If there is room to extend the sphincterotomy, this may need to be done. If not, the stone should be crushed with the lithotripter as outlined below to allow complete retrieval.

7. One tip to help gauge if the stone will be easily removed is to inflate the balloon to the size of the stone and to pull through the sphincterotomy. If the balloon does not pass easily, further intervention as noted above may need to be considered. Avoid impacting the stone in the distal bile duct as this may make further attempts at extraction more difficult.

**Mechanical Lithotripsy**

This device is generally used for stones greater than 1.5 cm to 2 cm in diameter, as stones below this threshold can usually be retrieved with balloons or baskets after sphincterotomy. Complete duct clearance rates of >90% have been reported from experienced centers (2–4). Through-the-scope basket lithotripsy systems are now available that are relatively easy to use, work very well for the majority of stones, and should be a part of the therapeutic biliary endoscopist's armamentarium. The use of the Soehendra lithotripter is described first, though the principle upon which it works is the basis for most basket lithotripsy systems. Every endoscopy lab should have this system available not only for potential lithotripsy but also, more importantly, for removal of entrapped baskets.

*Procedure*

Soehendra lithotripter, the prototypic mechanical lithotripter, is used for rescuing impacted baskets as well as for crushing large, difficult stones that cannot be removed by standard basket or balloon techniques. Images from the Wilson-Cook Medical GI Endoscopy Web site may be accessed to enhance this description. The procedure begins as above with passage of a standard basket and subsequent impalement of the basket wires into the stone. At this point, the basket is prepared so that the duodenoscope can be removed and the mechanical lithotripter employed.

1. First, the basket is kinked, as shown in Fig. 29.2, just below the handle and shrink tube to prevent the cable from sliding inside the tube.

2. The basket cable is cut, as shown in Fig. 29.3 using wire cutters, below the 10-Fr sheath and above the previously made kink. Care must be taken to avoid removing the 7-Fr sheath from the basket wire as this could result in basket fragmentation and the need for surgery to remove the device.

3. Once the basket cable has been cut, the duodenoscope is removed while monitoring the position of the basket fluoroscopically. The lithotripsy cable is then threaded over the basket sheath and advanced until it reaches the basket in the duct.

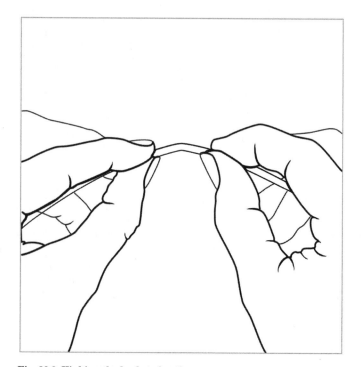

**Fig. 29.2. Kinking the basket sheaths.**

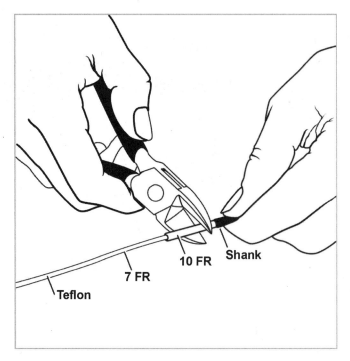

**Fig. 29.3. Cutting the plastic sheath.**

4.  The basket wire and sheath are then passed through the Luer-lock adapter of the lithotripter handle, through the hole in the rotating rod, and wrapped several times around the rod until secure. See Fig. 29.4.

5.  The handle is then rotated while monitoring the stone fluoroscopically for evidence of fracture. See Fig. 29.5 and Fig. 29.6.

Once fractured, the stone fragments will generally require balloon extraction for complete duct clearance. In the setting of a dilated duct with multiple remaining small fragments, however, a stent or nasobiliary catheter may need to be placed until future duct clearance can be performed when the duct has decompressed.

Through-the-scope basket lithotripsy systems are composed of a heavy-gauge wire basket that runs through a plastic or Teflon catheter along with a spiral metal catheter that is then advanced over the inner plastic/Teflon catheter. If a through-the-scope basket lithotripsy system is not routinely used, it is good practice to go through the steps of setting up and using the device on the bench top first if use of this system is anticipated.

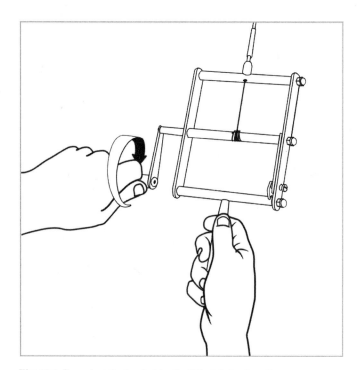

**Fig. 29.4. Securing the basket to the lithotripter handle.**

A dimly lit room under stressful conditions is not the place to "learn" to use this system.

1. Pass the system though the working channel of the therapeutic duodenoscope, use the plastic inner catheter to cannulate the common bile duct, and then capture the stone in the basket as with a standard retrieval basket.

2. Advance the metal sleeve over the catheter and up to the basket.

3. Apply pressure slowly from the device handle (usually a wheel and ratchet or screw-type device), drawing the basket/stone into the metal catheter, resulting in fragmentation of the stone.

4. Use the basket to remove the fragments. Alternatively, a standard retrieval basket or balloon can be used to clear the bile duct in the usual fashion.

## Biliary Stents

Plastic endoprostheses or stents are useful for the management of choledocholiths that are unable to be removed by basket,

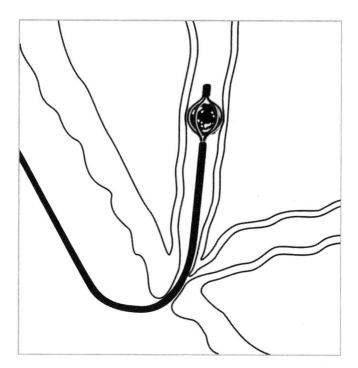

**Fig. 29.5. Entrapped stone.**

balloon, or lithotripter. Stents allow unobstructed bile flow while preventing stones from impacting at the papilla until definitive removal occurs. This strategy is most commonly used to temporarily alleviate obstruction while preparing for other modalities such as extracorporeal shockwave lithotripsy (ESWL), while awaiting surgery or pending transfer to a tertiary referral center, or to allow for repeat attempt at ERCP with stone extraction at a later date. Studies have demonstrated a reduction in size of choledocholiths over time in the presence of an indwelling stent alone (5) or with concomitant ursodeoxycholic acid (6). This strategy offers a possible repeat endoscopic management option for patients who are not surgical candidates or whose medical condition may warrant a delay in more definitive therapy. The patient should be made aware that subsequent ERCP will need to be performed. For simple short-term decompression while awaiting further care, a 7-Fr stent is generally sufficient to breach the papilla. For longer-term management, a 10-Fr stent will provide superior patency over a 7-Fr stent, but sizes larger than 10-Fr are generally not incrementally better as the literature has not demonstrated any significant advantage with an 11.5-Fr stent (7). For dilated ducts, we prefer the double pigtail

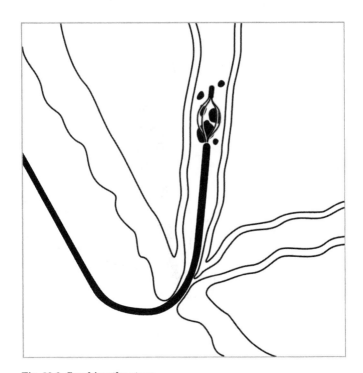

**Fig. 29.6. Crushing the stone.**

stent. Some endoscopists may choose to place several stents in this instance to increase the fragmentation of residual stones. In general, we do not recommend long-term stenting as the only therapy for CBD stones unless faced with a terminal situation, since the risk of cholangitis over time is significant.

*Procedure*

1. Endoscopic retrograde cholangiopancreatography and sphincterotomy will have already been performed.

2. Pass a 0.035-in. guidewire through the previously employed ERCP catheter/sphincterotome, and, using fluoroscopic guidance, position the proximal end at the bifurcation of the common hepatic duct.

3. Slowly remove the catheter from the bile duct, keeping the wire in place (exchange) and maintaining just a short distance of wire between the papillary orifice and the duodenoscope tip to prevent accidental dislodgement of the wire. Stabilize the wire by holding it firmly with the elevator.

4. For 7-Fr stents, the stent may be pushed over the guidewire using the sphincterotome or catheter used previously for

ERCP, taking care not to impact the tapered tip of the catheter or sphincterotome into the stent with too much force as this may result in an inability to successfully disengage the stent from the device used to push it into place.

5. For stents larger than 7 Fr, a guiding catheter is passed over the guidewire. Introduce the catheter, tapered end first, over the wire, passing it to the desired level of stent insertion, while maintaining the tip of the guidewire beyond the guiding catheter.

6. Introduce the tapered end of the stent over the guiding catheter first, and advance the stent halfway into the instrument port.

7. Place the pushing catheter over the wire guide and guiding catheter to push the stent through the duodenoscope channel and into position with the bile duct. Keep the scope in a short position, and have the assistant maintain tension on the guiding catheter and wire guide. Periodically raise and lower the elevator to help maneuver the stent up the duct until it is in proper position.

8. Withdraw the wire, maintaining pressure on the stent with the pushing catheter.

9. Withdraw the guiding catheter next and then withdraw the pushing catheter.

**ADVANCED TECHNIQUES**

These techniques will not be described in detail, as they should only be performed in expert referral centers. The therapeutic biliary endoscopist should be familiar with these techniques; however, a description of their employment is beyond the scope of this chapter.

1. Electrohydraulic lithotripsy (EHL). This tecnique works on the principle that sparks discharged in a water medium generate high-frequency hydraulic pressure waves. These shock waves are powerful enough to destroy normal tissue (to include the bile duct wall); therefore, direct visualization via mother-daughter ERCP is required to apply the electrohydraulic shock waves directly to the stone(s). The therapeutic duodenoscope (mother) is passed into the duodenum as usual. The cholangioscope (daughter) is then passed through the working channel of the duodenoscope and into the bile duct, allowing the operator to guide the EHL probe through the working channel of the cholangioscope to the stone. Since EHL is only possible when the stone can be directly visualized, inability to cannulate the major papilla or failure to visualize the stone due to stricture or anatomic deformity precludes its successful application.

2. Extracorporeal shock wave lithotripsy (ESWL). This technique is used for large stones that have failed other methods of extraction, especially intrahepatic stones and stones in the setting of biliary strictures. It is also used in frail, elderly patients or in situations in which the risk of further

conscious sedation, endoscopy, or surgery is prohibitive. Complete duct clearance rates of 64% to 100% (mean = 66%) are reported with first-generation machines (8). The procedure requires either ERCP with nasobiliary tube placement, percutaneous transhepatic cholangiography with percutaneous biliary drainage catheter, or a surgically placed T-tube to enable contrast localization of the stone(s) under fluoroscopy. Ultrasound guidance may also be used to target the stone(s). Conscious sedation with electrocardiograph monitoring is often used during the ESWL procedure. Possible complications include cholangitis, acute cholecystitis, perinephric hematoma, and macroscopic hematuria. While not a complication, a potential disadvantage is that ERCP is again necessary afterward to remove remaining stone fragments.

3.  Laser lithotripsy. This is similar in concept to EHL in that shock waves are generated under water. Three types of lasers have been used including the quality-switched Nd:YAG laser, flash lamp pulsed dye laser, and pulsed dye laser with automatic stone recognition. Again, retrograde cholangioscopy (mother-daughter endoscopy) or fluoroscopic guidance using a laser basket, centering balloon, or laser sleeve is required to ensure the quartz fiber that delivers the laser is in direct contact with the stone. Automatic stone recognition technology has improved the accuracy and safety of the procedure by enabling the laser to target only the stone and automatically disengage from firing if nonstone tissue is encountered. The equipment is quite expensive and therefore only available in expert referral centers.

4.  Rendezvous procedure. The rendezvous procedure is a cooperative venture undertaken between an interventional radiologist and a therapeutic biliary endoscopist. It is considered in situations wherein cannulation of the major papilla has failed, yet therapeutic biliary endoscopy (e.g., biliary decompression via balloon dilation or stent placement, stone retrieval, brush cytology, etc.) is still required. The aim of this procedure is to insert a guidewire (passed percutaneously by a radiologist) down through the biliary tree and across the papilla, with its distal end lying in the duodenal lumen. The endoscopist passes a therapeutic duodenoscope orally and subsequently uses the guidewire for assisted cannulation. Once access to the biliary tree is obtained, ERCP is performed as usual.

**SUMMARY**

Despite advances in laparoscopic biliary surgery, the therapeutic biliary endoscopist has an important role in the evaluation, diagnosis, and management of patients with choledocholithiasis. Endoscopists who perform ERCP for the management of patients with choledocholithiasis and common duct stone-related disease such as acute biliary pancreatitis must not only be facile in the techniques described above, but should also be cognizant of the risks and limitations of therapeutic biliary endoscopy. The expertise that is required to perform the advanced techniques mentioned and the expense of the equipment necessary for these procedures usually mandates the referral of patients with difficult bile duct stones requiring advanced techniques to expert centers that have frequent experience with this higher level of care.

## CPT Codes

**43264** – Endoscopic retrograde cholangiopancreatography (ERCP); with endoscopic retrograde removal of stone(s) from biliary and/or pancreatic ducts.

**43265** – Endoscopic retrograde cholangiopancreatography (ERCP); with endoscopic retrograde destruction, lithotripsy of stone(s), any method.

**43268** – Endoscopic retrograde cholangiopancreatography (ERCP); with endoscopic retrograde insertion of tube or stent into bile or pancreatic duct.

## REFERENCES

1. Soetikno RM, Montes H, Carr-Locke DL. Endoscopic management of choledocholithiasis. *J Clin Gastroenterol* 1998;27:296–305.
2. Shaw MJ, Mackie RD, Moore JP, et al. Results of a multicenter trial using a mechanical lithotripter for the treatment of large bile duct stones. *Am J Gastroenterol* 1993; 88:730–733.
3. Chung SCS, Leung JWC, Leong HT, et al. Mechanical lithotripsy of large common bile duct stones using a basket. *Br J Surg* 1991;78:1448–1450.
4. Committee ATA. Biliary lithotripsy. *Gut* 1996;44:771–773.
5. Chan AC, Ng EK, Chung SC, et al. Common bile duct stones become smaller after endoscopic biliary stenting. *Endoscopy* 1998;30:356–359.
6. Johnson GK, Geenen JE, Venu RP, et al. Treatment of non-extractable common bile duct stones with combination ursodeoxycholic acid plus endoprostheses. *Gastrointest Endosc* 1993;39:528–531.
7. Kadakia SC, Starnes E. Comparison of 10 French gauge stent with 11.5 French gauge stent in patients with biliary tract diseases. *Gastrointest Endosc* 1992;38:454–459.
8. Ellis RD, Jenkins AP, Thompson RPH, et al. Clearance of refractory bile duct stones with extracorporeal shockwave lithotripsy. *Gut* 2000;47:728–731.

# Management of Biliary and Pancreatic Ductal Obstruction: Endoprosthesis and Nasobiliary/Nasopancreatic Drain Placement

Nalini M. Guda and Martin L. Freeman

Endoscopic intervention is an effective strategy in relieving both benign and malignant obstructions of the biliary and pancreatic ducts and has relatively few risks when compared to either surgery or percutaneous drainage procedures. The principal aim of any endoscopic biliary or pancreatic drainage procedure is to relieve obstructive jaundice, pancreatitis, or infection; decompress stone disease; close duct disruptions; and/or relieve symptoms. In addition, pancreatic stents are increasingly placed to reduce the risk of postendoscopic retrograde cholangiopancreatography (ERCP) pancreatitis. Collaboration with surgeons and interventional radiologists may be appropriate.

## INDICATIONS

Duct drainage may be achieved by sphincterotomy, stent, or both. Sphincterotomy alone may be sufficient in some situations such as clearance of bile duct stones (see Chapter 29). In other situations, placement of one or more stents is indicated (see Chapter 28). Indications are listed according to the endoprosthesis used.

### Plastic Biliary Endoprosthesis

1. Treatment of benign strictures (postsurgical, chronic pancreatitis, sclerosing cholangitis, etc.)

2. Relief of jaundice in malignant strictures (due to distal and proximal biliary, pancreatic, periampullary, and metastatic tumors)

3. Incomplete removal of bile duct stones

4. Relief of obstructive cholangitis

5. Closure of bile leaks (postcholecystectomy, etc.)

### Nasobiliary Drain

1. Same as for plastic endoprostheses when temporary drainage or ability to repeat a cholangiogram is desired

2. Prior to definitive biliary stent placement

### Self-Expanding Metallic Biliary Stent

1. Palliative relief of jaundice resulting from biliary, pancreatic, periampullary, or metastatic tumors that are unresectable due to tumor stage or the patient's poor surgical condition

2. Benign biliary strictures only in the few patients who have refractory strictures and are not surgical candidates

3. Removable covered metallic stents will be indicated in all of the same situations as plastic stents

### Plastic Pancreatic Endoprosthesis

1. Pancreatic strictures (chronic pancreatitis, other)

2. Pancreatic stones prior to endoscopic removal or extracorporeal shock-wave lithotripsy

3. Pancreatic duct disruption/fistula

4. Transpapillary drainage of pseudocysts

5. Part of therapy of relapsing acute pancreatitis

6. Palliation of inoperable malignant pancreatic obstruction with pancreatic complications such as pancreatic fistula, relapsing pancreatitis, or obstructive pain (latter rarely indicated)

7. Part of therapy of symptomatic pancreas divisum

8. Prevention of post-ERCP pancreatitis (high-risk cases such as sphincter of Oddi dysfunction, difficult cannulation, precut sphincterotomy, pancreatic sphincterotomy, endoscopic ampullectomy)

### Nasopancreatic Drain

1. Same as for pancreatic endoprostheses, when short-term drainage is desired, or to aid targeting for extracorporeal shock-wave lithotripsy

### Metallic Pancreatic Endoprosthesis

1. Palliation of inoperable malignant pancreatic obstruction with pancreatic complications such as pancreatic fistula, relapsing pancreatitis, or obstructive pain (latter rarely indicated)

### CONTRAINDICATIONS (RELATIVE)

Contraindications are similar to those for diagnostic ERCP. Please refer to Chapter 7.

In patients with suspected sphincter of Oddi dysfunction and intact papilla, placement of biliary stents as a therapeutic trial is not recommended due to the very high risk of causing pancreatitis. Extended pancreatic stenting is not recommended solely as a therapeutic trial in patients with relatively normal ducts due to the risk of pancreatic duct injury.

### PREPARATION

Please also refer to the general principles of ERCP in Chapter 7 and the use of antibiotics in gastrointestinal (GI) procedures in Chapter 1.

## EQUIPMENT, ENDOSCOPES, DEVICES, ACCESSORIES

A completely equipped and highly sophisticated ERCP unit with high-resolution fluoroscopy and staffed by experienced GI assistants is necessary. As for all endoscopy units, electrophysiologic monitoring must include monitoring devices for electrocardiography (EKG), blood pressure and pulse oximetry, oxygen delivery systems, oral suction, and emergency resuscitation equipment.

1. A standard diagnostic duodenoscope (3.2-mm channel) is adequate for deploying an endoprosthesis up to 8.5 Fr in diameter. A therapeutic duodenoscope (4.2-mm channel) is required for larger endoprostheses. For pediatric or infant patients or patients with high-grade luminal stenosis, pediatric duodenoscopes may be required, but these allow only 5- to 7-Fr stents.

2. Cannulas ranging from 5 Fr standard-tip down to ultra-tapered 5-4-3 Fr

3. Guidewires 0.018 to 0.035 in. wide, including hybrid and hydrophilic, straight and angle-tip

4. Papillotome (double or triple lumen to allow guidewire and contrast injection)
    a. standard 6- to 7-Fr diameter traction-type
    b. small-caliber (5-Fr) wire-guided traction-type (rotatable papillotomes may facilitate difficult cannulation)
    c. needle-knife

5. Water-soluble contrast (standard plus nonionic contrast for patients allergic to iodinated contrast)

6. Electrosurgical generator

7. Biliary endoprostheses
    a. Plastic: straight-type (Amsterdam) stents, typically with an inner and outer retention flange, in 7-, 8.5-, 10-Fr diameter (11.5 Fr optional), 3 to 15 cm long; double-pigtail stents, typically 7- and 10-Fr, 4 to 10 cm long. Simple pusher tubes for up to 7-Fr stents, and two-stage introducer systems for 8.5-Fr stents and larger stents are required (consisting of inner catheter and pusher tube).
    b. Nasobiliary drains: typically 6- or 7-Fr, with a single pigtail on the inner end.
    c. Self-expanding metallic stents: uncovered stents (bare mesh) and covered stents (silicone membrane-covered), in 8- or 10-mm diameter and 4- to 10-cm lengths.

8. Pancreatic stents
    a. Plastic: Plastic pancreatic stents differ from biliary stents in that multiple side-holes are usually standard, French sizes are smaller (3, 4, 5, 7 Fr), and the inner end is always straight with one, two, or no flanges. In addition, to prevent inward migration, the outer end is either straight with two flanges or has a single partial

pigtail. Lengths range from 2 to 15 cm. Pusher tubes or appropriately sized cannulas are used as pusher tubes. Introducer systems are not necessary.

b. Nasopancreatic catheters: similar to nasobiliary drains except for smaller caliber (4 or 5 Fr), multiple side holes, and straight inner end with one or two retention flanges.

c. Self-expanding metallic stents: same as biliary stents.

9. Dilating catheter 3- to 10-Fr diameter

10. Dilating balloons (low profile) 4 mm, 6 mm, 8 mm, 10 mm

11. Screw-type dilators (or stent extractors)

12. Snares, rat-tooth grasping forceps, and stone-retrieval baskets (standard and wire-guided) for removal of existing /migrated endoprostheses

13. Sclerotherapy needles, thermocoagulation (bipolar or heater probe) probes, and endoscopic clips for hemostasis

14. Wire-guided cytology brush

15. Biopsy forceps (small caliber without a pin)

16. Mechanical lithotripter (through-the-scope preferable)

## PROCEDURE

Please see Chapter 7 for information on sedation and Chapter 28 for details on insertion of the instrument and selective duct cannulation.

### Biliary Stent Placement

1. If the likelihood of performing a sphincterotomy is high, cannulate with a double or triple lumen papillotome pre-loaded with a guidewire. This is cost-effective and may facilitate cannulation by varying the angle of approach.

2. Once the papillary orifice is engaged, inject contrast under fluoroscopic guidance. Opacify the duct to adequately visualize the anatomy. In patients with suppurative cholangitis, minimize injection of contrast in ducts, and aspirate bile above the stricture to avoid causing cholangitis. When draining hilar strictures, it is important to avoid initially injecting contrast above the hilum into multiple obstructed segmental ducts that cannot all be drained (see Step 17 and Step 18). The pancreatic duct should be opacified only enough to identify the course of the duct and any relevant pathology. Depending on the indication, only the biliary duct may be opacified, or the pancreatic duct may be opacified via major papilla and/or via minor papilla.

3. Secure the cannulation using a guidewire (0.018 to 0.035 in.). Larger wires may be used for biliary or large-caliber pancreatic stents. Small-caliber wires (0.018 to 0.025 in.) may be required for pancreatic stent placement (necessary for 3- and 4-Fr stents, respectively [Fig. 30.1]).

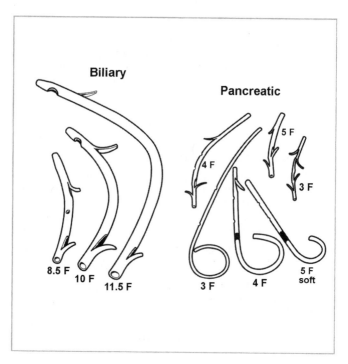

**Fig. 30.1. Various stents.**

4. Perform deep cannulation by traversing the sphincter and any stricture with a guidewire (hydrophilic wire may be necessary for tight stenoses).

5. Perform biliary sphincterotomy, preferably prior to placement of large-caliber biliary stents, to facilitate forceps biopsy, repeated instrumentation, and future stent exchange and possibly to reduce the risk of pancreatitis in high-risk patients.

6. If a malignant biliary stricture is suspected but has not been confirmed, pass a wire-guided cytology brush through the stricture. Take forceps biopsies by passing a small forceps into the bile duct beside the guidewire (multiple biopsies for higher yield). Sphincterotomy may facilitate biopsies. Similar techniques apply for pancreatic duct lesions, although risk may be higher, and pancreatic stenting may be necessary.

7. Highly stenotic strictures may require predilation prior to placement of a stent (typically hilar cancers, primary sclerosing cholangitis [PSC], and postoperative strictures; distal malignant tumors seldom require predilation). A hydrostatic wire-guided balloon is optimal to dilate the

stricture, but the inflated diameter of the balloon should not exceed the native duct diameter above or below the stricture. The balloon is dilated to the specified atmospheres of pressure or until the waist is seen to disappear on fluoroscopy. For extremely stenotic strictures, a balloon (with catheter diameter of 5 Fr) often cannot be passed through the stenosis; in this case graduated dilators must be passed in increasing diameters from 3 Fr up to 7- to 10-Fr. If these cannot be passed, a corkscrew-type dilator or stent extractor can be used to bore a path through an otherwise undilatable stricture. Once the lumen of the stricture is at least 5-Fr in diameter, a hydrostatic balloon dilator can be passed across the stricture and inflated to the specified atmospheres of pressure. Stents are generally inserted after stricture dilation to maintain stricture patency and drainage, with the possible exception of primary sclerosing cholangitis, in which stents may promote bacterial colonization and recurrent cholangitis.

8. Measure the length of the intended stent after adjustment for magnification. Two methods are most accurate to measure strictures. To perform the first method, place the end of the wire-guided catheter at the top of the stricture, pinch the catheter tightly at its entry point into the endoscope, pull the catheter back to just outside the papilla, then measure the length of catheter pulled out of the endoscope. To perform the second method, measure the length of guidewire pulled from the top to the bottom of the stricture instead. New guidewires with graded markings facilitate measurement of stricture length, although they are visible only endoscopically and not fluoroscopically.

9. Plastic endoprostheses should extend at least 2 cm above the proximal end of the stricture and 1 cm beyond the papilla. Metallic stents typically must extend at least 1 to 2 cm above and below the stricture and traverse the papilla for distal strictures but may remain entirely intraductal for hilar strictures.

10. For long (12- to 15-cm), large-caliber (8.5 Fr or greater) plastic endoprostheses placed above the hilum, straight plastic stents will not conform to the shape of the duct, particularly if placed deep into the left hepatic duct and thus potentially result in stent malfunction or distal migration. Heat-molding is necessary to shape the stent so that it will stay in place. This is done by immersing the proximal end of the stent in boiling sterile water or saline (heated in a microwave or other device) or holding it above a steam kettle (careful to avoid burns), then bending the stent into a right or other angle to conform to the course of the duct. Another alternative is to use a double-pigtail stent, and place the proximal pigtail in a straightened configuration deep into the left or right hepatic duct.

11. For smaller endoprostheses (< 7 Fr), introduce the prosthesis into the channel with the tapered end in first, pushed by the pushing catheter, which should ideally be a different

color from the stent to facilitate endoscopic visualization of stent placement. Several new delivery systems from a number of manufacturers allow rapid insertion of stents using a monorail system that minimizes the length of guidewire required. For 8.5 Fr and larger endoprostheses, backload the stent onto a two-stage introducer system, and pass the assembly over a guidewire.

12. Since most varieties of plastic endoprosthesis introducers do not allow retrieval once the stent is passed into the endoscope, it is advisable to have the papilla in view prior to insertion of the device into the channel.

13. Once the prosthesis is out of the scope, the assistant pulls back on the guidewire for smaller stents or on the guide catheter for larger stents. In case of straight endoprostheses, the stent is pushed into the duct until the second flange is visible. For pigtail stents it is helpful to mark the point on the shaft at which the loop begins with a permanent marker, so that once the stent is out of the scope, it can be easily identified. Push the prosthesis over the guidewire, through the channel, and into the stricture using steady pressure, with added force by lifting the elevator, and with even greater force by dialing the big wheel of the endoscope and pulling back on the shaft of the endoscope. Highly stenotic strictures can be traversed by adding repeated left/right torquing motions.

14. Once the stent is into position, pull back the guide catheter and/or guidewire.

15. For metallic stents, position a 7.5- to 8-Fr delivery system containing the compressed stent across the stricture using fluoroscopy. The assistant then slowly withdraws the outer sheath, while the endoscopist simultaneously pulls back on the outer sheath to compensate as expansion begins from the proximal end. Wallstents foreshorten substantially after deployment but can be reconstrained and repositioned even after two-thirds of the stent has been deployed. Zilver stents and other stents do not foreshorten, but cannot be reconstrained or repositioned once deployment has been initiated.

16. For temporary drainage of unremovable bile duct stones, either straight or double-pigtail stents can be placed. We generally recommend placing two double-pigtail stents with the upper pigtail above the top of the uppermost stone. This configuration allows drainage between the stents long after the lumens occlude, and distal migration will be minimized. The upper pigtail will form into a pigtail in the duct best if the guidewire is pulled back into the pigtail as soon as the tip passes above the stone, allowing further pushing to complete formation of the pigtail inside the duct.

17. For hilar tumors, special techniques are advised to avoid contamination of undrainable ducts and resultant cholangitis (Fig. 30.2). Magnetic resonance cholangiopancreatography (MRCP) should be obtained prior to ERCP to stage

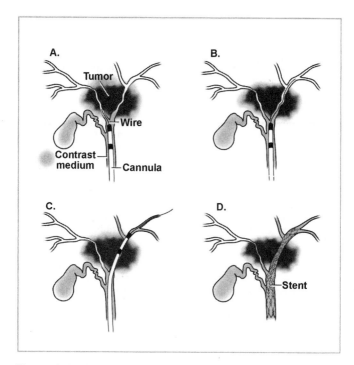

**Fig. 30.2A–D. Passage of the stent into the duct.**

the tumor and plan drainage, generally of the largest inter-communicating segmental ducts. Although bilateral drainage has been widely advocated, recent data support that unilateral stenting using selective access and opacification techniques results in equally effective palliation with fewer complications, and certainly greater technical success and ease of repeat intervention. Selective cannulation and opacification of targeted intrahepatic ducts is performed as follows: initially inject contrast only to the bottom of the stricture. Access the desired intrahepatic duct using a hybrid guidewire, or if necessary, a straight or angle-tip "glide" wire. Once the wire passes freely and deeply into the liver in the direction of the desired intrahepatic duct, advance the cannula deep into that lobe. Remove the guidewire, and aspirate as much bile as possible to decompress the duct. If a satisfactory duct has been accessed, only then is contrast injected through the catheter deep into the liver, filling peripherally and tracking back toward the hilum. It is important not to overfill as cholangitis may occur, and multiple other undrainable segmental ducts may "backfill". If at least 25% of the liver parenchyma appears to be drained, perform balloon dilation of the stricture, followed by placement of a single stent (preferably metallic). If a large-caliber stent cannot be placed due to extreme stenosis or difficult angulation, place a 5-Fr straight nasopancreatic-type drain through the hilar stenosis for a few days to decompress the duct and open up the stricture and assess for improvement in jaundice. This will usually allow placement of a larger stent at subsequent ERCP.

18. Bilateral stents may be necessary for hilar tumors in the following situations: a) significant contamination of multiple obstructed segmental ducts by previously placed stents or excessive contrast injection; b) failure to respond to single stents (usually placed in nonoptimal ducts); or c) for placement of bilateral stents for intraductal photodynamic therapy or brachytherapy. Bilateral stents are placed similarly to the procedure described in Step 17, except that dual wires should generally be placed prior to placing the first stent. In general, the left hepatic duct stent should be placed first as it is more angulated and difficult to place, and the right hepatic duct placed second in a side-by-side configuration. For plastic stents, it may not be feasible to place dual 10-Fr stents, especially if the distal duct is small caliber, or the hilar stricture highly stenotic. In that case, 8.5- or even 7-Fr stents may be placed at the first ERCP, with an early (2- to 3-week) repeat procedure to upsize the stents. For metal stents, the second stent may not pass beyond the expanded bottom of the first expanded stent; alternatives are to place long (10-cm) transpapillary Wallstents, or to place a wide-mesh stent, such as the Zilver stent, in the left hepatic duct, and then pass a wire through the lumen of the mesh of the left hepatic duct into the right duct, dilate the tract, and place a second stent in a "Y" configuration.

**Pancreatic Stent Placement**

1. Pancreatic stent placement is similar to biliary stent placement except for a number of features including the following: a) stents are generally much smaller (3 to 7 Fr); b) the stents are placed directly over a wire without an introducer system; c) pancreatic ducts are much smaller and more tortuous than bile ducts, and thus are more difficult to pass a wire into deeply; d) the pancreatic duct has side branches into which the tip of the guidewire tends to exit; and e) there is potential for pancreatic duct injury from a stent that is too large or malpositioned, especially in a normal small duct. Three- or 4-Fr stents cause less ductal injury than larger stents and are increasingly recommended for prevention of post-ERCP pancreatitis in patients with normal pancreatic ducts.

2. We recommend small-caliber wires (0.018 to 0.025 in.) for pancreatic stent placement in normal ducts, as they are the largest wires that will allow 3- and 4-Fr stents, respectively. Hybrid-type biliary wires may work but tend to exit side branches and sometimes cannot be passed deeply enough into the duct to obtain a sufficient anchor. Nitinol-tipped 0.018-in. (Roadrunner) wires have a very soft tip that will

usually knuckle within the main duct; if the tip exits a side branch, pushing deeper will usually flip the knuckle forward into the main duct which will almost always follow the main duct and stay out of side branches. If the goal of pancreatic stenting is reduction of post-ERCP pancreatitis in a normal duct and the wire passes easily to the body or tail of the pancreatic duct, either a short (2- to 3-cm) or long (8- to 10-cm) small-caliber stent can be placed. Long, unflanged, very small-caliber (3-Fr) stents with a single pigtail in the duodenum are increasingly used, as they are relatively atraumatic to normal ducts, will stay in place for at least a few days, and often pass spontaneously so that repeat endoscopy is not required. With small or tortuous ducts, it is often difficult or impossible to advance a guidewire deep into the duct. In that case, only 1 to 2 cm of a 0.018 Nitinol-tipped wire need be advanced beyond the pancreatic sphincter, and a short (2-cm), straight, single inner-flanged, 3- to 5-Fr stent delivered (depending on size of duct and duration of stenting required). Many straight-type pancreatic stents come with two inner flanges, at least one of which should be removed with a scalpel as inward migration may otherwise occur.

## Nasobiliary Catheter Placement

1. Perform ERCP with or without biliary sphincterotomy. After deep cannulation, insert a 0.025-in. or 0.035-in. guidewire deep into the duct (larger wires allow easier insertion of the pigtail). If the goal is placement of the drain in the common hepatic duct, placement in either the left or right hepatic duct is adequate; if the goal is anchoring the drain deep in the intrahepatic ducts for closure of a bile leak or other reason, then the left hepatic duct may be preferable. Once the wire is in place, advance the nasobiliary catheter over the guidewire, maintaining endoscopic and fluoroscopic control for proper location and avoiding slack on the wire by applying gentle traction. Pigtail-type catheters are most widely used, and the straightened tip is advanced directly over the guidewire by the assistant. Straight-tipped drains with retention flanges may occasionally be required to pass through tight strictures but are more likely to fall out. Alternately, the nasobiliary catheter may be preloaded on a guidewire and may be inserted into the biliary duct after a sphincterotomy. This is a one-step maneuver and might be preferred by some endoscopists. After the insertion of the nasobiliary catheter, withdraw the guidewire to form the pigtail to lock it in place. Then, in a coordinated fashion, the assistant withdraws the endoscope while the endoscopist advances the catheter shaft, taking care to avoid excessive loop or traction under fluoroscopic observation. Once the endoscope is withdrawn from the mouth, the assistant should hold the nasobiliary catheter in place while the endoscope is removed.

2. Conversion of the drain from the mouth to the nose is performed in the following manner. The guidewire is best left in place because if it is removed, the catheter may kink and be rendered nonfunctional. Insert a small nasogastric catheter

(16-Fr) without a guidewire into the patient's nose, advance it so that it exits into the posterior pharynx, and then retrieve it by reaching a finger deep into the patient's mouth. Pull the tip of the nasogastric tube out of the mouth and through the mouthpiece (otherwise the mouthpiece will be "jailed" in the loop), then feed the tip of the guidewire and nasobiliary catheter through the tube, and pull the nasal end of the tube back. Then remove the nasogastric catheter, and pull the nasobiliary catheter back until the pharyngeal loop is straightened, and without pulling the distal end in the biliary tree. It is critical to make sure there is no residual "alpha" loop of nasobiliary tube in the posterior pharynx and that there is a gentle loop of catheter in the stomach and duodenum (assessed fluoroscopically). Once proper position is confirmed, tape the nasobiliary catheter to the patient's nose, loop it around the ear, and pin it to the patient's gown. Cut any excess tubing. Attach a Touhy-Borst adapter to the end of the catheter so that it will accept a syringe or biliary drainage collection bag. Inject contrast through the catheter to reconfirm the position of the catheter in the biliary system. Optimal drainage from a nasobiliary tube will occur if the drainage bag is placed below the level of the patient to create negative pressure and act as a "siphon".

### Nasopancreatic Drain Placement

This technique is similar to placement of the nasobiliary drain except that straight-type 4- or 5-Fr drains with one or two inner retention flanges are generally used; a guidewire must be passed to at least the mid-body of the pancreas and the drain passed over the guidewire.

## POSTPROCEDURE MANAGEMENT AND COMPLICATIONS

### Early Complications

1. Pancreatitis can occur in 1% to 30%. The frequency varies with definition, patient-related and procedure-related factors.

   a. Prevention: Avoid unnecessary or marginally indicated ERCP and limit pancreatic duct instrumentation and injection. Placing pancreatic stents for high-risk cases (prior to precut sphincterotomy or during high-risk cases such as suspected sphincter of Oddi dysfunction, difficult cannulation, balloon dilation of biliary sphincter, ampullectomy or pancreatic sphincterotomy) reduces risk of overall and severe pancreatitis; stents should generally be removed within two weeks. Pure cutting current is safer than blended current; the effect of automated generators is unclear.

   b. Management is as for any other pancreatitis, consisting of analgesia, intravenous (IV) hydration, fasting, and management of any local or systemic complications.

2. Hemorrhage occurs in <1% to 2% and is mostly related to sphincterotomy. It presents within 0 to 10 days after the procedure as hematemesis or melena, with or without hemodynamic changes and hemoglobin drop.

a. Prevention is aided by avoiding sphincterotomy in high-risk patients including those with coagulopathies, correcting coagulopathy prior to sphincterotomy, withholding anticoagulation (especially heparin or coumadin [warfarin]) for at least 2 to 3 days after sphincterotomy (the at-risk interval), avoiding "zipper" cuts, possibly injecting the edges of the sphincterotomy with epinephrine for oozing bleeding at time of sphincterotomy, or even adding thermal coagulation or placing endoscopic clips for severe bleeding during the procedure. The risk of taking aspirin and nonsteroidal antiinflammatory agents is unclear; therefore, withholding these prior to and following the procedure for at least a few days is generally recommended unless the indication is critical.

b. Management is the same as for any other upper GI bleeding.

3. Perforation occurs in <1%. Perforations are seen either retroduodenally due to sphincterotomy, through the bowel wall due to the endoscope or stent, or at any location due to guidewire/endoprosthesis. It presents with abdominal pain, fever, or leukocytosis and can be difficult to distinguish from pancreatitis which can occur simultaneously. If perforation is suspected during ERCP, define it by injecting contrast through ducts and/or any sphincterotomy and examining for extravasated contrast or extraluminal air with flouroscopy. After the procedure, perforation is best diagnosed by a spiral computed tomography (CT) scan looking for extraluminal air, fluid, or contrast because abdominal x-ray alone may miss small leaks (postsphincterotomy leaks are generally retroperitoneal, hence free air is rarely seen).

a. Prevention: The endoscopist should avoid excessive length of sphincterotomy and needle-knife precut sphincterotomy, unless he or she is experienced and the patient has an appropriate anatomy and indication; avoid forceful scope manipulation if luminal anatomy is not clear, and avoid excessive force when passing guidewires or stents.

b. Management: For duct leaks or small sphincterotomy perforations recognized immediately, place a stent or nasobiliary plus/minus nasopancreatic drain (depending on which sphincter was cut) across site of leak or the sphincterotomy. Consider immediate closure of sphincterotomy or ampullectomy leaks with endoscopic clips. Then place a nasoduodenal and/or nasogastric tube. The patient should be kept NPO and broad-spectrum IV antibiotics started, and a surgery consult and CT scan should be obtained. Duct perforations and small sphincterotomy leaks will almost always close when recognized early and treated with appropriate ductal drainage and decompression. However, large sphincterotomy leaks and bowel perforations should be considered for emergent surgery. Perforations that are recognized late often result in complex infection and poor outcomes.

4. Cholangitis is recognized by fever, chills, rising liver chemistries, and leukocytosis.

a. Prevention centers on avoiding excessive injection or manipulation of obstructed or infected ducts and on achieving thorough drainage. Antibiotics should be given prophylactically to patients with biliary obstruction to reduce bacteremia, but their efficacy in preventing clinical cholangitis is less clear.

b. Management: This is best done by use of broad-spectrum antibiotics, fluid resuscitation, and biliary drainage (endoscopic, percutaneous, or surgical).

5. Cardiopulmonary and other complications related to sedation and analgesia

a. Prevention is achieved by careful assessment of risk and use of the anesthesia department if the patient is at a high risk.

b. Management is achieved as for any other cardiopulmonary emergency.

**Late Complications and Management**

1. Occluded/migrated biliary endoprosthesis: This complication presents as recurrent cholestasis, jaundice, and/or cholangitis. The median time of occlusion is 3 months for plastic biliary stents, 6 months for uncovered metal stents, and longer for covered metal stents; early occlusion (as soon as 1 month or earlier) is not unusual for plastic prostheses. This can be treated by replacement of a plastic stent with a plastic or a metal stent, or placement of new plastic or metal stent through previous metal stent. Migration occurs mostly with plastic prostheses, and can be inward (short stents) or outward (hilar tumors). This is treated by stent removal; inwardly migrated plastic stents often require balloon dilation of the sphincter, passage of wire beyond the stent, and extraction with a wire-guided balloon, snare, or basket, or with a forceps. Migration seldom occurs with uncovered metal stents but may occur with covered metal stents. Outwardly migrated covered stents can usually be removed with a snare.

2. Occluded/migrated pancreatic endoprostheses: Typically these occlude earlier than biliary stents and may present with pain, pancreatitis, or pancreatic infection. Many pancreatic stents are intended to pass spontaneously and seldom cause clinical problems. Migration is treated by removal of the migrated stent, with or without replacement of a new stent depending on the clinical situation. Inwardly migrated pancreatic stents are removed by the same techniques as biliary stents but can be very difficult to manage due to small/tortuous ducts and require use of miniature baskets, wire-guided snares, or biopsy forceps; pancreatic sphincterotomy and/or balloon dilation are usually required. If the stent cannot be retrieved, a wire and stent or nasopancreatic drain should be placed beyond the prosthesis to dilate and straighten the duct, with stent retrieval reattempted at a later date by a highly experienced endoscopist.

3. Cholangitis: This is managed by reestablishing endoscopic drainage.

4. Stenosis of the sphincterotomy: Perform a repeat sphincterotomy.

5. Recurrent choledocholithiasis: Repeat endoscopic intervention or surgery.

6. Cholecystitis: This occurs due to retained gallbladder stones or from the placement of a stent (usually plastic) across the cystic duct in patients with tumors involving the takeoff of the cystic duct, especially if contrast has been instilled into the gallbladder. This should be managed by surgical cholecystectomy or by percutaneous or endoscopic gallbladder drainage in high-surgical-risk patients.

## CPT Codes

**43260** – Endoscopic retrograde cholangiopancreatography (ERCP); diagnostic, with or without collection of specimen(s) by brushing or washing (separate procedure).

**43261** – With biopsy, single or multiple.

**43262** – With sphincterotomy/papillotomy.

**43263** – With pressure measurement of sphincter of Oddi (pancreatic duct or common bile duct).

**43264** – With endoscopic retrograde removal of stone(s) from biliary and/or pancreatic ducts.

**43265** – With endoscopic retrograde destruction, lithotripsy of stone(s), any method.

**43267** – With endoscopic retrograde insertion of nasobiliary or nasopancreatic drainage tube.

**43268** – With endoscopic retrograde insertion of tube or stent into bile or pancreatic duct.

**43269** – With endoscopic retrograde removal of foreign body and/or change of tube or stent.

**43271** – With endoscopic retrograde balloon dilation of ampulla, biliary and/or pancreatic duct(s).

**43272** – With ablation of tumor(s), polyp(s), or other lesion(s) not amenable to removal by hot biopsy forceps, bipolar cautery or snare technique.

## SUGGESTED READINGS

Shah SK, Mutignani M, Costamagna G. Therapeutic biliary endoscopy. *Endoscopy* 2002; 34:43–53.

Siegel JH. Decompression techniques. In: Siegel JH, ed. *Endoscopic Retrograde Cholangiopancreatography*. New York: Raven Press, 1992:272–363.

Davids PHP, Groen AK, Rauws EA, et al. Randomized trial of self-expanding metallic stents versus polyethylene stents for distal malignant biliary obstruction. *Lancet* 1992;340:1488–1492.

De Palma GD, Galloro G, Sicilliano S, et al. Unilateral versus bilateral endoscopic hepatic duct drainage in patients with malignant hilar biliary obstruction: results of a prospective, randomized and controlled study. *Gastrointest Endosc* 2001;53: 547–553.

Freeman ML, Overby C. Selective MRCP and CT-targeted drainage of malignant hilar biliary obstruction with self-expanding metallic stents. *Gastrointest Endosc* 2003;58:41–49.

Neuhaus H. Therapeutic pancreatic endoscopy. *Endoscopy* 2002;34:54–62.

Tarnasky PR, Palesch YY, Cunningham JT, et al. Pancreatic stenting prevents pancreatitis after biliary sphincterotomy in patients with sphincter of Oddi dysfunction. *Gastroenterology* 1998;115: 1518–1524.

Freeman ML, Overby CS, Qi DF. Pancreatic stent insertion: consequences of failure, and results of a modified technique to improve success. *Gastrointest Endosc* 2003 (*in press*).

Freeman ML. Adverse outcomes of ERCP. *Gastrointest Endosc* 2002; 56:S273–S282.

Cotton PB, Lehman G, Vennes Ja, et al. Endoscopic sphincterotomy complications and their management: an attempt at consensus. *Gastrointest Endosc* 1991;37:383–391.

# Management of Fluid Collections

Richard A. Kozarek

## PANCREATICOBILIARY FLUID COLLECTIONS

The approach to pancreaticobiliary fluid collections depends upon the clinical context and is subsumed by the following broad questions: Whom to drain? When to drain? How to drain? A corollary to these questions is whether and how to approach the ductal disruption that caused the fluid collection in the first place.

Most biliary fluid collections are iatrogenic, either as a consequence of bile duct injury at time of cholecystectomy or duct reconstruction, or from penetrating or blunt abdominal trauma (1–3). Pancreatic leaks, in turn, are not unusual in the setting of acute pancreatitis, exacerbation of chronic pancreatitis, or ductal obstruction from pancreatic calculi, as well as trauma (4). Whereas the former most commonly result in bilomas in the gallbladder fossa or bilious ascites in the setting of large or chronic leaks, the consequence of pancreatic duct collections are myriad and include acute and potentially spontaneously resolving fluid collections, pseudocysts, pancreatic ascites, and high amylase pleural effusions (4). Leaks are also often associated with smoldering pancreatitis and have been documented in up to two-thirds of patients with pancreatic necrosis (5).

Enlarging biliary fluid collections or bile ascites requires percutaneous or laparoscopic drainage and insertion of one or more indwelling Jackson-Pratt (JP) drains. Endoscopic retrograde cholangiopancreatography (ERCP) also is required to define whether there is an endoscopically amenable anatomy (e.g., cystic duct or nontransected common bile duct leak). These latter situations can be handled with placement of one or more transpapillary stents, (1–3) the insertion technique of which is covered in Chapter 30.

Pancreatic duct leaks, in turn, can also be managed by a transpapillary prosthesis, provided the gland has not been severed completely by necrosis or blunt trauma (6,7). This will control the leak but may not treat the consequences of the leak, and frequently large volume thoracentesis and paracentesis will be required in pancreatic pleural effusion and pancreatic ascites, respectively. In contrast, multiple large-caliber JP drains may need to be inserted percutaneously or surgically to treat the consequences of ductal disruption secondary to pancreatic necrosis.

Pseudocysts, one form of pancreatic duct leak, may be resolved after occluding the leak with a stent or decreasing intraductal pressure with a transpapillary prosthesis (7). Large pseudocysts or those in which an ongoing ductal connection has been lost, may require surgical, interventional radiologic, or endoscopic drainage. The focus of this chapter will be on transgastric or transduodenal endoscopic drainage of an amenable pancreatic pseudocyst.

## ENDOSCOPIC CYST-GASTROSTOMY/DUODENOSTOMY (8,9)

### Indications

1.  An enlarging or symptomatic pseudocyst with symptoms to include pain, biliary obstruction with cholestasis or cholangitis, gastric outlet obstruction, or infection

### Contraindications

Contraindications can be divided into clinical and anatomic. Clinical contraindications include the following:

1.  Inadequate endoscopic experience or lack of surgical or interventional radiologic backup

2.  Significant coagulopathy

3.  A significant fall in hematocrit or sudden rapid pseudocyst enlargement suggesting development of a pseudoaneurysm

4.  Any patient without an antecedent history of pancreatitis or those with imaging criteria raising the possibility of cystic tumor of the pancreas

From an anatomic standpoint, the following should be considered as relative exclusions to endoscopic drainage:

1.  A poorly circumscribed fluid collection occurring in the setting of acute pancreatitis

2.  An acute pseudocyst of less than 4 to 6 weeks' duration which has not developed an adequate "rind" or adherence to the stomach or duodenal wall

3.  A fluid collection occurring in the setting of pancreatic necrosis that has significant solid or semisolid debris

4.  A pseudocyst that is distant from the gut wall through which drainage is planned

5.  The presence of gastric varices at the site of transgastric puncture (relative)

### Preparation

1.  Patients being considered for endoscopic pseudocyst drainage should have adequate abdominal imaging prior to the procedure. This most commonly consists of a pancreas protocol computed tomography (CT) scan but might also consist of abdominal or endoscopic ultrasound because CT notoriously underestimates the amount of solid debris within a cystic cavity. In some centers, secretin-magnetic resonance cholangiopancreatography (MRCP) is used to define the site of ductal disruption as well as to plan combined transpapillary and transgastric/enteric drainage approach.

2.  Clotting parameters should be checked and optimized.

3.  Broad spectrum antibiotics are infused preprocedure.

### Equipment

1.  A variety of scopes should be available contingent upon the ability to delineate the pseudocyst with or without endoscopic ultrasound (EUS) localization.

2. Fluoroscopy is desirable and mandatory if EUS is not utilized.

3. Multiple accessories are required (see Fig. 31.1).

    a. Sclerotherapy-type needle
    b. Needle-knife sphincterotome and cautery equipment
    c. 5- to 10-Fr catheter and 6- to 10-mm balloon dilators
    d. 0.035-in. slippery guidewire(s)
    e. 5- to 7-Fr straight and 7- to 10-Fr double pigtail stents
       in a variety of lengths
    f. 6- or 7-Fr nasobiliary/nasopancreatic drains
    g. hemostasis capability

**Procedure**

As most commonly undertaken today, pseudocyst drainage consists of the following steps:

1. Baseline ERCP to define the presence or absence of ongoing ductal disruption

    a. Transpapillary stent placement (if feasible) beyond the leak for head and body leaks
    b. Short transpapillary stent for demonstrable tail leak
    c. Transpapillary stent alone for complete disruption in absence of upstream ductal stricture or stone

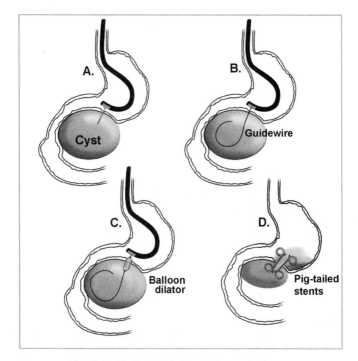

Fig. 31.1A–D. Transgastric pseudocyst drainage.

2. Pseudocyst localization via

    a. Pancreatography

    b. A visible cyst bulge on the stomach or duodenal wall

    c. EUS. This is particularly helpful to define debris in the setting of necrosis and the presence of intervening vascularity with concomitant splenic vein thrombosis, by application of Doppler ultrasound (US).

    d. Transmural contrast injection using a sclerotherapy needle. The latter is mandatory if not using EUS.

3. Pseudocyst puncture using one of the following:

    a. Needle-knife sphincterotome using pure cut current

    b. A Seldinger-type needle with internal stylet

4. Aspiration of fluid for Gram stain, culture, amylase, and cytology

5. Control of the fistula by placing one or preferably two guidewires curled deeply within the pseudocyst tract

6. Dilation of the tract to 6 to 10 mm using hydrostatic balloons

7. Placement of at least two pigtail stents into the pseudocyst cavity with proximal ends residing in stomach or duodenum (Fig. 31.1)

Alternatively, if EUS is used, the following drainage techniques can be used:

1. Cyst localization with therapeutic linear array echoendoscope

2. Direct needle puncture and guidewire placement into pseudocyst cavity

3. Endoscopic pigtail stent placement into pseudocyst

4. If placing more than one stent, Steps 1 through 3 need to be repeated.

**Postprocedure**

1. Patients should be kept NPO, receive broad spectrum antibiotics, and be observed for exacerbation of pancreatitis or peritoneal signs.

2. Minimize acid-reducing drugs in patients with a transgastric drain to avoid bacterial overgrowth in the stomach and bacterial translocation in the lesser sac.

3. Obtain a follow-up pancreas protocol CT at 24 hours to assure partial pseudocyst decompression and absence of local complications.

4. Begin refeeding.

5. Administer three days of oral antibiotics if no bacteria exist in aspirate or longer if there is a baseline pseudocyst infection.

**Interpretation**

Perhaps the best single institution publication has been that of Baron, et al., in which he reviewed use of the above techniques in three types of patients with pancreatic fluid collections; they are "pseudocysts" in the setting of acute or chronic pancreatitis or pancreatic necrosis (10). Drainage was successful in 74% to 95% of patient groups but statistically less successful in necrosis. Moreover, drainage of the fluid collections associated with necrosis had a twofold complication rate, a two- to sixfold increase in hospital stay, and a two- to threefold recurrence rate. Although successful pseudocyst drainage was more common in chronic as opposed to acute pancreatitis (92% versus 74%), there was no statistical difference in other commonly defined outcome parameters.

## Complications

*Periprocedure Complications*

1. Bleeding with puncture. This can be minimized with Doppler EUS, initial transgastric injection with contrast to avoid gastric varices in patients with splenic vein thrombosis, and dilating rather than incising the tract after initial puncture.

2. Free perforation. This occurs most commonly in patients with immature fluid collections not adherent to contiguous gut. Alternatively, endoscopists may misinterpret extrinsic gallbladder, liver, or colon impressions as the compression caused by the pseudocyst. The latter can be minimized by use of EUS and/or transmural injection of contrast material prior to formal fistulation (11).

*Postprocedure Complications*

1. Iatrogenic infection is by far and away the most common postprocedure complication of endoscopic pseudocyst drainage. This can be minimized by avoiding fluid collections with thick debris, by adding an additional percutaneous drain, or by placing a nasocystic drain to effect chronic irrigation, if there is inadvertent puncture of a pseudocyst with considerable debris.

2. Postprocedure pancreatitis is unusual unless the pancreatic duct is manipulated but not adequately stented.

3. Transpapillary stent placement complications include the following: iatrogenic ductitis, and occasionally, induction of pancreatic sepsis in the setting of stent occlusion, pancreatic necrosis, or the disconnected gland syndrome (12).

## Other Uses for this Technique

As noted above, some endoscopists have attempted to utilize the above-mentioned pseudocyst drainage techniques to treat pancreatic necrosis (9,13,14). From personal experience, iatrogenic infection is inevitable without constant irrigation, and because of the size and consistency of the necrotic debris, most practitioners handle these patients either with surgery or by placement of multiple, percutaneous, large-diameter JP drains.

## CPT Codes

Contingent upon concomitant ERCP and stent placement
**43262** – Endoscopic retrograde cholangiopancreatography (ERCP); with sphincterotomy/papillotomy.

**43268** – Endoscopic retrograde cholangiopancreatography (ERCP); with endoscopic retrograde insertion of tube or stent into bile or pancreatic duct.

**43240** – Upper Gastrointestinal Endoscopy with transmural drainage of pseudocyst.

## REFERENCES

1. Csendes A, Navarrete C, Burdiles P, Yarmuch J. Treatment of common bile duct injuries during laparoscopic cholecystectomy: endoscopic and surgical management. *World J Surg* 2001;25: 1346–1351.
2. Bhattacharjya S, Puleston J, Davidson BR, Dooley JS. Outcome of early endoscopic biliary drainage in the management of bile leaks after hepatic resection. *Gastrointest Endosc* 2003; 57:526–530.
3. De Palma GD, Galloro G, Iuliano G, et al. Leaks from laparoscopic cholecystectomy. *Hepatogastroenterology* 2002;49:924–925.
4. Kozarek RA. Pancreatic fistulas and ascites. In: Brandt JL, ed. *Clinical Practice of Gastroenterology.* Current Medicine, Inc. Philadelphia, 1999; 1175–1180.
5. Lau ST, Simchuk EJ, Kozarek RA, Traverso LW. A pancreatic ductal leak should be sought to direct treatment in patients with acute pancreatitis. *Am J Surg* 2001;181:411–415.
6. Kozarek RA, Ball TJ, Patterson DJ, et al. Transpapillary stenting for pancreaticocutaneous fistulas. *J Gastrointest Surg* 1997;1:357–361.
7. Kozarek RA. Endoscopic therapy of complete and partial pancreatic duct disruptions. *Gastrointest Endosc Clin North Am* 1998;8:39–53.
8. Kozarek RA. Endoscopic treatment of pancreatic pseudocysts. *Gastrointest Endosc Clin North Am* 1997;7:271–283.
9. Pitchumoni CS, Agarwal N. Pancreatic pseudocysts. When and how should drainage be performed? *Gastroenterol Clin North Am* 1999;28:615–639.
10. Baron TH, Harewood GC, Morgan DE, Yates MR. Outcome differences after endoscopic drainage of pancreatic necrosis, acute pancreatic pseudocysts, and chronic pancreatic pseudocysts. *Gastrointest Endosc* 2002;56:7–17.
11. Giovannini M, Pesenti C, Rolland AL, et al. Endoscopic ultrasound-guided drainage of pancreatic pseudocysts or pancreatic abscesses using a therapeutic echo endoscope. *Endoscopy* 2001;33:473–477.
12. Kozarek R, Hovde O, Attia F, France R. Do pancreatic duct stents cause or prevent pancreatic sepsis? *Gastrointest Endosc* 2003;58:505–509.
13. Seifert H, Wehrmann T, Schmitt T, et al. Retroperitoneal endoscopic debridement for infected peripancreatic necrosis. *Lancet* 2000;356:653–655.
14. Giovanni M, Binmoeller K, Siefert H. Endoscopic ultrasound-guided cystgastrostomy. *Endoscopy* 2003; 35:239–245.

# Argon Plasma Coagulation

Ian S. Grimm

Argon plasma coagulation (APC) is a form of monopolar electrocautery. Used both for hemostasis and for tissue destruction, the argon plasma coagulator has several advantages over laser and other forms of thermal therapy. First, APC does not require the safety precautions necessary for medical laser therapy. Second, the argon plasma beam can be rapidly sprayed over relatively large areas of the gastrointestinal (GI) tract, using a non-contact method. Third, the depth of the thermal injury is self-limited, allowing for treatment of lesions in the cecum and other thin-walled structures.

## INDICATIONS

1. Fulgurization of polyps. Argon plasma coagulation is particularly useful for treatment of residual adenomatous tissue following snare polypectomy and for broad sessile lesions (1).

2. Cauterization of vascular lesions, such as angioectasias, radiation-induced neovascularity, and gastric antral vascular ectasias (GAVE) (or watermelon stomach)

3. Treatment of nonvariceal bleeding lesions, including duodenal and gastric ulcers, Mallory-Weiss tears, and both benign and malignant tumors

4. Debulking of obstructing neoplasms

5. Unclogging of occluded self-expanding metal stents

## CONTRAINDICATIONS

An inadequately evacuated colon, due to the risk of explosion (2).

## PREPARATION

Preparation is the same as for esophogogastroduodenoscopy (EGD) or for colonoscopy.

## EQUIPMENT

1. APC generator, such as the ERBE APC 300 Plasma Coagulator system, which includes the ICC 200E/A generator, or the Conmed System 7500 ABC

2. Disposable probes (2.3-mm outer diameter [OD], in 220- or 440-cm lengths; 3.2-mm OD, 220 cm; 2.3-mm OD side-fire probe)

3. Patient return electrode pad

4. Medical argon gas (two tanks are situated in the rear of the unit)

## PROCEDURE

1. Advise the nursing staff that the APC equipment will be needed. It is helpful to have an assistant set up the equipment before it is actually required.

2. Place a patient return electrode pad on the patient; plug it into the electrocautery unit.

3. Turn on both the electrocautery unit and the argon unit.

4. Cycle the mode setting to APC at 40 W. On the ERBE unit, this is designated "A40" on the right side of the control panel, color-coded in blue. The "blue" functions are activated by the blue footswitch.

5. Attach the power cord that connects the electrocautery unit to the APC unit.

6. Check to see that the argon tank valves are open.

7. Attach the grounding wire from the electrocautery unit to the endoscope, at its connection to the video processor. Failure to do so will result in video interference.

8. Check the gauges to verify that there is argon gas in the tanks.

9. Replace the gas filter before each procedure. This is a clear plastic disc attached between the argon gas source and the probe tubing.

10. Choose a probe. Side-fire probes may be preferable when a broad beam is desired.

11. Attach the probe to the connecting tube. Attach the other end of the connecting tube to the air filter. Since the connecting tube requires disinfection between procedures, it is advisable to have an extra tube available.

12. Purge the catheter with argon gas by pushing the purge button for several seconds.

13. Adjust the power setting. Forty watts is considered a reasonably safe upper limit for the cecum and other thin-walled structures. The depth of the thermal injury with APC is a function of both the power setting (typically in the range of 40 to 100 W) and the application time; treatment duration is a more important predictor of depth of injury than the power setting (3). In general, keeping the power settings at the lowest effective level is the safest approach. High power settings are rarely necessary, except for tumor debulking.

14. Select the argon flow rate, usually set in the range of 0.5 to 1.0 L/min for end-firing probes. For lateral APC probes (side-firing), the argon flow should be increased to between 1.0 and 2.0 L/min.

15. Insert the probe through the working channel of the scope until the first black ring of the catheter appears in the visual field.

16. Begin by activating the probe in short bursts, typically 0.5 to 2.0 seconds in duration. With the ERBE unit, activation is controlled by the blue footswitch. Longer bursts can be used in a "spray-painting" technique.

17. Adjust the power and flow settings, as well as the distance between the probe and the target tissue to produce the desired effects; these are visible electrical arcs and tissue whitening. The operative distance ranges from 2 mm to 8 mm, with shorter distances corresponding to lower power settings.

18. Avoid touching the mucosal surface. It is easiest to simply touch the target tissue with the probe tip and then withdraw slightly prior to activating the footswitch. If the probe is activated in contact with the tissue, a bleb of submucosal argon gas may suddenly appear. This is typically an innocuous event.

19. Remove the catheter for manual cleaning if a coagulum forms on the tip.

20. Aspirate often to avoid overdistention with argon gas. In certain cases, such as treatment of extensive GAVE, use of a double channel endoscope is helpful for removal of insufflated argon.

## POSTPROCEDURE

1. Obtain abdominal films for localized abdominal pain, peritoneal signs.

2. Consider proton pump inhibitor therapy following treatment of upper GI lesions to promote healing.

3. Arrange for appropriate postpolypectomy follow-up colonoscopy, typically in 3 to 6 months for large sessile lesions.

## COMPLICATIONS

1. Gaseous bloating and transient abdominal pain occurs in about 10% of procedures (4).

2. Anal pain may occur after treatment of distal rectal lesions.

3. Barotrauma: Submucosal emphysema is considered a benign event. Pneumoperitoneum can occur from dissection of air through a tiny perforation. Surgery may be unnecessary if there are no clinical signs of peritonitis (5).

4. Perforation can occur rarely, with a reported frequency of 0.27%.

5. Ulcers occur commonly following treatment for radiation proctopathy (6,7). Most have a clinically benign course. To reduce the risk of ulceration, spot treatments may be preferable to extensive spray painting of rectal mucosa following radiation therapy for prostate cancer.

6. Stricture formation

7. Fistulization

8. Fever

## OTHER USES FOR THIS TECHNIQUE

1. Ablation of small, superficial cancers in patients at prohibitive operative risk

2.   Treatment of Zenker's Diverticulum

3.   Ablation of metaplastic mucosa in Barrett's esophagus

4.   Ablation of esophageal varices following ligation or sclerotherapy

**CPT Codes**

**43227** – Esophagoscopy, rigid or flexible; with control of bleeding.

**43228** – Esophagoscopy, rigid or flexible; with ablation of tumor(s), polyp(s), or other lesion(s), not amenable to removal by hot biopsy forceps, bipolar electrocautery, or snare technique.

**43255** – Esophagogastroduodenoscopy with control of bleeding, any method.

**43258** – Esophagogastroduodenoscopy with ablation of tumor(s), etc.

**43272** – ERCP with ablation of tumor(s), etc.

**44366** – Enteroscopy; with control of bleeding.

**44369** – Enteroscopy; with ablation of tumor(s), etc.

**44378** – Enteroscopy including ileum; with control of bleeding.

**44391** – Colonoscopy through stoma with control of bleeding.

**44393** – Colonoscopy through stoma with ablation of tumor(s), etc.

**45317** – Proctosigmoidoscopy, rigid; with control of bleeding

**45320** – Proctosigmoidoscopy, rigid; with ablation of tumor(s), etc.

**45334** – Sigmoidoscopy, flexible; with control of bleeding.

**45339** – Sigmoidoscopy flexible; with ablation of tumor(s), etc.

**45382** – Colonoscopy with control of bleeding.

**45383** – Colonoscopy; with ablation of tumor(s), etc.

**46614** – Anoscopy; with control of bleeding

**46615** – Anoscopy; with ablation of tumor(s), etc.

**REFERENCES**

1. Brooker JC, Saunders BP, Shah SG, et al. Treatment with argon plasma coagulation reduces recurrence after piecemeal resection of large sessile colonic polyps: a randomized trial and recommendations. *Gastrointest Endosc* 2002;55:371–375.

2. Soussan EB, Mathieu N, Roque I, Antonelli M. Bowel explosion with colonic perforation during argon plasma coagulation for hemorrhagic radiation-induced proctitis. *Gastrointest Endosc* 2003;57:412–413.

3. Norton ID, Wang L, Levine SL, et al. In vivo characterization of colonic thermal injury caused by argon plasma coagulation. *Gastrointest Endosc* 2002;55:631–636.

4. Grund KE, Zindel C, Farin G. Argon plasma coagulation (APC) in flexible endoscopy. Experience with 2193 applications in 1062 patients. *Gastroenterology* 1998;114:A603.

5. Hoyer N, Thouet R, Zellweger U. Massive pneumoperitoneum after endoscopic argon plasma coagulation. *Endoscopy* 1998;30:S44–45.

6. Ravizza R, Fiori G, Trovato C, et al. Frequency and outcomes of rectal ulcers during argon plasma coagulation for chronic radiation-induced coagulopathy. *Gastrointest Endosc* 2003;57:519–525.

# Photodynamic Therapy for Barrett's High-Grade Dysplasia

Bergein F. Overholt, Masoud Panjehpour, and Mary Phan

Photodynamic therapy (PDT) is a photochemical process for the ablation of Barrett's high-grade dysplasia (HGD). Photodynamic therapy requires three components for effective therapy. The first is a photosensitizing drug. The only photosensitizer approved by the Food and Drug Administration for use in Barrett's HGD is porfimer sodium (Photofrin). Second, light of proper power and wavelength is required. Lasers are typically used to provide light for PDT. Diode lasers are less expensive, are portable, and are durable but produce low-power output, requiring longer treatment time. Potassium-titanyl-phosphate (KTP)-pumped dye lasers and argon-pumped dye lasers can produce high-power outputs and therefore shorter treatment times but are more expensive, are not portable, and often require special electrical power and water cooling. Third, tissue oxygen is required.

## INDICATIONS

Prior to any treatment of HGD, the diagnosis should be confirmed by an expert gastroenterologic pathologist. For confirmed HGD, indications include the following:

1. Focal HGD. If only a few HGD glands are found, the patient could be treated with twice-daily proton pump inhibitor (PPI) therapy and undergo another biopsy in 3 months. If HGD persists, PDT is indicated.

2. Multifocal HGD. If several areas of confirmed HGD exist, PDT is indicated.

3. Nodular HGD. Endoscopic ultrasound followed by mucosal resection is generally recommended, although PDT is highly effective for small nodular areas. After mucosal resection, it is best to wait 6 weeks for the mucosal defect to heal and then to treat the remainder of the Barrett's mucosa with PDT.

4. Persistent HGD. If HGD persists after PDT and is unifocal, either aggressive thermal ablation or repeat PDT can be attempted. However, if HGD persists after thermal ablation, PDT is indicated. PDT is also indicated for multifocal HGD persisting after PDT.

An important guideline for Barrett's HGD: The first goal is to eliminate the HGD. The second goal is to eliminate Barrett's completely.

## CONTRAINDICATIONS

Contraindications include the following:

1. Generally those associated with contraindications for endoscopy

2. Limited life expectancy secondary to other diseases

## PATIENT PREPARATION

1. Other than administration of the photosensitizer, no special preparation is needed for PDT other than that associated with endoscopy.

2. The destruction of esophageal mucosa after PDT can be significant, resulting in poor oral intake, nausea and vomiting, and chest pain. Therefore, for all elderly patients and most young patients, lab work is obtained, including a complete blood count, serum electrolytes, and a chemical profile. A chest x-ray and electrocardiogram are usually obtained.

## EQUIPMENT

1. Porfimer sodium, (2 mg/Kg)

2. Lasers. Several lasers are available for delivery of light including the KTP-pumped dye laser (low-power and high-power models) manufactured by Laserscope (San Jose, CA), the Lambda plus argon-pumped dye laser manufactured by Lumenis (Santa Clara, CA), and a diode laser manufactured by Diomed (Andover, MA) (1).

3. Balloons and diffusers. The appropriate lengths of cylindrical diffusers and balloons should be available prior to the injection of the patient with porfimer sodium (1). Balloons are available with window lengths of 3 cm, 5 cm, and 7 cm with corresponding cylindrical diffusers of 5 cm, 7 cm, and 9 cm in length. An inflation device (with gauge) to inflate and monitor the pressure in the balloon during light delivery is needed along with a 10-cc luer-lock syringe of saline or sterile water to flush the balloon catheter immediately prior to starting the laser treatment.

## PROCEDURE

### Day 1

Porfimer sodium administration and photosensitivity precautions: Administer Porfimer sodium (Photofrin), 2 mg/Kg intravenously (IV) over 5 to 10 minutes as per labeling instructions. Carefully instruct patients on photosensitivity.

### Day 3

Preparation of PDT balloon: Prior to the endoscopy, prepare the appropriate-length balloon and cylindrical diffuser depending on the length of Barrett's segment to be treated and according to the manufacturer's instructions (2).

Laser treatment parameters: Patients should receive an energy dose of 130 J/cm regardless of the length of window on the balloon. The power settings and duration of laser treatment are related to the type of laser and the length of windowed balloon used (Tables 1–3 in Appendix A).

PDT Treatment:

1. Attain adequate conscious sedation.

2. Deliver oxygen, 2 to 4 L/min to maintain oxygen saturation at or above 95%.

3. Pass a regular video-endoscope, and obtain distances for the squamocolumnar junction, gastric folds, and diaphragmatic squeeze. Obtain a gastric aspirate pH. If it is < 4.0, the proton pump inhibitor medication is doubled.

4. Pass a guidewire into the antrum, and then pass the deflated balloon over the guidewire.

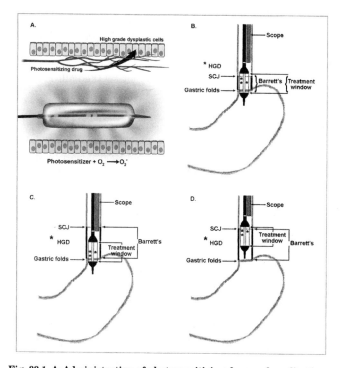

Fig. 33.1. A: Administration of photosensitizing drug and application of laser therapy. B: If the Barrett's is 6 cm or less, treat the entire segment. The balloon window extends 0.5 cm distal the gastroesophageal junction (beginning of the gastric folds) and 0.5 cm proximal to the squamocolumnar junction providing complete treatment of the Barrett's. C: If the Barrett's is greater than 6 cm to 7 cm, treat the high-grade dysplasia (HGD) area first. The HGD is in the distal segment of the BE here. D: Here the HGD is in the proximal BE. This area is treated with the proximal balloon window margin extending 0.5 cm to 1 cm proximal to the squamocolumnar junction (SCJ).

5. Reinsert the scope. Using endoscopic guidance, withdraw the balloon shaft to the point that the yellow marker on the shaft is 3 cm proximal to the proximal margin of the treatment field (Fig. 33.1A and Fig. 33.1B).

6. Withdraw the guidewire, and reattach the balloon/fiber adaptor.

7. Inflate the balloon to 80 mm Hg pressure, and then quickly deflate to 20 mm Hg. Maintain the balloon pressure at 20 mm Hg or less. If excessive motility causes wide fluctuations in the pressure readings, reduce the pressure to 10 to 20 mm Hg.

8. Once the balloon is properly positioned, fully insert the cylindrical diffuser into the balloon and luer-locke it into the balloon assembly.

9. Flush the fiberoptic channel with 4 to 5 cc saline to clear any gastric juices, blood, or bile from the channel. Leave the syringe attached to the adaptor to prevent any fluid from reentering the cleared channel.

10. Fix the scope and balloon position at the mouth with your hand. Minor position changes of either the balloon or the scope are common, so continue endoscopic monitoring of the positions of the scope and the balloon shaft to adjust for any position change. If motility is prominent, Glucagon 0.5 mg can be given IV at the start of the treatment and the remaining 0.5 mg given halfway through the treatment.

11. Initiate the laser treatment. The duration of laser treatment is determined by the amount of light dose to be delivered to the esophageal mucosa (Table 33.1 and Table 33.2). After the laser light has been delivered, the balloon is fully deflated, and the scope and the balloon assembly are removed.

12. If the patient has a nodule within the treatment field, perform pretreatment of the nodule with 50 J/cm using a 1- to 2.5-cylindrical diffuser passed through the scope prior to the balloon treatment (Table 33.3).

**Table 33.1. Laser parameters for different balloons using a high power laser and an external power meter. The laser is considered high power if a minimum power of 2,430 mw can be measured from a 9-cm cylindrical diffuser.**

| Length of balloon window (cm) | 3 cm | 5 cm | 7 cm |
|---|---|---|---|
| Length of cylindrical diffuser (cm) | 5 cm | 7 cm | 9 cm |
| Power density (mw/cm) | 270 mw/cm | 270 mw/cm | 270 mw/cm |
| Power (mw) | 1,350 mw | 1,890 mw | 2,430 mw |
| Treatment time (seconds) | 480 seconds | 480 seconds | 480 seconds |
| Energy density (J/cm) | 130 J/cm | 130 J/cm | 130 J/cm |

**Table 33.2. Laser parameters for different balloons using a low-power laser and an external power meter. The laser is considered low power if a minimum power of 2,430 mw cannot be measured from a 9-cm cylindrical diffuser.**

| Length of balloon window (cm) | 3 cm | 5 cm | 7 cm |
|---|---|---|---|
| Length of cylindrical diffuser (cm) | 5 cm | 7 cm | 9 cm |
| Power density (mw/cm) | 270 mw/cm | 200 mw/cm | 200 mw/cm |
| Power (mw) | 1,350 mw | 1,400 mw | 1,800 mw |
| Treatment time (seconds) | 480 seconds | 650 seconds | 650 seconds |
| Energy density (J/cm) | 130 J/cm | 130 J/cm | 130 J/cm |

13. Patients are treated in the outpatient environment, but patients are required to stay in close proximity to the treatment center. During the day of PDT, 1000 to 1500 cc of IV fluid is usually given to maintain hydration. Medications for pain and nausea are also given as needed. A sample regime includes the following:

   a. Oxycontin 10 to 20 mg q 12 hours beginning the evening of PDT and continuing for 7 to 10 days
   b. Meperidine 50 mg p.o. q 3 to 4 hours for breakthrough pain
   c. Lidocaine 2%. 2 oz mixed in a 12-oz bottle of Mylanta and sipped or taken as needed for retrosternal burning and hiccups
   d. Promethazine (Phenergan) 25 mg p.o. q 6 hours for nausea
   e. Prochlorperazine (Compazine) suppositories, 25 mg q 8 hours as needed for nausea

**Table 33.3. Laser parameters for different length cylindrical diffusers for pretreatment of nodules and skip areas.**

| Length of cylindrical diffuser (cm) | 1 cm | 1.5 cm | 2 cm | 2.5 cm |
|---|---|---|---|---|
| Power density (mw/cm) | 400 mw/cm | 400 mw/cm | 400 mw/cm | 400 mw/cm |
| Power (mw) | 400 mw | 600 mw | 800 mw | 1000 mw |
| Treatment time (seconds) | 125 seconds | 125 seconds | 125 seconds | 125 seconds |
| Energy density (J/cm) | 50 J/cm | 50 J/cm | 50 J/cm | 50 J/cm |

f. Sucralfate suspension 15 cc 1 hour after meals (or mealtime) for patients with severe PDT effect; proton pump inhibitor medication, bid

**Day 5**

Perform repeat endoscopy at 48 hours to evaluate tissue damage. In the majority of patients, it will be circumferential and severe, and no additional therapy will be needed. For a few, a skip area in the treatment field will be found which can be retreated with a fiber diffuser, 50 J/cm of light dose. For example, if a skip area of 1.5 cm is found on the left wall, a 2.5-cm diffuser can be used with the treatment field including the skip area and covering an additional 0.5 cm proximal and distal to the skip area (Table 33.3).

## POSTPROCEDURE

1. Generally, patients do not drink well for 24 to 48 hours. They are encouraged to increase oral fluids and nutritional supplements as soon as possible after PDT.

2. Once their oral intake is satisfactory (at least 6 to 8 glasses daily) and they take in some calories, they are ready to return home, usually 4 to 5 days after PDT.

## COMPLICATIONS

Almost all patients experience side effects of mucosal ablation including the following:

1. Chest pain is typically described as moderate but controllable with medication.

2. Anorexia is common, and nausea and occasionally vomiting can occur.

3. Hiccups can be problematic for some patients but are usually controlled using the lidocaine suspension and sucralfate.

4. Esophageal strictures occur in approximately 20% of patients and usually become symptomatic with dysphagia at 3 weeks after PDT. About half can be managed with three to four dilations, but half are severe and require multiple dilations. The principals of management of the severe post-PDT stricture therapy include early diagnosis and intervention, as well as frequent and progressive dilations beginning with a Savary #33 or #36 and progressing over several weeks to a Savary #51 or #54 and then lengthening the dilation intervals. The post-PDT stricture is a thick-walled structure and requires moderately deep tears from dilations to accomplish adequate effect. Local depomedrol injection (20 mg in 4 sites) into the inflamed stricture once weekly during the first 3 weeks of dilations appears to be helpful. Dilating twice weekly until Savary #48–#51 is reached, then weekly for several weeks with a Savary #51 or #54, and then monthly for several months, is advised. Stricturotomy can be used for persistent fibrotic strictures (2).

## FOLLOW-UP AFTER PHOTODYNAMIC THERAPY

Endoscopy and biopsies are conducted about 3 months after PDT. Healing of the mucosa post-PDT requires 2 to 3 months. Endoscopy or biopsies conducted before healing will show severely inflamed mucosa with patches of healed and nonhealed mucosa. Cobblestoned mucosa will commonly be found. Biopsies taken prior to healing are difficult to interpret due to the inflammation.

## CPT Codes

**96570 -** Photodynamic therapy by endoscopic application of light to ablate abnormal tissues via activation of photosensitive drug(s); first 30 minutes (list separately in addition to code for endoscopy or bronchoscopy procedures of lung and esophagus).

**96571 -** Photodynamic therapy by endoscopic application of light to ablate abnormal tissues via activation of photosensitive drug(s); each additional 15 minutes (list separately in addition to code for endoscopy or bronchoscopy procedures of lung and esophagus).

## REFERENCES

1. Panjehpour M, Overholt BF, Haydek JM. Light sources and delivery devices for gastrointestinal photodynamic therapy. *Gastrointest Endosc Clin North Am* 2000;10:513–532.
2. Overholt BF, Panjehpour M. Photodynamic therapy techniques for ablation of Barrett's esophagus. *Techniq Gastrointest Endosc* 2000;2:203–208.

## SUGGESTED READINGS

Overholt BF, Lightdale CJ, Wang K, et al. International, multicenter, partially blinded, randomized study of the efficacy of photodynamic therapy (PDT) using porfimer sodium (POR) for the ablation of high-grade dysplasia (HGD) in Barrett's esophagus (BE): results of 24 month follow-up. *Gastroenterology* 2003;124 (Suppl 1):A–20.

Overholt BF, Panjehpour M, Halberg D. Photodynamic therapy for Barrett's esophagus with dysplasia and early carcinoma: long term results. *Gastrointest Endosc* 2003;58:183–188.

Overholt BF, Panjehpour M, Haydek J. Photodynamic therapy for Barrett's esophagus: follow up in 100 patients. *Gastrointest Endosc* 1999;49:1–7.

Panjehpour M, Overholt BF, Haydek JM, Lee SG. Results of photodynamic therapy for ablation of dysplasia and early cancer in Barrett's esophagus and effect of oral steroids on stricture formation. *Am J Gastroenterol* 2000;95:2177–2184.

Wang KK. Photodynamic therapy of Barrett's esophagus. *Gastrointest Endosc Clin North Am* 2000;10:409–419.

Wolfson, HC, Woodwar TA, Raimondo M. Photodynamic therapy for dysplastic Barrett esophagus and early esophageal adenocarcinoma. *Mayo Clin Proc* 2002;77:1176–1181.

# Infrared Coagulation of Hemorrhoids

Sidney E. Levinson

Infrared coagulation of hemorrhoids (IRC) is an outpatient procedure used in the treatment of symptomatic internal hemorrhoids. Other treatment options include topical therapy, radio frequency coagulation, sclerotherapy, cryosurgery, rubber band ligation, and surgery (1–5). Therapy is usually reserved for internal hemorrhoids that prolapse with defecation and reduce spontaneously (grade II), that prolapse and require manual reduction (grade III), and that cannot be reduced (grade IV) (2–4). However, grade I hemorrhoids can also be treated if sufficiently symptomatic (e.g., recurrent bleeding), and grade IV hemorrhoids are optimally treated by other methods, including surgery. Significant symptoms from hemorrhoids include recurrent bleeding, sensation of pressure or fullness, discomfort of an aching or pruritic nature, and pain following defecation. While some patients may ultimately require surgery for recalcitrant symptoms, most patients will benefit from initial treatment regimens which can improve or control the patient's symptoms. Infrared coagulation is a relatively simple and minimally painful procedure that can be performed in an outpatient setting with little disruption to the patient's lifestyle and work schedule.

## INDICATIONS (1–7)

1. Recurrent bleeding documented to be from internal hemorrhoids
2. Discomfort, including pain and itching
3. Symptoms of rectal oozing which may be associated with large hemorrhoids

## CONTRAINDICATIONS

1. Recurrent rectal bleeding that has not been evaluated endoscopically
2. Active, brisk bleeding
3. Active pain from fissure
4. Presence of acute thrombosis
5. Presence of perirectal abscess

## EQUIPMENT

1. IRC unit (manufactured by Redfield Corporation) with clean IRC probe
2. Disposable sheath suction apparatus

3. Tray to include the following:

   a. Operating anoscope
   b. Long cotton swabs
   c. Water-soluble lubricant
   d. Basin
   e. 2-x-2-in. and 4-x-4-in. cotton gauze pads
   f. Saline solution

**PREPARATION**

1. Fleet's enema should be administered one hour prior to the appointment (may be omitted).

2. No sedation is necessary; therefore, no driver is required.

3. Patients who are in pain or have experienced significant pain during prior exams may premedicate with acetaminophen (Tylenol). Nonsteroidal medications may be effective but may increase bleeding risk.

4. Patients should give informed consent.

**PROCEDURE**

1. After the patient changes into a gown, place him or her in the left lateral decubitus position.

2. Perform visual inspection of the anal verge and perineum.

3. Lubricate the anal verge generously with water-soluble lubricant, and perform a thorough digital examination to exclude any local masses or areas of significant tenderness.

4. Introduce an operating anoscope, and carefully examine the anal verge and distal rectum for rectal mucosal abnormalities, the presence of fissures and hypertrophied anal papillae, and the location and size of hemorrhoids. For patient comfort, it is useful to completely remove the anoscope following the initial examination and to reintroduce the instrument using the obturator before beginning treatment.

5. Once you have chosen the area for initial treatment, position the anoscope to expose the mucosa proximal to the target hemorrhoids. Place the IRC against the mucosa, apply pressure with the tip of the instrument, and pull the trigger. A timed light pulse will occur, and the resultant coagulation is apparent within 2 seconds. Gauge patient discomfort as an assistant wipes the end of the coagulator with a 2-x-2-in. cotton pad soaked in saline solution. Determine the next location of application of the IRC, and repeat the procedure as described above. The location of the individual applications should form a pattern that will obliterate venous flow beneath the areas coagulated. This pattern may be arranged in alternating rows or a diamond-like pattern (Fig. 34.1A) or may take the form of a crescent of contiguous applications (Fig. 34.1B). Anywhere from six to 12 applications may be applied in a single treatment. Avoid treatment of more than one-third of the circumference of the anal verge.

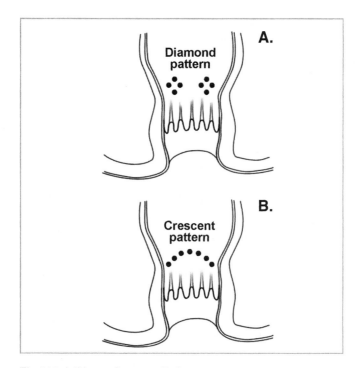

**Fig. 34.1. A: Diamond pattern. B: Crescent pattern.**

**POSTPROCEDURE**

1. Immediately after the procedure, evaluate the patient for signs of bleeding and for significant discomfort.

2. Instruct the patient to contact the operating physician for any untoward symptoms, including bleeding, local anal pain, fever, or chills.

3. A course of suppositories with hydrocortisone, one used nightly for 7 days, is helpful in reducing postprocedure discomfort and bleeding and may speed healing of the coagulation sites.

4. For discomfort, the patient may take analgesics, which may include acetaminophen, ibuprofen, or in rare instances low-dose narcotics.

5. The patient may return to normal activity, though it is wise to counsel the patient to avoid strenuous activity for 24 to 48 hours. A course of bulk agents and fluids should be encouraged.

## INTERPRETATION OF RESPONSE

The assessment of success from infrared coagulation requires combined observations by the patient and physician. Patients may report diminished episodes or extent of bleeding, diminished sense of pressure or pruritus, and less overall discomfort. Commonly, significant reduction in symptoms requires a second or third treatment, and frequently at least three treatments in monthly intervals are necessary. Patients who require a second course of treatment months or years after initial therapy frequently respond to one or two additional treatments.

## COMPLICATIONS

1.  The major complication following IRC is bleeding with bowel movements. On rare occasions, hemorrhage from ulcers at the coagulation sites may require clinical observation and possibly hospitalization.

2.  Postprocedure discomfort may persist for several hours, and in a small percentage of patients, pain may require treatment with analgesics.

3.  Thrombosis of external hemorrhoids is a theoretical possibility but is not seen in practice, perhaps because of the limited depth of tissue injury.

4.  The limited depth of injury may also explain the exceedingly low incidence of local or distant postprocedure infectious complications, which are more likely to occur following band ligation (1,3,4–7). This lesser depth of injury and clinical response compared to other treatments may explain the need to retreat up to 10% of patients within 3 months (1,4,6,7). The instrument's disposable sheath limits concerns regarding cross-contamination.

## OTHER USES FOR THIS PROCEDURE

Infrared coagulation of hemorrhoids has particular utility in the treatment of hemorrhoids. The instrument may be used in the treatment of other medical conditions, including the removal of warts or tattoos as well as control of superficial bleeding during dermatologic procedures.

## CPT Codes

**46934** – Destruction of hemorrhoids, any method; internal.

## REFERENCES

1.  Johanson JF, Rimm A. Optimal nonsurgical treatment of hemorrhoids: a comparative analysis of infrared coagulation, rubber band ligation, and injection sclerotherapy. *Am J Gastroenterol* 1992;87(11):1600–1606.
2.  Janick DM, Pundt MR. Anorectal disorders. *Emerg Med Clin North Am* 1996;14(4):757–788.
3.  Pfenninger JL, Surrell J. Nonsurgical treatment options for internal hemorrhoids. *Am Fam Physician* 1995;52(3):821–834, 839–841.
4.  MacRae HM, McLeod RS. Comparison of hemorrhoidal treatment: a meta-analysis. *Can J Surg* 1997;40(1):14–17.

5. Accarpio G, Ballari F, Puglisi R, et al. Outpatient treatment of hemorrhoids with a combined technique: results in 7850 cases. *Tech Coloproctol* 2002;6(3):195–196.
6. Gupta PJ. Infrared coagulation versus rubber band ligation in early stage hemorrhoids. *Braz J Med Biol Res* 2003;36(10): 1433–1439.
7. Linares Santiago E, Gmez Parra M, Mendoza Olivares FJ, et al. Effectiveness of hemorrhoidal treatment by rubber band ligation and infrared coagulation. *Rev Esp Enferm Dig* 2001;93(4): 238–247.

# Endoscopic Management of Foreign Bodies of the Upper Gastrointestinal Tract

Craig J. Cender

Ingestion of foreign bodies or food impaction is a frequent cause of gastrointestinal emergency resulting in significant morbidity and up to 1,500 fatalities per year. The majority of foreign bodies pass through the alimentary tract uneventfully, but endoscopic intervention is required in 10% to 20% of instances. Generally, food bolus disimpaction or foreign body retrieval by endoscopic means is successful in over 90% of cases. Surgical intervention is required in no more than 1% of instances but is mandated by a failure of an object to progress over several days or the development of symptoms of obstruction or peritoneal irritation (1).

The preponderance of foreign body ingestions occur in the pediatric population, with the peak incidence between 6 months and 6 years, although this is also often observed in adults with psychiatric disorders or mental impairment or in those seeking secondary gain with access to a medical facility. Food bolus impaction is most often observed in those with underlying esophageal pathology (2).

## INDICATIONS

Foreign objects requiring removal include smooth objects and disc batteries lodged in the esophagus, long objects (> 10 cm), sharp objects in the stomach or proximal duodenum, and objects that fail to pass out of the stomach within 3 to 4 weeks. The precise timing of intervention, however, is dependent on both the nature of the object as well as its particular location as outlined below (3,4).

### Emergent

1. High-grade esophageal obstruction with any object
2. Sharp object or disk battery lodged in the esophagus

### Urgent

1. Sharp object within stomach or proximal duodenum that can be safely removed
2. Esophageal impaction with any object (under no circumstances should a foreign body be allowed to remain in the esophagus beyond 24 hours from presentation)

### Routine

1. Foreign body of greater dimension than known to pass safely
   a. Adult: > 6 to 10 cm in length, > 25 mm in diameter
   b. Pediatric: > 3 cm in length, > 20 mm in diameter

2. Disc battery when signs/symptoms of gastric mucosal injury are present, larger than 20 mm in diameter, or if not expelled from the stomach within 48 hours

3. Blunt objects that fail to pass out of stomach within 3 to 4 weeks (1)

## CONTRAINDICATIONS

### Absolute

1. Evidence of free mediastinal or peritoneal air

2. Narcotic packets. Endoscopic recovery should not be attempted due to the risk of rupture, as leakage of contents can be fatal.

3. Same as standard upper endoscopy

### Relative

1. Upper esophageal stricture

2. Zenker's diverticulum

3. Postligament of Treitz position of foreign body (as the majority of these will pass spontaneously)

4. Same as standard upper endoscopy

### Special Considerations

1. High esophageal impaction

2. Esophageal impaction of unknown duration (prolonged impaction may result in tissue necrosis, increasing the risk of major complications)

In both instances consider anesthesia and surgical consultation. General endotracheal anesthesia is helpful for airway protection in these cases. Laryngoscopy or rigid esophagoscopy is the preferred method for impacted sharp objects at the level of the cricopharyngeus (1).

## PREPARATION

### Historical Considerations

1. Assess circumstances (e.g., object, timing) of suspected ingestion.

2. Obtain a replica of a foreign body for inspection if it is a non-food object.

3. Determine the presence of known esophageal pathology (anatomic or dysmotility).

4. Characterize prior symptoms of dysphagia or a history of any previous food impaction.

5. Determine the presence of any neurologic impairment (e.g., cerebrovascular accident, multiple sclerosis) that may increase risk of aspiration.

### Physical Examination

1. Assess swelling, tenderness, or crepitus in the neck region to exclude esophageal perforation.

2. Assess the abdomen for evidence of peritonitis or small bowel obstruction.

3. Assess ventilation, airway compromise, and risk of aspiration.

**Anatomic Considerations**

1. Impaction or obstruction most often occurs at areas of acute angulations or physiologic narrowing.
   a. Cricopharyngeus muscle
   b. Aortic arch
   c. Esophagogastric junction
   d. Pylorus
   e. Ligament of Treitz
   f. Ileocecal valve

**Radiologic Considerations**

1. Identify and localize the object with biplane radiographs.
   a. Most foreign bodies, including steak bones, are radiopaque, but some commonly encountered that are radiolucent include fish/chicken bones, wood (e.g., toothpicks), plastic, and most glass.
   b. Localization of the foreign body within the intestinal tract
      i. Flat objects (e.g., coins) lodged in the esophagus are most often oriented in the coronal plane resulting in visualization of the full diameter on anterioposterior projections and on-edge view in the lateral projection. Tracheal foreign bodies usually align in the sagittal plane reversing this orientation.
      ii. An object within the left upper quadrant (LUQ) is more likely to be located within the stomach if the lateral view reveals an anterior position. If the object is located more posteriorly, it may be positioned at the splenic flexure.

2. Exclude perforation by assessing for the presence of mediastinal, subdiaphragmatic, or subcutaneous air.

3. Contrast radiography should not be routinely performed due to the risk of aspiration and because coating of the foreign body and mucosal lining often compromises subsequent endoscopy (3,4).

4. In certain circumstances when symptoms are absent or nonspecific and routine radiographs are nonrevealing, cautious administration of contrast or computed tomography may be useful.

5. Nonvisualized objects are frequently encountered and still warrant endoscopic evaluation.

**Food Impaction**

1. Encourage physical activity to promote the influence of gravity (i.e., jumping up and down, drinking liquids).

2. Glucagon 1 mg intravenously. This may allow spontaneous passage of an impacted food bolus by relaxation of the lower esophagus (3).

3.   Proteolytic enzymes (e.g., papain). This should not be used because it has been associated with hypernatremia, erosion, and esophageal perforation.

**EQUIPMENT**

1.   Endoscopes
    a.   Standard or Therapeutic
        i.   Single channel, larger diameter channel
        ii.   Dual channel, instances when two devices may be required to manipulate object
2.   Retrieval Devices (5) (Refer to Table 35.1 for additional details; this includes representative manufacturers but is not intended to be comprehensive.)
    a.   Grasping forceps
    b.   Retrieval baskets
    c.   Loop snares
    d.   Roth Net retrieval device (U.S. Endoscopy, Mentor, OH)
    e.   Ligation cap from Stiegmann-Goff endoscopic ligator (Bard, Tewksbury, MA)
    f.   Magnetic extractor (Olympus, Melville, NY)

### Table 35.1. Retrieval devices.

| Instrument | Available sizes OW (mm) / MCS (mm) | Special features / uses | Manufacturer |
|---|---|---|---|
| Rat Tooth ± Alligator Jaw(AJ) (Fig. 35.3A) | 4.7 / 2.8<br>8.3 / 3.7<br>11.3 / 2.8 (AJ)<br>14.9 / 2.8 (AJ)<br>15.5 / 2.8<br>19.5 / 2.8 (AJ) | Wide variety of opening widths to accommodate the majority of foreign bodies regardless of size | Ballard Olympus FLEX |
| Shark Tooth ± Alligator Jaw(AJ) | 4.7 / 2.8<br>6.9 / 2.8 (AJ) | Rotatable in alligator jaw form, intended for removal of stents | Olympus |
| Alligator Jaw | 7.5 / 2.8<br>11.3 / 3.7 | Intended for sharp-edged objects | FLEX Olympus |
| 3-Prong (Fig. 35.3B) 4-Prong | 15 / 1.8<br>15 / 2.3 | Barbed tips to allow for grasping of edge or end of foreign body | ACMI Annex Medical Ballard Olympus Wilson Cook |
| Tripod Pentapod | 20.0 / 2.8 | Smooth rounded tips primarily designed for polyp retrieval, but may accommodate foreign bodies which could be enclosed within forceps | FLEX Olympus |

**Table 35.1. (continued)**

| Instrument | Available sizes OW (mm) / MCS (mm) | Special features / uses | Manufacturer |
|---|---|---|---|
| V-Shape/ Forked Jaw | 13.0 / 2.0 | W-shaped, wide opening prongs, retractable into sheath for thin and flat objects (e.g., coins) | FLEX Olympus |
| Rubber Tip | 4.8 / 2.0 <br> 7.3 / 2.8 | Rubber tips for slippery flat objects, needles, or nails | Olympus |
| 4-Wire Baskets Hexagonal (Fig. 35.3C) Spiral Circular Flower | OBD <br><br> 15 × 35 <br> 20 × 40 <br> 25 × 50 <br> 30 × 60 <br><br> 20 × 25 (N-Circle) <br> 35 × 60 (USE Rotatable) <br><br> MCS = 2.0 / 2.8 / 3.2 | Multiple Configurations Hexagonal Spiral/Helical Trapezoid Circular (N-Circle, WC) Flower (Olympus) 6 & 8 wire (WC) <br><br> Available in: Sterile-Disposable Sterile-Reusable Autoclave Rotatable (USE) | Ballard Boston Scientific Mill-Rose Olympus US Endoscopy Wilson Cook |
| Snares Oval (Fig. 35.3D) Duckbill Hexagonal Crescent | OW <br> 11 (X-Small) <br> 16 (Mini) <br> 23 (Medium) <br> 32 (Large) | Multiple Configurations Oval Crescent Hexagonal Duckbill Available in: Sterile-Disposable Rotatable (USE, BS) | Bard Ballard Boston Scientific Mill-Rose US Endoscopy Wilson Cook |

OW – opening width
MCS – minimum channel size
FLEX – First Line Endoscopic Accessories
ACMI – American Cytoscope Makers, Inc.

3.  Foreign Body Hood Protector (Ballard, Draper, UT)

4.  Overtubes. Esophageal and gastric lengths which allow for the following:

    a.  Airway protection
    b.  Multiple passes for piecemeal extraction
    c.  Protection of esophageal mucosa during retrieval of sharp objects

5.  Suction equipment

    a.  One wall-unit suction canister each for the endoscope and patient

6.  Fluoroscopic equipment (optional)

    a.  Helpful for extracting large radiopaque objects from stomach or duodenum

## PROCEDURE

### Simulation

1.  Perform a "dry run" by simulating the extraction prior to endoscope insertion.

2.  Using a replica (if available), experiment with various devices and grasping methods to determine the optimal approach.

### Intubation

1.  Assure proper functioning of suction equipment.

2.  Place the patient in the left lateral position with either head-of-bed elevation to 30° to 45° or reverse Trendelenburg position.

3.  Advance the endoscope into the hypopharynx, and note possible obstruction at the level of the cricopharyngeus, which might require endotracheal intubation or laryngoscopy for extraction.

4.  As the patient swallows, gently insert the endoscope into the esophageal lumen during relaxation of the cricopharyngeus.

5.  Once the endoscope has passed the upper esophageal sphincter, advance it under direct vision with minimal air insufflation or fluid lavage until the foreign body/food impaction is reached. Direct visualization is necessary at all times in order to avoid inadvertently striking the object, resulting in further impaction or penetration into the mucosal wall.

### Overtube Insertion

1.  Overtubes can be backloaded onto the endoscope and then advanced forward after esophageal intubation.

2.  As a result of inherent stiffness and diameter discrepancy (compared to the gastroscope), attempts to advance the overtube (especially the esophageal length) beyond the

hypopharyngeal shelf may be met with considerable resistance and have even resulted in perforation.

    a.  Softening the overtube by running it under warm water can be helpful to reduce the stiffness element.

    b.  Passage of a 42-Fr Maloney dilator backloaded with the overtube can eliminate the diameter discrepancy making for less traumatic insertion.

The endoscopic equipment used to remove upper intestinal foreign bodies varies by the type of object and is discussed in further detail below.

## Esophageal Food Impaction

1. Avoid excessive fluid lavage to prevent aspiration, especially with large amounts of retained food debris or high-grade esophageal obstruction. Use an air-filled syringe to clear debris from the suction channel of the endoscope instead.

2. If retrograde removal of the food bolus appears to be necessary, then one of the following approaches should be pursued:

    a.  Use a friction-fit adaptor from a single band ligation kit (Bard) attached to the tip of the endoscope, which can then facilitate aspiration of food fragments into the "cap" for withdrawal.

    b.  Use the Roth Net (U.S. Endoscopy) to collect food particles for withdrawal.

    c.  Place an esophageal-length overtube to protect the airway and to facilitate piecemeal extraction.

    d.  Request endotracheal intubation to provide airway protection during withdrawal of the foreign body.

3. Otherwise, attempt to advance endoscope around the food impaction to exclude underlying esophageal pathology after which the food bolus can be gently pushed into the stomach. Recent evidence suggests that judicious application of pressure on the bolus, even in the absence of excluding distal pathology, can safely relieve a majority of food impactions (6).

4. Consider performing esophageal dilation after disimpaction if there are no obvious contraindications. It may be wise to avoid this if prolonged impaction has led to significant mucosal irritation.

## Blunt Objects

Blunt objects should be removed with devices that are best suited for the shape of the object.

1. Extraction of coins can be accomplished with any number of devices, including grasping forceps (e.g., V shape, rat tooth), a Roth Net, retrieval baskets, or loop snares.

2. Disc batteries, as well as smooth rounded objects, are most effectively removed using the Roth Net (7).

3. Blunt objects longer than 6 to 10 cm (e.g., toothbrushes, spoons) can be grasped with a snare close to the cephalad

end of the object such that it will align itself with the long
axis of the esophagus during withdrawal. Other options
include the following:

   a.  Use of a gastric length overtube followed by withdrawal
      of the entire apparatus

   b.  Double wire-loop snare technique (Fig. 35.1) with a
      dual-channel therapeutic endoscope to manage the ori-
      entation of the object during withdrawal (8)

4.  Objects within the esophagus that cannot be secured may be
    advanced into the stomach to facilitate a position that may
    allow for easier grasping.

5.  Consider use of an overtube to provide airway protection in
    the event the foreign body is dislodged during withdrawal
    through the hypopharynx.

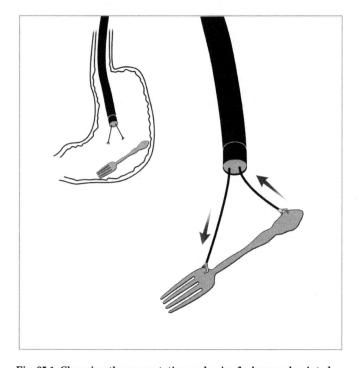

**Fig. 35.1. Changing the presentation and axis of a long and pointed
ingested object. Use a double wire-loop snare or double forceps to
rotate the foreign body by pulling on one end of the object and
pushing on the other; correct orientation is with the sharp end
trailing on withdrawal.**

## Sharp Objects

1. Determine the optimal device for grasping the object and the optimal orientation to allow for removal.

   a. Polypectomy snares may be superior for removal of both toothpicks and tacks, although grasping forceps and retrieval basket are also successful (7).

   b. The Roth Net may be less effective than other instruments in retrieval of sharp objects such as a tack or toothpick (7).

2. Use maneuvers or equipment intended to minimize mucosal trauma during extraction.

   a. Distend the esophagus with full insufflation to minimize mucosal contact.

   b. Always orient the object with the pointed end or sharp edge trailing during extraction.

   c. Fit a protector hood on the tip of the endoscope as depicted (Fig. 35.2). The hood maintains its inverted position during insertion of the endoscope; during withdrawal the bell portion then flips back to its original shape enclosing the sharp object within the hood protector.

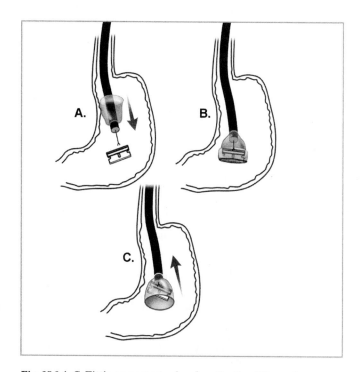

**Fig. 35.2 A–C. Fitting a protector hood on the tip of the endoscope.**

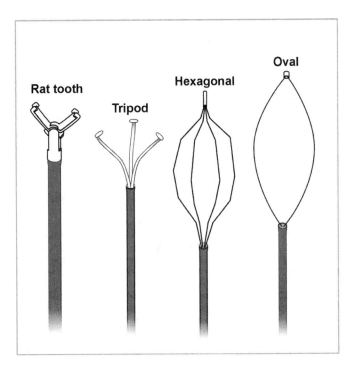

**Fig. 35.3. Types of snares.**

d. Use an overtube to protect the esophageal mucosa and to provide airway protection in the event the foreign body is dislodged during withdrawal of the hypopharynx.

e. Use the cut-off fingertip of a glove as a satchel in which to deposit multiple sharp objects, and then grasp both sides of the open end to close and withdraw (9).

f. A novel technique to grasp a safety pin with forceps and subsequently close with a snare has been described (10).

## POSTPROCEDURE

1. Monitor the patient for signs or symptoms of perforation following the intervention for an acceptable recovery period.

2. Perform immediate contrast study (e.g., gastrograffin) if there is clinical suspicion of perforation, especially if the extraction was difficult or complicated.

3. Restrict diet to clear liquids or pureed foods when appropriate depending on the amount of intervention and the timing of the next intervention.

4. Determine disposition and an appropriate follow-up plan, such as repeat endoscopy for dilation of identified esophageal pathology.

## COMPLICATIONS

1. Failure rate is generally considered to be very low, probably 1% to 4%, although one study reports a failure rate of 24% (1,11).

2. Rigid endoscopy was associated with a higher complication rate than flexible endoscopy in one review where both modalities were used (10% versus 5%) (1).

3. Reported complication rates from endoscopy for ingested foreign body range from 0% to 5.1%. However, many large series indicate negligible (< 0.5%) risk, as many report no morbidity or mortality associated with the endoscopic procedure (1).

4. Specific complications associated with endoscopic disimpaction/retrieval include the following:
   a. Mucosal laceration
   b. Hemorrhage
   c. Aspiration
   d. Mediastinitis
   e. Perforation
   f. Death

5. No complications have been specifically attributable to retrieval devices, although bleeding and perforation have been reported with overtube insertion.

### CPT Codes

**43215** – Esophagoscopy, rigid or flexible; with removal of foreign body.

**43247** – Upper gastrointestinal endoscopy including esophagus, stomach, and either the duodenum and/or jejunum as appropriate; with removal of foreign body.

**44363** – Small intestinal endoscopy, enteroscopy beyond second portion of duodenum, not including ileum; with removal of foreign body.

### REFERENCES

1. Webb WA. Management of foreign bodies of the upper gastrointestinal tract: update. *Gastrointest Endosc* 1995;41:39–51.
2. Brady PG. Esophageal foreign bodies. *Gastro Clinics North Am* 1991;20:691–701.
3. ASGE. Guideline for the management of ingested foreign bodies. *Gastrointest Endosc* 2002;55:802–806.
4. Ginsberg GG. Management of ingested foreign objects and food bolus impactions. *Gastrointest Endosc* 1995;41:33–38.
5. ASGE. Endoscopic retrieval devices. *Gastrointest Endosc* 1999;50:932–934.
6. Vicari JJ. Outcomes of acute esophageal food impaction: success of the push technique. *Gastrointest Endosc* 2001; 53:178–181.
7. Faigel DO, Stotland BR, Kochman ML, et al. Device choice and experience level in endoscopic foreign object retrieval: an in vivo study. *Gastrointest Endosc* 1997;45:490–492.
8. Yong PTL. Removal of a dinner fork from the stomach by double-snare endoscopic extraction. *HKMJ* 2000; 6:319–321.

9. Whelan RL. Retrieval of five razor blades from the stomach using a new endoscopic technique. *Gastrointest Endosc* 1995; 41:161–163.

10. Karjoo M. A novel technique for closing and removing an open safety pin from the stomach. *Gastrointest Endosc* 2003;57: 627–629.

11. Mosca S. Endoscopic management of foreign bodies in the upper gastrointestinal tract: report on a series of 414 adult patients. *Endoscopy* 2001;33:692–696.

# Capsule Endoscopy

Blair S. Lewis

An endoscopic capsule (Given Imaging Limited, Yoqneam, Israel) obtains images from the entire small bowel (1). Individual digital images are transmitted out of the body by radio frequency to a recording device worn about the patient's waist. The images are viewed as a video on a computer workstation at a later date.

## INDICATIONS

Capsule endoscopy is indicated as a procedure for evaluation of suspected disease of the small intestine including the following:

1. Obscure gastrointestinal (GI) bleeding (2): These are patients with GI bleeding in whom no diagnosis has been made despite colonoscopy and upper endoscopy. Capsule endoscopy has been shown to be superior to push enteroscopy and to x-ray studies of the small bowel in the evaluation of these patients (3).

2. Known or suspected Crohn's disease: In one study capsule endoscopy detected all the lesions seen on small bowel series and computed tomography scanning and detected additional lesions in 47% of cases (4).

3. Other suspected small bowel pathology. A growing body of literature supports the superiority of capsule endoscopy over other imaging modalities of the small bowel (5).

## CONTRAINDICATIONS

1. Swallowing disorders (though the capsule can be placed endoscopically)

2. Implanted pacemakers and defibrillators

3. Small bowel obstruction

## PREPARATION

The typical timing of a capsule exam is to begin the study at 8 a.m. and disconnect the patient from the recorder at 4 p.m. This allows 8 hours of image acquisition during one working day.

1. Instruct the patient to present on the morning of the exam after a 12-hour fast.

2. Discontinue oral iron supplementation 3 days prior to the exam.

3. Instruct patients not to smoke cigarettes since this may cause a change in the color of the stomach lining.

4. Advise them not to take medications or antacids; medications such as sucralfate can coat the intestinal lining limiting visualization. Narcotics and antispasmodics can delay both

gastric and intestinal emptying, making it difficult to visualize the entire small bowel during the 8-hour acquisition time.

5.   Instruct patients to bring their medications with them to take during the day, if necessary. If a patient is diabetic, insulin doses may need to be adjusted.

6.   Anticoagulants do not need to be stopped prior to the exam.

7.   Instruct the patient to wear loose clothing on the day of the exam. Dresses should be avoided. A buttoned shirt and loose-fitting pants work best.

8.   Charge the recorder's battery pack through a standard outlet the evening prior to the study.

**EQUIPMENT**

1.   The capsule (Fig. 36.1): Measuring $11 \times 26$ mm, this contains 6 light-emitting diodes, a lens, a color camera chip, two silver oxide batteries, a radio frequency transmitter, and an antenna. The camera is a complementary metal oxide semiconductor chip. This chip requires less power than charged coupled device chips presently found on video endoscopes and digital cameras, and it can operate at very low levels of illumination. The capsule obtains 2 images per second and transmits the data via radio frequency to the recording device worn about the patient's waist. The capsule is disposable and does not need to be retrieved by the patient. It is passed naturally in a bowel movement.

2.   The recording device: This is a mini-computer worn on a belt with 5 gigahertz of memory, allowing for storage of the 57,600 images obtained during a typical 8-hour examination. Once the study is completed, the recording device is downloaded to a computer workstation with software that provides the images to the computer screen.

3.   The workstation: This contains software that interprets several aspects of the data obtained. In addition to the video images, the system is designed to grossly identify the capsule's location within the small bowel. There is an algorithm in the workstation software that determines the capsule's location in two dimensions based on the signal strength at the individual sensors of the sensor array (6). A drawing of the small bowel passage is produced that provides a location for each of the images obtained during the 8 hours. This localization is an estimate since not only does the capsule move within the intestine, but the small bowel also moves within the abdominal cavity. Thus the proximal jejunum can be located in the right lower quadrant or the left upper quadrant. In addition, the bowel's location is related to the position of the patient. For example, the small bowel can sag to the pelvis while a patient is standing. Still, when the diagram produced is combined with the knowledge of the length of time the capsule has been in the small bowel, along with the time between pyloric passage and an identified lesion, and the amount of visible bowel traversed to the lesion and

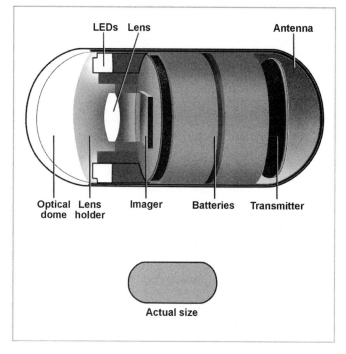

**Fig. 36.1. The Video Capsule.**

from a lesion to the ileocecal valve, an approximation of the location of the lesion can be made.

In addition to localization software, the system also contains an image recognition algorithm that identifies red pixels in the data. This identifies possible areas of bleeding or the possible presence of vascular lesions (7).

**PROCEDURE**

1. Enter the patient's personal data into the computer workstation.

2. Initialize the recording device to the patient. This ensures that once completed the recording device data cannot be confused with that of any other patient.

3. Apply the sensor array to the patient's abdomen. This will capture the signals from the capsule and carry them to the recording device. The sensor array leads are attached by adhesive to the patient's abdomen. Some patients may need to be shaved prior to sensor attachment.

4. Place the empty belt around the patient's waist.

5. Place the recording device and battery pack into the belt pockets.

6. Attach the sensor leads to the recording device.

7. Attach the recording device to the battery pack. The powered recorder will illuminate its light for a short period of time. The light will go out once the hard drive has successfully booted.

8. Remove the capsule from its blister pack. Removing the capsule from the magnet in the pack turns the capsule on, and it begins to flash and transmit its images twice per second. The recorder's light flashes in synchrony with the capsule, attesting to successful transmission of each image.

9. Instruct the patient to swallow the capsule, followed by a full glass of water. We ask patients to drink two additional glasses of water to assure that the capsule does not simply lie in the esophagus.

10. Advise the patient that he or she may then leave the facility and carry on a normal day. The patient should a) refrain from exercising and heavy lifting during the exam, b) avoid large transmitters and magnetic resonance imaging (MRI) machines, c) not stand directly next to another patient undergoing capsule endoscopy, d) not touch the recorder or the antenna array leads, e) not remove the leads, and f) not take the belt or the shoulder straps off; in addition, the patient should be very careful when bringing up underwear over the sensors to avoid disconnection. The patient may a) walk, sit, and lie down; b) drive a car; c) return to work; d) use a computer, radio, stereo, or cell phone; e) loosen the Velcro on the belt to facilitate going to the bathroom; f) eat beginning 4 hours after swallowing the capsule; and g) take his or her medications at that time.

**POSTPROCEDURE**

1. When the patient returns after 8 hours, remove the belt and the sensor arrays.

2. Instruct the patient to avoid having an MRI until the capsule passes. Should passage not be seen, an abdominal flat-plate can be obtained.

3. Discharge the patient.

4. Clear the download memory in the workstation.

5. Attach the recorder to the workstation. Generally downloads last two and one-half hours.

6. Once the download is complete, disconnect the recorder from the workstation, or it can be initialized for a new patient.

7. Review the images on the workstation.

**INTERPRETATION**

Prior to reading a capsule study, physicians should be familiar with the patient's medical history, not only including the indication for the study but also any surgical history. Prior knowledge of a surgical small bowel anastomosis can aid or simplify the interpretation of the study. In addition, physicians must have experience in interpreting endoscopic images. The reader must be able to make a diagnosis based on the images. This will allow the dismissal of normal variants and nonpathologic lesions and the identification of specific pathologies requiring specific therapies. The images obtained at capsule endoscopy are slightly different from traditional endoscopy, since there is no air distention of the bowel wall and the capsule is at times located within millimeters of the mucosa. This is so-called "physiologic endoscopy". The bowel is not altered by the process of the examination. There is no sedation used, and thus there are no hemodynamic effects. There is no trauma caused by the capsule. There is no air insufflation to affect the microvasculature.

There are very specific steps that can be taken to ease the process of reading a capsule exam. A pattern of practice must be developed by the physician. The following is recommended:

1.  Examine the very last image to assure that the colon has been entered. The presence of stool will confirm this finding.

2.  After returning to the very first image, activate blood detection software (if the exam was performed in the setting of obscure gastrointestinal bleeding). To scan the entire study including the stomach, the first image is falsely identified as the first duodenal image on a thumbnail edit. This turns on the Suspected Blood Indicator (SBI) software. Any positive findings can be quickly examined and thumbnails created. Once completed, the first image thumbnail is deleted.

3.  Identify the three specific locations needed to determine both the gastric and small bowel emptying times. Increase the image rate to 25 frames/second, and play the images forward in an automatic mode. The esophagogastric junction is quickly seen, and the first gastric image is duly noted on a thumbnail edit. Using the time bar, quickly advance the images forward and backward until the first image of the duodenum is identified. This too is noted on a thumbnail edit. It should be remembered that the capsule can move backward and forward through the pylorus several times prior to its final passage and further advancement into the small bowel. Again, use the time bar to identify the ileocecal valve. This landmark proves to be quite difficult for many physicians. The presence of formed stool is a definite indicator of the colon. It can take some time for the beginning reader to reliably identify this landmark, and then note it on a thumbnail edit.

4.  Calculate transit times. The average gastric time is approximately 60 minutes, the average time in the small bowel is 240 minutes, and the average passage time to the colon is 300 minutes (8). An 8-hour acquisition time assures that most capsules will reach the colon, allowing for complete inspection of the small bowel.

5.  Once the landmarks have been thumbnailed, view the images. The gastric portion of the exam should be examined,

but it can be viewed at a rapid rate. In the small bowel, starting at the first image of the duodenum, use the multi-viewer function to scan two images side by side at a total rate of 20 frames/second or 10 frames/second of the individual images A mouse with a jogwheel is always kept at the ready. If reading is performed on a laptop computer, a mouse should be attached, since this greatly eases the reading process. When an area moves by too quickly or if a possible abnormality is seen, movement of the jogwheel will stop the progress of the images and allow review of the passed images. The capsule moves extremely quickly in the proximal small bowel as compared to the distal sections. In the duodenum, the frame-to-finding ratio is quite high, and thus the duodenum often requires using the jogwheel to examine each individual image. The frame-to-finding ratio in the ileum is quite low, and the use of the jogwheel diminishes distally. When an abnormality is identified, a thumbnail is created. Routinely creating thumbnails for every 30 minutes of images viewed is recommended. This allows the reader to stop, to read, and to find where the reading stopped and also prevents having to start over should the reader lose his or her place.

6. Review localization data. This allows the physician to know if an identified abnormality is within reach of a push entero-scope. The information can also guide subsequent surgery. Generally, the localization drawing well identifies the duodenum and ligament of Treitz. The physician derives location of an abnormality within the jejunum or ileum from a compilation of data. This includes the quadrant location provided by the localization drawing, the time of passage from the pylorus to the lesion, the amount of bowel visually traversed by the capsule en route to the lesions, and the amount of bowel traversed from the lesion to the ileocecal valve. This information is difficult to quantify, but qualitative judgments by an experienced physician can be quite accurate in providing a location and thus a differentiation between those patients treated with enteroscopic therapy and those requiring surgical intervention. Lesions found within one hour of passage from the pylorus and those located in the left abdomen are generally within reach of a 2.5-m-long push enteroscope. This statement is based on a typical small bowel passage time of 4 hours and a normal progression of the capsule within the proximal small bowel. Occasionally, a capsule may remain for a prolonged time in the duodenal bulb, altering the above generalizations. Lesions more than 1 hour beyond the pylorus may occasionally be reached by a push enteroscope, but those beyond the 2-hour mark generally require surgical intervention for management.

## COMPLICATIONS

1. Capsule retention. Experience reveals that this occurs in approximately 1% of examinations. The capsule is typically retained at a site of pathology that is likely to require

surgery such as nonsteroidal antiinflammatory drugs or Crohn's stricture or a partially obstructing tumor. It does not routinely become lodged in colonic diverticula or in the appendiceal orifice. Retention only rarely causes symptoms of obstruction. A normal small bowel series does not mean that a capsule cannot become retained.

## OTHER USES FOR THIS TECHNIQUE

1. Suspected Crohn's disease
2. Celiac disease
3. Chronic abdominal pain

### CPT Codes

**91110 -** Gastrointestinal tract imaging, intraluminal (e.g., capsule endoscopy), esophagus through ileum, with physician interpretation and report.

The diagnosis codes associated with capsule endoscopy are dependent on the indication and findings. The most common codes are those for GI bleeding, once colonoscopy and upper endoscopy are nondiagnostic.

### REFERENCES

1. Meron G. The development of the swallowable video capsule (M2A). *Gastrointest Endosc* 2000;6:817–819.
2. Lewis B, Goldfarb N. The advent of capsule endoscopy — a not-so-futuristic approach to obscure gastrointestinal bleeding. *Aliment Pharmacol Ther* 2003;17:1085–1096.
3. Costamagna G, Shah S, Riccioni M, et al. A prospective trial comparing small bowel radiographs and video capsule endoscopy for suspected small bowel disease. *Gastroenterology* 2002;123: 999–1005.
4. Eliakim R, Fischer D, Suissa A, et al. Wireless capsule video endoscopy is a superior diagnostic tool in comparison to barium follow-through and computerized tomography in patients with suspected Crohn's disease. *Eur J Gastroenterol Hepatol* 2003;15:363–367.
5. Scapa E, Jacob H, Lewkowicz S, et al. Initial experience of wireless-capsule endoscopy for evaluating occult gastrointestinal bleeding and suspected small bowel pathology. *Am J Gastroenterol* 2002;97:2776–2779.
6. Fischer D, Shreiber R, Meron G, et al. Localization of a wireless capsule endoscope in the GI tract. *Gastrointest Endosc* 2001;53: AB126.
7. Liangpunsakul S, Mays L, Rex D. Performance of given suspected blood indicator. *Am J Gastroenterol* 2003;98:2676–2678.
8. Appleyard Glukhovsky A, Jacob H, et al. Transit times for the capsule endoscope. *Gastrointest Endosc* 2001;53:AB122.

# Stretta

Douglas Corley

The goal of developing endoscopic and endoluminal treatments for gastroesophageal reflux disease (GERD) is to safely improve gastroesophageal reflux symptoms while decreasing the need for daily medication use. Radiofrequency energy delivered to the gastroesophageal junction and cardia (a.k.a. the "Stretta procedure") is one of several such treatments recently introduced. A randomized trial demonstrated that patients receiving the Stretta procedure had fewer GERD symptoms and a higher overall quality of life than patients receiving a sham procedure (1). Other results, however, were mixed; only about half of the treated patients had a substantial response, and although the treated responders decreased their acid exposure compared with baseline values, on average the treated patients as a whole did not have a lower acid exposure than did the sham group and did not have less medication use. These results differed from those of open-label trials that demonstrated improvements in acid exposure and medication use compared with baseline values (2). Evaluation of the long-term effectiveness of all endoscopic and endoluminal techniques is pending, and no comparative trials of the different techniques currently exist.

The net results of open-label and randomized trials suggest the Stretta procedure is effective at improving symptoms in some patients but that it is not appropriate for patients with complicated GERD. The results also emphasize the critical need for sham-controlled trials of all new gastrointestinal procedures prior to widespread clinical use.

We present here both the technique used in the randomized and open-label trials and the technique currently recommended by Curon Medical (the manufacturer of the Stretta equipment). This document serves as a general guide but should be supplemented by formal training, since the procedure is not a direct extension of common gastrointestinal techniques.

## INDICATIONS

1. Typical GERD symptoms (e.g., heartburn, reflux, acid regurgitation) that are at least partially responsive to antisecretory medications. Until adequate data are available, endoscopic procedures for GERD are not indicated for atypical manifestations of GERD such as asthma, pharyngitis, etc.

2. A 24-hour pH monitor that confirms the presence of increased esophageal acid exposure.

## CONTRAINDICATIONS

1. Complicated GERD (e.g., esophageal ulcerations, esophageal strictures)

2. Substantial anatomical defects (e.g., hiatal hernia >2 cm in size)

3.   Prominent dysphagia

4.   Unless supportive data becomes available, exclude patients with substantial disorders of esophageal motility, such as achalasia or esophageal aperistalsis.

5.   Unstable cardiac, pulmonary, or other life-threatening conditions

6.   Significant bleeding diathesis or need for continuous anticoagulation

7.   Pregnancy

**PREPARATION**

1.   Patients should be NPO for at least 6 hours prior to the procedure.

2.   Obtain written consent (see potential complications section for rates unique to this procedure). Also consult with patients about the standard cardiopulmonary risks of conscious sedation and for postprocedure retrosternal discomfort.

3.   Start an intravenous (IV) line to administer conscious sedation. Given that the procedure may last up to an hour, consider giving supplemental long-acting agents such as diphenhydramine.

4.   Place a grounding pad.

**EQUIPMENT**

1.   Standard diagnostic upper endoscope

2.   Stretta catheter, generator, grounding pad. The catheter consists of a flexible balloon-basket assembly with four electrode needle sheaths (the Stretta system, Curon Medical, Sunnyvale, CA). The generator includes a monitor that permits measurement of electrode temperature and impedance and uses a computer algorithm that will shut off electrodes that reach an excessive temperature or have the incorrect impedance (suggesting that the electrodes are not imbedded in tissue).

3.   2 to 4 L of chilled, sterile water (not saline) in standard IV-type bags

4.   Lubricant

5.   Gloves

6.   Suction set-ups for the endoscope and the Stretta catheter

**PROCEDURE**

1.   Set up and test the Stretta equipment. Confirm placement of the grounding pad on the patient, and attach the catheter and foot pedal to the generator. Insert the floppy disk into the generator, and boot the computer. Attach the irrigation and suction lines (keep suction turned off until the catheter is in the patient) to their respective ports on the catheter. Confirm that any flow restriction devices on the irrigation line are in the full open position. Connect the

syringe to the balloon's inflation port, and test it by fully inflating the balloon with 25 cc of air. The syringe comes with an optional pressure relief valve.

2.  With the balloon inflated, test the needle deployment by fully advancing the deployment slide lever. Do not test the needle deployment with the balloon deflated; this may result in the puncture of the balloon. Ensure that the balloon is deflated and the needles are retracted during catheter insertion, movement between treatment positions, and instrument withdrawal.

3.  Elevate the head of the bed to minimize aspiration risk.

4.  Perform a standard diagnostic upper endoscopy. Evaluate the esophagus for the presence of potential contraindications (e.g., large hiatal hernia, substantial esophagitis, etc.).

5.  Carefully measure the distance from the teeth to the squamocolumnar junction, and confirm that the squamocolumnar junction approximates the muscular pinch of the gastroesophageal junction; this distance will be used to approximate the distance needed for probe placement of the radiofrequency delivery catheter.

6.  Introduce the radiofrequency delivery catheter by mouth. The introduction technique is similar to the method used for introducing a dilator. The clinical trials used direct passage similar to the introduction of a Maloney dilator; subsequently, the catheter has been modified to permit the optional use of a guidewire. The catheter balloon assembly is stiff; a gloved hand can be used to assist the passage of the assembly past the curvature of the hard palate. Generously lubricate the balloon assembly, and slightly hyperextend the patient's neck to permit easier passage of the catheter assembly.

7.  Using the measurements obtained in Step 5, advance the catheter to the gastroesophageal junction. Because the catheter is stiffer than the endoscope, it has less bending in the oropharynx, and the measurements from the teeth to the gastroesophageal junction are typically 0.5 to 2 cm shorter for the catheter assembly than those obtained using the endoscope. Thus, it may be advisable to place the first set of treatments approximately 1 cm more proximally than the endoscopically measured distance to the gastroesophageal junction. For example, if the measured distance from the teeth to the gastroesophageal (GE) junction using the endoscope is 40 cm, place the first treatment set at 39 cm from the teeth using the measurements on the Stretta catheter.

8.  Inflate the balloon until mild resistance is met (called a "push back" of 3 to 4 cc of air in the syringe); the feel for this mild resistance will become apparent after several inflations and can be practiced prior to insertion of the catheter by inflating the balloon against mild resistance in

a closed hand (Fig. 37.1A). If the balloon is not adequately inflated, the esophageal wall tension will not be sufficient to permit needle puncture; if the balloon is excessively inflated, it will migrate out of its desired position, particularly when it is within the narrower region of the gastroesophageal junction (similar to the movement of a wet seed when squeezed between a thumb and forefinger). Once this pressure is achieved, disconnect the syringe (the balloon will now stay inflated at this pressure).

9. Fully deploy the electrode needles (22 gauge, 5.5 mm long) to puncture the esophageal mucosa, and then withdraw the needles to the treatment position on the catheter slide lever. Depressing the foot pedal will initiate energy delivery and irrigation; the device will continue delivering energy until the preset time is completed or until the limits on impedance or tissue temperature are exceeded. Pressing the pedal a second time will also stop both processes. The initial trials delivered radiofrequency energy for 90 seconds; Curon Medical currently presets the delivery time to 60 seconds (Fig. 37.1B).

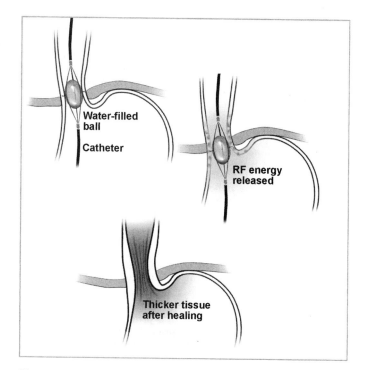

Fig. 37.1. A: Correct position of balloon. B: Demonstration of treatment area. C: Postprocedure appearance.

10. Immediately after energy delivery is completed (or if the patient is moving, or if you feel there is any reason it is unsafe to continue with the needles deployed), retract the needles fully and deflate the balloon. Rotate the catheter to the right 45°, reinflate the balloon, redeploy the needles as described above, and repeat the procedure.

11. Once the second (or third, if you are following the protocol of the trial) set of lesions at this level is completed, again retract the needles and deflate the balloon. Advance the catheter 0.5 cm to a new level and repeat two additional treatments in the same manner.

12. After placing two levels of treatments (a total of four needle deployments, two at each level), introduce a well-lubricated endoscope alongside the catheter (with the balloon deflated), and confirm the location of the treatments. These will appear as small puncture marks often with small surrounding white areas of tissue coagulation.

13. Adjust the position of the catheter for the next set of treatments, withdraw the endoscope, and repeat this process serially every 0.5 cm in the desired distribution (see item 17 below for details). Now deliver two levels of "pull back" lesions.

14. To deliver the "pull back" lesions, advance the catheter into the stomach, then fully inflate the balloon to 25 cc, and gently pull back on the catheter to pull the balloon against the gastric cardia until slight resistance is felt. This treatment level usually measures at approximately the distance to the GE junction. Fully extend the needles as described above, and deliver a treatment. Retract the needles, advance the catheter slightly into the stomach to free the balloon from the mucosa, rotate the catheter 45° to the right, again retract the inflated balloon against the cardia, deploy the needles, and repeat the treatment. Now, again retract the needles, rotate the device 90° to the left (this will be 45° to the left of the original first treatment at this level), pull the balloon against the cardia a third time, redeploy the needles, and repeat another treatment. This will result in three treatments at this level of the cardia.

15. Now, advance the catheter into the stomach again, deflate the balloon, reinflate it with 22 cc of air, and withdraw the catheter against the cardia until it meets slight resistance; due to retraction of the stomach, this level usually measures 0.5 to 1 cm above the GE junction by the scale.

16. Repeat three treatments at this level of the cardia (a total of six treatments, three at each of two levels in the cardia). At the end of the procedure, it is prudent to reintroduce the well-lubricated endoscope prior to catheter removal to again confirm the desired areas have been appropriately treated (Fig. 37.1C).

17. For the randomized trial, there were a total of 22 total lesion sets. There were eight levels of lesions with two sets

per ring; the most proximal ring was 2 cm above the Z-line, the most distal ring was 1.5 cm below the Z-line with a 5-mm separation between rings plus an additional two sets of "pull-back" lesion sets, each with three sets of lesions per ring. Curon Medical currently recommends patients be treated with 14 lesion sets; this regimen uses two sets every 0.5 cm from 1 cm proximal to the gastroesophageal junction to 0.5 cm below the gastroesophageal junction, plus two levels of "pull back" lesions; this represents a total of four levels, with two sets at each level, plus six "pull back" lesion sets. These regimens have not been compared against each or tested against other regimens.

## POSTPROCEDURE

1. Monitor vital signs.

2. Keep the head of the bed elevated to minimize aspiration risk.

3. Some patients experience transient dysphagia postprocedure; thus, it is prudent to advise patient to take only liquids and soft solids for 1 to 2 days postprocedure.

4. Much of the treatment effect is not immediate but likely occurs after remodeling of the GE junction lesions. Thus, patients should continue their current medications for 3 to 4 weeks after treatment. If symptoms return, medications can be restarted and another attempt at discontinuation can be attempted 2 to 3 months after treatment.

5. Patients can take acetaminophen for mild retrosternal/epigastric discomfort but should be cautioned to report substantial pain, fever, or other symptoms concerning perforation or another major complication and avoid aspirin and nonsteroidal antiinflammatory drugs.

## COMPLICATIONS

1. No perforations, deaths, or postprocedure esophageal motility abnormalities occurred in the open-label or randomized trials; one treated patient had self-limited bleeding, and one patient in the sham group developed an aspiration pneumonia (2).

2. Radiofrequency energy treatment has not been reported to interfere with the subsequent performance of antireflux surgery (3).

3. During the first 6 months of general commercial use after approval by the United States Food and Drug Administration, ten complications occurred in 453 cases (2.2%) consisting of four perforations, two bleeding episodes, two mucosal injuries, one fatal aspiration a week postprocedure, and one effusion. The treatments for the perforations are not fully documented; some required open surgery, and some were treated without open surgery. In the next two 6-month intervals, an additional 1,331 cases were performed, with significant adverse event rates for these intervals of 0.6% and 0.1%, respectively (4).

## CPT Codes

**43257** – Upper gastrointestinal endoscopy including esophagus, stomach, and either the duodenum and/or jejunum as appropriate; with delivery of thermal energy to the muscle of lower esophageal sphincter and/or gastric cardia, for treatment of gastroesophageal reflux disease, for the Stretta procedure.

## REFERENCES

1. Corley DA, Katz P, Wo JM, et al. Improvement of gastroesophageal reflux symptoms after radiofrequency energy: a randomized, sham-controlled trial. *Gastroenterology* 2003;125(3): 668–676.
2. Triadafilopoulos G, DiBaise JK, Nostrant TT, et al. The Stretta procedure for the treatment of GERD: 6 and 12 month follow-up of the U.S. open label trial. *Gastrointest Endosc* 2002;55(2): 149–156.
3. Triadafilopoulos G, Utley DS. Temperature-controlled radiofrequency energy delivery for gastroesophageal reflux disease: the Stretta procedure. *J Laparoendosc Adv Surg Tech A* 2001;11(6): 333–339.
4. Fleischer D. The Stretta procedure: technique optimization and complication rates. *Gastrointest Endosc* 2002;55:AB256.

# Enteryx Injection for Gastroesophageal Reflux Disease

David A. Johnson

Enteryx (Microvasive) is a bioinert polymer (ethylene vinyl alcohol copolymer) which has a radiopaque marker (tantalum) in a liquid solvent (dimethyl sulfoxide [DMSO]). This low viscosity solution precipitates as a spongy material that becomes a permanent implant. This device was approved by the Food and Drug Administration in April 2003 for the treatment of symptomatic gastroesophageal reflux disease (GERD).

## INDICATIONS

Enteryx is indicated for use in the endoscopic injection into the region of the lower esophageal sphincter in patients with symptomatic GERD who have had a good response to proton pump inhibitor therapy but continue to require daily medical therapy.

## CONTRAINDICATIONS

1. Patients who are poor candidates to undergo the sedation and endoscopy required for the implantation of this device
2. Patients with portal hypertension, where injection of the implant device into the distal esophagus might have incremental risk
3. Patients with suspected GERD who were nonresponders to medical therapy. The efficacy data was confined to only those patients with typical GERD symptoms of heartburn and regurgitation, who were responsive to medical therapy.
4. There are no data yet on the use in the treatment of extraesophageal GERD.

## PATIENT PREPARATION

1. The patient should be fully apprised of the indications, contraindications, efficacy, and safety data on Enteryx and informed that this is not a removable device.
2. The patient should be informed of the published peer reviewed publication data to date with specific annotation of the length of follow-up.
3. The preprocedural patient preparation is standard for upper endoscopy.
4. Patients are kept on their proton pump inhibitors (PPIs) up to and 10 days after their procedure.
5. Preprocedural prophylactic antibiotics are given at the discretion of the physician but are not required.

## EQUIPMENT

The upper endoscope used for this procedure must have a working channel lined with polytetrafluorethylene (PTFE), polyethylene, or polypropylene which are all compatible with DMSO which is the liquid primer solution. The operator should check with the original manufacturer of the gastroscope or the reconditioner (if reconditioned) to ensure compatibility. Similarly, the injection needles used for this must be DMSO-compatible, and only the Enteryx injection needles should be used. Provision for fluoroscopy during the procedure is required.

The component parts of the sterile Enteryx procedure kit include the following:

| | |
|---|---|
| Enteryx solution (1) | 10 mL |
| DMSO primer solution (1) | 10 mL |
| Enteryx injector (1) | 2.4 mm × 165 cm |
| Syringes (2) | 1 mL |
| Needles (2) | 18 gauge × 1.5 in. |

## PREPARATION

1.  Read all of the instructions for use.

2.  Inspect the kit, and make sure there is no damage to the component parts.

3.  The Enteryx and primer solutions should be at or above 65° F (19° C). If the product freezes, it should be warmed and thawed at room temperature before use.

4.  Begin shaking the Enteryx vial for at least 10 minutes. This is to ensure that the tantalum radiopaque marker is uniformly distributed in the colorless Enteryx solution. This is critical to ensure appropriate direction of the implant under fluoroscopy.

5.  Remind the nurses and technical staff that the Enteryx solution to be injected must be kept in constant motion (rocking back and forth) to ensure even distribution of the components.

6.  Remove the injection catheter, and uncoil the Enteryx injector needle prior to deploying and testing needle extension and retraction. Failure to test the catheter before use may cause damage, and if this occurs, the needle catheter should be discarded and replaced.

7.  Draw 1 mL of primer into the syringe, and flush injection catheter.

8.  Draw 1 mL of Enteryx solution into syringe, and prime catheter with 0.75 mL at 0.1 mL/second. The black-colored Enteryx/tantalum solution should be injected to 1 in from the tip of the catheter after priming. This shortened level of priming is to ensure that there is not a dripping out of the needle into the injection needle sheath. If that occurs, the Enteryx solution becomes sticky and may impede the

needle retraction/advance mechanism or impede the flow of the injection. Premature precipitation of the Enteryx solution may also occur if the liquid comes in contact with saline, blood, or mucosal fluid.

9. Draw 1 mL of Enteryx solution into the second syringe, and attach to the catheter. Confirm that the needle is retracted.

10. Refill the priming syringe with a full 1 mL of Enteryx solution, and have it ready for exchange when the first syringe is fully injected.

11. Patient sedation should be more than that used for a standard upper endoscopy. A slightly deeper sedation level of moderate sedation (more on par with what would be done for endoscopic retrograde colangiopancreatography [ERCP]) is advised. Use of standard sedative agents such as meperedine, fentanyl, or benzodiazepines is advised. Propofol may be used at the discretion of the physician. Intravenous use of a preprocedural supplemental antiemetic may be helpful, such as prochlorperazine (compazine) or promethazine (phenergan); this seems to reduce patient movements during the procedure.

## PROCEDURE

1. Following appropriate informed consent and sedation of the patient, introduce the gastroscope in standard fashion. Perform upper endoscopy with particular attention to the squamocolumnar junction, diaphragmatic hiatus, and the cardia of the stomach.

2. Pass the Enteryx injector (primed and loaded with the Enteryx solution) down the working channel, and advance it until the tip of the sheath is seen in the lumen of the stomach. Advance the needle out so the operator can see the deployment of the needle relative to the end of the catheter. Retract the needle, and reposition the endoscope just above the squamocolumnar junction.

3. Select an injection site at or slightly below the squamocolumnar junction, and redeploy the injector needle. Have the operator position the endoscope close to the tip of the needle catheter to well visualize the puncture site at the time of injection. Puncture the mucosa in an antegrade direction, and advance the needle into the muscle. This frequently requires angling the catheter at around 45° or more to get the needle into the deep muscle. A perpendicular injection (or use of an ERCP scope) is not recommended as this may increase the likelihood of a transmural injection. Injecting from a retrograde position is extremely difficult and not recommended. Do not push too firmly on the catheter as it may also increase the risk of perforation. It is suggested that the needle be positioned in the wall with the catheter causing no indentation or a slight indentation at the insertion into the mucosa.

4. Always have a second syringe loaded with Enteryx ready for use at all times during the procedure.

5. Preserve a small amount of DMSO solvent in a small cup or on a 4 × 4 gauze to use to clean the needle if there is any occlusion problem.

6. Begin injection of the Enteryx solution at a rate no faster than 0.1 mL every 6 seconds (it is helpful for the nurse to count out loud slowly).

7. Direct immediate attention to the puncture site. There should be no back extrusion of the solution, signs of mucosal bulge, or bluish/black discoloration at the site (secondary to the black tantalum powder in the Enteryx solution). This would indicate a submucosal injection and would be evident with the first 0.1 to 0.2 mL of injection. If submucosal injection is evident, the injection should be stopped immediately. A light grayish or no mucosal discoloration coupled with no mucosal bulge is the typical endoscopic appearance for an injection into the deep muscle.

8. Use endoscopic and fluoroscopic guidance to confirm intramural implant location (see Fig. 38.1A and Fig. 38.1B). On fluoroscopy, when appropriately placed within or along the muscle layer, the implants show as blebs which often have arcuate extension or coalesce to form a ring-like pattern. If

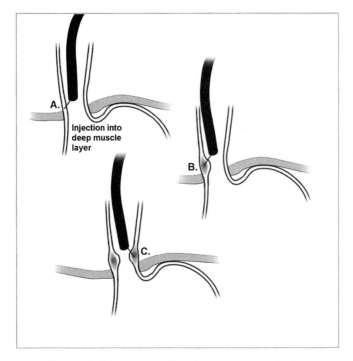

**Fig. 38.1.A–C. Appropriate location for Enteryx injection.**

the material forms an arc or ring, continue to use multiple syringes to add material at the same injection site/position. Multiple injections of 1 to 1.5 mL each for a total of approximately 6 to 8 mL total injected into the intramuscular layer (Fig. 38.1C).

9. Transmural injections are often identified as a sharp thin vertical radiodensity line that dissipates quickly. In distinction, injections into the muscular layer coalesce and allow for a more contrasted appearance. If a transmural injection occurs, stop immediately, and choose a new injection site. Studies in animal models have shown that material explanted beyond the esophagus does not have any significant risk.

10. Upon completion of injection at each site, instruct the nurse to remove his/her thumb from the plunger of the syringe to release the injection pressure. Next, do not withdraw the needle immediately, but rather maintain the position for 30 seconds. This allows the polymer to solidify and minimizes extrusion back through the injection tract.

11. Keep a log to record the total volume of Enteryx injected.

12. Take a PA/lateral chest x-ray following the procedure to assess the appearance of the implant and allow comparison with future assessments.

## POSTPROCEDURE

1. Patients should be told to expect some chest pain or substernal sensation of warmth for the first 24 to 48 hours following the procedure.

2. Routine dosing of acetaminophen for the first 24 hours is strongly recommended. Alternatively, some patients may require short-term use of mild narcotic analgesics as needed.

3. Patients will notice (as will their families, nurses in recovery, and anyone around them) a garlic smell or taste that typically abates in 24 hours following the procedure. This is due to the DMSO solvent that is absorbed, excreted into the lungs, and subsequently exhaled.

4. Patients should continue their PPIs for 10 days after the procedure.

5. A mechanically soft diet is suggested for the first several days with a subsequent advance in diet as tolerated.

6. Some patients do well for several days or weeks and then develop chest pain; this most likely reflects a submucosal injection and a slough of the implant. Transient esophageal mucosal ulceration will develop, and patients should be placed back on their PPIs for at least 4 to 8 weeks to facilitate healing.

## COMPLICATIONS

1. There have been no major (serious infection, perforation, hemorrhage, death) adverse events or complications in the

pivotal trials reported to date. Complications have been reported, albeit rarely, in the more widespread usage. These complications include: mediastinal abscess, pericardial effusion, pleural effusion, renal arterial embolization, aortic-esophageal fistula, and death.

2. Patients should be told to expect retrosternal chest pain, which occurs in most patients and was the most common device-related adverse event reported in the pivotal studies.

3. Dysphagia may occur but is typically transient. No strictures have been reported from any of the patients treated to date.

4. Typical procedure-related adverse events secondary to the endoscopy (but not the implantation device) may be seen. Pharyngitis and nausea were the most common adverse events reported in the pivotal studies.

5. Patients should be told to immediately report to their physician any postprocedural symptom of severe chest pain, dysphagia, or fever.

## CPT Codes

**C9704 –** Injection or insertion of intert substance for the submucosal/intramuscular injection(s) into the upper gastrointestinal tract, under fluoroscopic guidance.

**43234 –** Upper gastrointestinal endoscopy, simple primary examination (e.g., with small diameter flexible endoscope).

**43235 –** Upper gastrointestinal endoscopy including esophagus, stomach and either the duodenum and/or jejunum as appropriate; diagnostic, with or without collection(s) of specimen(s).

1. None of the GERD endoscopic therapies are on the Medicare list of covered procedures for ambulatory surgical centers (ASCs).

2. Effective January 1, 2004, Centers for Medicare and Medicaid (CMS) recommends that hospitals use the following codes to report Enteryx for Medicare patients in the hospital setting:

    C9704 + CPT code 43234 or C9704 + CPT code 43235

3. Effective January 1, 2004, CMS recommends that hospitals use 43234 or 43235 to bill for the endoscopy portion of the Enteryx procedure. These codes will be used instead of 43499. Hospitals will also bill C9704 that is intended to include payment for the device and fluoroscopy.

4. Physician billing. The current Medicare guidelines have no bearing on the physician reimbursement. Physicians should select the code that is most appropriate for the Enteryx procedure. It is recommended that at present, physicians use CPT 43499, unlisted procedure, esophagus.

5. Before scheduling the procedure it is suggested that the physician contact the individual payer to determine whether the procedure is covered, how much the patient will pay, and

how the patient wants the service billed. For Medicare patients, it is advisable that the patient be given a completed Advanced Beneficiary Notice (ABN) to sign prior to scheduling the procedures. In this way, if Medicare payment is denied as "not medically necessary", the practice can bill the patient for the procedure.

## REFERENCES

1. Johnson DA, Ganz R, Aisenberg J, et al. Endoscopic deep mural injection of Enteryx for the treatment of GERD: 6 month follow-up of a multicenter trial. *Am J Gastroenterol* 2003;98(9):250–258.
2. Johnson DA, Ganz R, Aisenberg J, et al. Endoscopic implantation of Enteryx for GERD treatment: 12 month results of a prospective multicenter trial. *Am J Gastroenterol* 2003; 9:1921–1930.

## SUGGESTED READINGS

Deviere J, Pastorelli A, Louis H, et al. Endoscopic implantation of a biopolymer in the lower esophageal sphincter for gastroesophageal reflux disease: a pilot study. *Gastrointest Endosc* 2002:98: 250–258.

Lehman GA. The history and future of implantation therapy for gastroesophageal reflux disease. *Gastrointest Endosc Clin North Am* 2003;13:191–200.

Louis H, Deviere J. Endoscopic implantation of Enteryx for the treatment of gastroesophageal reflux disease: technique, pre-clinical and clinical experience. *Gastrointest Endosc Clin North Am* 2003; 13:191–200.

# Endoscopic Sewing— EndoCinch

## David A. Johnson

Although laparoscopic and open fundoplication are effective in skilled hands, there remain drawbacks to surgery, in particular with regard to issues related to morbidity, mortality, durability, and cost-effectiveness. An endoscopic procedure, if comparable (to some degree) with surgical or medical intervention, might offer a less invasive alternative to patients with chronic symptoms due to gastroesophageal reflux disease. Potentially, if the procedure were safe, less invasive, and more effective, this might offer significant advantage to those patients who are seeking alternatives to chronic medical therapy and who do not desire to pursue the option of surgery. In 2000 the Food and Drug Administration approved EndoCinch (Bard) as an endoscopic option for the treatment of symptomatic gastroesophageal reflux disease (GERD). In prospective, yet uncontrolled and nonrandomized studies, this endoscopic intervention has been shown to be effective for the control of symptomatic GERD. Studies have demonstrated variable, if any, improvement in the lower esophageal sphincter pressure, however (6 to 12 months). The primary efficacy seems to be more consistently explained by improvement in transient lower esophageal sphincter relaxations.

## PREPROCEDURAL PREPARATION

1.  Both the endoscopist and the assistant should read the instructions and be familiar with all aspects of the procedure.

2.  Lay the gastroscope flat, and stretch it out so the flexible component is fully straightened.

3.  Insert the flexible end of the guidewire into the biopsy channel, and advance it until this extends out of the distal end of the endoscope.

4.  Backload the suturing needle assembly over the guidewire. Once the needle exits from the proximal end of the scope, remove the guidewire leaving the needle in the endoscope. Remove the needle protector.

5.  Notice that the green pusher wire has a 1-cm marker band at the tip. Insert this end into the needle device and advance until it exits from the tip of the needle. Manipulation may be necessary to pass the pusher wire through the needle assembly past the bifurcation in the biopsy channel of the endoscope.

6.  Advancement of the needle wire and pusher unit together as a unit will allow the flexible needle sheath to guide the pusher wire past the bifurcation of the endoscope.

7.  Remove the capsule and suction tubing from the package. Confirm that the endcap is attached to the capsule. Slide the capsule sleeve over the needle and pusher wire, keeping the bevel of the needle up. The capsule only goes on one way. Continue sliding the capsule until it is seated in the biopsy channel and is against the scope tip.

8.  Ensure that the needle has not been pushed back into the biopsy channel. If it has, with the scope straight, remove the capsule, advance the needle, and repeat the placement of the capsule.

9.  Once the capsule is in place, remove the suture loader from the kit. The end that has two small "fingers" is the operating end of the capsule attachment tool. Within the two fingers is a ridge. Align this ridge with the notches on the spring loader wedge that is located on the proximal end of the capsule.

10. Keeping the tool level, firmly slide the wedge proximally to secure it against the scope tip. Remove the suture loader from the capsule, being careful not to dislodge the wedge. Save the loader for future use.

11. Pull firmly on the capsule to ensure that it is securely affixed to the scope tip.

12. Take the handle and loosen the collar and black and silver knobs. The silver knob requires a "push and rotate" maneuver for both loosening and tightening, similar to a child safety cap. The handle may be in the full forward position. Slip the handle over the pusher wire and needle assembly. It may be necessary to rotate the handle in order for the wire to pass through the handle completely.

13. Advance the handle fully onto the biopsy port and tighten the collar. With the handle fully forward and the endoscope straight, lock the black knob on the handle to prevent the pusher wire from moving while you adjust the needle. Unscrew the capsule endcap. Using forceps or a Kelly clamp, adjust the needle so the marker band is even with the distal face of the capsule.

14. When in position, to deploy, press the side knob on the handle, slide knob forward, and turn clockwise to tighten. The knob will pop back up and move freely, but the needle remains secure.

15. Loosen the black knob on the handle, and using a pair of Kelly clamps, adjust the pusher wire so the proximal end of the marker band is even with the needle tip. Once in place, tighten the black knob

16. Check the system by briskly actuating the handle several times. Reassess the capsule, location of the needle tip, and pusher wire. The system should line up exactly as it did during the initial setup. It may be necessary to readjust the needle or pusher wire by following the same steps as originally performed.

## SUTURE LOADING TAG

1. The 3.0 monofilament has a metallic tag at the end. This tag allows the suture to be captured in the capsule endcap after a suture has been made. To load the suture tag into the needle, the capsule endcap must be removed.

2. With the handle fully advanced, pull back the black handle to retract the pusher wire, leaving the needle advanced in the capsule.

3. Insert the tapered end of the tag into the slot on the flat end of the suture loader. Place the suture loader onto the needle tip.

4. Align the slot of the loader with the slot of the capsule and needle. Transfer the tag from the suture loader into the needle until it is seated at the proximal end of the needle.

5. Without any tension on the suture, fully retract the handle. This withdraws the needle and suture from the capsule chamber. Reattach the capsule endcap.

6. The system is now ready for use. Place a piece of tape around the tubing at the proximal end of the scope. Attach the external vacuum to the suction tubing. Ensure that the three-way valve is attached to the suction tubing and is in the off position (off indicator should point toward the vacuum line).

## PROCEDURE

The endoscopist and the assistant must be familiar with all aspects of the procedure before starting; they will work as a synchronized team and each must understand his or her role in the procedure.

1. Following adequate sedation of the patient, perform routine upper endoscopy to become familiar with the specific anatomy. Remove any pooled secretions in the esophagus and stomach. This will help minimize aspiration risk during the procedure. Also suction oropharyngeal secretions during the procedure, as these may be difficult for the patient to clear spontaneously due to the presence of the overtube.

2. Backload the overtube onto a well-lubricated 45-Fr Maloney dilator. Pass it into the esophagus with special care to flex the patient's neck forward to facilitate passage and minimize trauma as the overtube passes through the cricopharyngeus. It is also helpful to have the patient initiate a swallow as the scope approaches the upper esophageal sphincter. This will facilitate passage and minimize the risk of an esophageal tear. If there is a lot of esophageal motility, use of an agent to decrease motility (e.g., glucagon or anticholinergics) may be helpful.

3. Choose a position along the lesser curvature for the first suture. Typically the best location is 1 to 1.5 cm below the squamocolumnar junction. Then place the capsule in apposition to the wall and apply suction. A vacuum pressure of at least 15 in. must be applied to adequately draw in the

tissue and consistently maintain the tissue in the suction chamber. Turn the three-way stopcock into the off position.

4. Tissue is drawn into the capsule chamber causing a " red-out" of the visual field. At this time have the assistant observe the suction tubing. If there is excessive agitation within the suction tubing, the suction should be broken and a new segment of tissue chosen and drawn into the suction capture maneuver. At this time the physician straightens the endoscope and relaxes the hand controls. Several seconds should follow to ensure that there is an adequate tissue purchase.

5. At this point actuate the EndoCinch handle by a quick and firm plunger-type motion.

6. After the stitch has been deployed, turn off the suction. Carefully rotate the capsule away from the stitch site, and advance the endoscope 5 to 10 cm to ensure it is clear of the mucosa.

7. Slowly and carefully withdraw the endoscope. Have the assistant ensure that as the scope is withdrawn, the suture material runs back through the overtube and through the stitched tissue. The stitch site may not be seen immediately upon withdrawal of the endoscope, but after a short distance, the suture site should be able to be seen distally.

8. Once the capsule is outside the patient's mouth, have the assistant reload the suture tag by removing the capsule endcap, advancing the needle, and reloading the same tag as was done originally with the suture loader device.

9. With a second pass of the endoscope, have the assistant take up the slack in the suture material in an equal fashion to match the distance that the scope is being advanced. Excess slack can result in the suture being tangled in the endoscope. Have the assistant carefully watch the video monitor to ensure that slack and entanglement are avoided. It is during this step that the communication between the physician and the assistant is most important.

10. Once in proper position, place a second stitch following the same procedure.

11. As the scope is withdrawn after the second stitch, the suture is now seen to be passing through two pieces of tissue. Accordingly, slightly more resistance may be felt on the withdrawal.

12. As the scope is withdrawn, have the assistant allow the suture to run freely through the tissue. Once the scope is outside of the patient's mouth, have the assistant cut the suture to remove the tag, and eliminate any excess suture length as desired.

13. Maintain light tension on both ends of the suture to avoid tangling or slippage back into the patient. Place a Kelly clamp on the two suture ends to secure these, and place it on the operating field alongside of the patient's mouth.

14. Next, prepare to secure the suture plication. Load the suture anchor delivery device into the endoscope via the biopsy channel distally. With the cage of the delivery device open, place one of the suture-anchoring, device-loading tools over the cage. Close the delivery device cage, encapsulating the suture anchor.

15. Actuate the loading tool to transfer the suture anchor into the delivery device. Remove the loading tool, and verify that the suture anchor is properly loaded.

16. Insert the suture threader into the slot at the distal end of the delivery device and advance until the wire exits from the distal tip. Thread the suture through the wire loop, and pull the suture threader in a lateral direction to start the suture drawing back into the delivery device.

17. Next, pull the suture threader in a direction perpendicular to the device until the ends of the suture exit the suture anchor and the delivery device; while maintaining light tension on both sutures, advance the endoscope and the delivery device to the stitch location.

18. Verify the plication location under endoscopic visualization, by extracorporeal measurement, or by feeling the tactile resistance.

19. Begin actuation of the delivery device by compressing the white and black portion of the handle firmly to cinch the suture within the anchor. Continue actuation by compressing and holding the red and white portions of the handle to cut the excess suture length. Release the suture from the delivery device.

20. After actuation, the plication should fall away from the delivery device, and the suture anchor should be visible. Confirm the plication's integrity by endoscopic visualization.

21. This plication can then be repeated in order to create a linear or circumferential pattern or a combination of both of these patterns, dependent on the amount of mucosa available at the esophagogastric junction as well as the preference of the endoscopist. Ideally, at least three plications are performed during the session.

### BREAKDOWN FOLLOWING THE PROCEDURE

1. To break down the system following completion of the procedure, first lay the scope on a flat surface.

2. Remove the tape from the suction tubing and endoscope.

3. Using the capsule attachment tool, fit the fingered end around the capsule wedge. Depress the wedge, and slide the capsule off the scope and the needle.

4. From the distal end of the scope, carefully withdraw the needle and pusher wire. Never pull the needle assembly out through the biopsy channel.

5. Loosen the handle collar, and remove the handle from the scope.

6.  The handle and overtube can be reused. Clean with an enzymatic cleaner to remove all tissue and blood. Sterilize using the 2% glutalraldehyde solution, and rinse with warm water. Do not use alcohol on the handle because it potentially can damage the small parts in the handle. All other parts are disposable and can be discarded according to institutional policy.

## TROUBLESHOOTING COMMON PROBLEMS

Knowing how to troubleshoot and intervene appropriately when a problem develops can be critical to the successful performance of the procedure.

1.  Problem: Suture tag pulls out of the needle prior to placing the stitch.

    Cause: There is too much tension on the suture.

    Recovery:

    a.  If before the first stitch, withdraw suture and replace tag in needle.
    b.  If before the second stitch, use snare or forceps to grasp and remove suture.
    c.  Tag and reload the needle.

2.  Problem: Suture tag is not captured either during or after stitching.

    Cause: Incorrect system setup and/or excessive bending of the scope tip.

    Recovery: Retrieve the tag using a snare or forceps. Check the needle/pusher-wire placement, and adjust if necessary. Straighten the scope and tip prior to handle actuation.

3.  Problem: Suture breaks.

    Cause: Suture may have been nicked and/or subjected to excessive tension.

    Recovery: For the first stitch, remove the suture and begin again. For the second stitch, if possible, retrieve the free end of the suture using the forceps.

4.  Problem: Tissue is not captured or stitched.

    Cause:

    a.  Tissue did not fill the capsule chamber.
    b.  Suture tag pulled out of the needle prior to stitching.

    Recovery:

    a.  Vacuum pressure must be at a minimum of 15 in of Hg and constant throughout the procedure.
    b.  Remove the suture and repeat the process.

5.  Problem: Tissue gapping or bridging is observed at the plication site.

    Cause: Too large a span between the first and second stitches.

    Recovery: Cut the stitch and begin again.

## COMPLICATIONS

1. Major complications have been reported, albeit rarely. There was one confined esophageal perforation (due to the placement of the overtube) in the original pivotal study. Subsequently, the reported trials have not described perforation, although major hemorrhage was described in 2 out of 27 patients in the one-year report from Europe.

## CPT Codes

**43499 -** Unlisted procedure, esophagus.

1. Category III CPT code 008T. The suturing device is reported using HCPCS C9703.

2. Physician billing. The current Medicare guidelines have no bearing on the physician reimbursement.

   Contact information: www.endocinch.com

3. For Medicare patients, it is advisable that the patient be given a completed Advanced Beneficiary Notice (ABN) to sign prior to scheduling the procedures. In this way, if Medicare payments is denied as "not medically necessary", the practice can bill the patient for the procedure.

## SUGGESTED READINGS

1. Filipi C, Lehman G, Rothstein RI, et al. Transoral endoscopic suturing for gastroesophageal reflux disease: a multicenter trial. *Gastrointest Endosc* 2001;53:416–422.
2. Swain CP, Park P. BARD EndoCinch: the device, the technique and pre-clinical studies. *Gastrointest Endosc Clin North Am* 2003;13:75–88.
3. Rothstein RI, Filipi CJ. Endoscopic suturing for gastroesophageal reflux disease: clinical outcome with the Bard EndoCinch. *Gastrointest Endosc Clin North Am* 2003;13:89–101.
4. Johnson DA. Endoscopic therapy for GERD—baking, sewing, or stuffing: an evidence based perspective. *Gastroenterologic Dis* 2003;3:142–149.
5. Mahmood Z, McMahon B, Weir D, et al. EndoCinch therapy for gastro-esophageal disease: a one year prospective follow-up. *Gut* 2003;52:34–39.
6. Fennerty MB. Endoscopic suturing for treatment of GERD. *Gastrointest Endosc* 2003;57:390–395.
7. Tam WCE, Holloway RH, Dent J, et al. Impact of endoscopic suturing of the gastroesophageal junction on lower esophageal sphincter function and gastroesophageal reflux in patients with reflux disease. *Am J Gastroenterol* 2004; 99(2):195–202.

# Esophageal Manometry

## Janice Freeman and Donald O. Castell

Esophageal manometry is a diagnostic test that measures changes in intraluminal pressure and the coordination of activity in the esophagus. Either a water-perfused catheter connected to external transducers or a solid-state catheter assembly containing small direct intraluminal transducers may be used.

## INDICATIONS

1. Evaluation of patients with dysphagia

   • Primary motility abnormality, such as achalasia
   • Secondary motility abnormality, such as scleroderma

2. Evaluation of possible gastroesophageal reflux disease. The test is useful to do the following:

   • Support the diagnosis in complex patients, patients who have failed treatment, or patients who have atypical symptoms
   • Evaluate for defective peristalsis (particularly prior to fundoplication)
   • Exclude scleroderma
   • Assist in placement of a pH probe

3. Patients with noncardiac chest pain

   • Identify primary esophageal motility abnormality
   • Pain response to provocative testing

## CONTRAINDICATIONS

1. High-grade esophageal strictures or esophageal obstruction

2. Postsedation state

3. Recent nasal surgery

## PREPARATION FOR STUDY

1. Prior to arrival of the patient everything should be assembled and prepared for the procedure. Connect the catheter to the manometry system, and complete calibration. The patient information may be entered into the computer at this time.

2. The patient is to be NPO for 6 hours prior to the procedure.

3. It is important to make the patient as comfortable as possible. Begin by explaining the procedure to the patient and clarifying what the patient can expect.

4. Answer questions the patient may have. It is important not to rush through this part of the study.

5. The use of music may aid in helping the patient relax during the procedure.

## PRIMARY EQUIPMENT

1. The solid state or water-perfused motility catheter

2. Water perfusion pump (either motor or gas driven), external transducers as necessary

3. Computer or physiograph

## SECONDARY EQUIPMENT

Secondary equipment includes a stretcher or bed, a pillow, towel, patient gown, 2% viscous lidocaine, oral topical anesthetic, lubricating jelly, cotton swab, tissue, 4-in. × 4-in. gauze, an emesis basin, 30-mL syringe, 360-mL disposable cup, straw, a container of room temperature water, tape, gloves, face shield, and soft music, which is always helpful to relax the patient.

## PROCEDURE

The procedure consists of five parts including the following: intubation of the patient, measurement of the gastric baseline, measurement of the lower esophageal sphincter (LES), measurement of esophageal body pressure, and measurement of the upper esophageal sphincter (UES).

### Intubation

1. Have the patient remove any eyeglasses.

2. Administer oral and nasal topical anesthetic.

3. Place the top of the catheter into the nose, and advance it slowly along the nasal passage until it stops at the upper esophageal sphincter.

4. Have the patient sip and swallow water rapidly through a straw, and quickly pass the catheter to the 60-cm marking on the catheter.

5. Once the catheter is in place, the patient should be lying flat with his or her head elevated on a pillow no more than 45 degrees.

### Measurement of the Gastric Baseline

1. Begin the procedure by making sure the data acquisition screen is displayed and the system is recording.

2. Start by asking the patient to take a deep breath (Fig. 40.1). Each of the pressure channels should show a rise in pressure on inspiration if sensors are in the stomach below the diaphragm. If the patient has a hiatal hernia or if the catheter is curled within the esophagus, the sensors may be located above the diaphragm, and a negative deflection will be seen on inspiration. If so, attempt to reposition the tube.

3. Measure gastric pressure through a series of quiet respirations. This value becomes the zero set for the subsequent LES pressure measurement. Thus, the LES pressure is not an absolute pressure but is relative pressure related to the gastric baseline pressure.

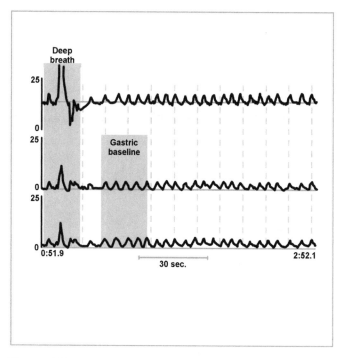

**Fig. 40.1. This tracing shows respiratory recording above and recordings from two transducers located in the stomach below. Note the increase in intragastric pressure with the deep inspiration. The gastric baseline pressure is obtained during a period of quiet respiration.**

## Measurement of the Lower Esophageal Sphincter

1. The LES is a tonically contracted smooth muscle, which relaxes in response to swallowing. In assessing LES function, the LES resting pressure is measured during a quiet "pull-through" or profile (Fig. 40.2). If the catheter contains directional sensors or water ports that are radially displaced, LES pressure must be measured with each port or sensor and the results averaged to get an accurate value for the LES resting pressure.

2. Obtain the LES pressure profile by slowly pulling a sensor 0.5 cm at a time through the LES. This allows identification of the distal border of the LES, the high-pressure zone of the LES, the PIP (Pressure Inversion Point or Point of Respiratory Reversal), and the proximal border of the LES (Fig. 40.2). If using a catheter that contains two circumferential or averaging sensors, the catheter is pulled upward in 1-cm increments until increased respiratory pressure

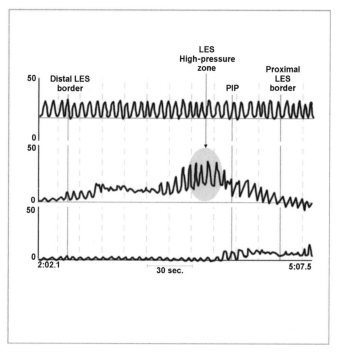

**Fig. 40.2. LES pressure.** Profile of the LES is obtained by a station pull-through of a transducer from the stomach, across the sphincter, to the esophagus (middle tracing).

changes are seen in the more proximal channel. At this point slow the catheter pulls to 0.5 cm per pull.

3. Wait 10 to 15 seconds between pulls (three or four respiratory cycles) to allow enough time for the pressure to stabilize. Note the probe depth at which the pressure is highest.

4. Assessing the LES function, continue to pull the catheter in 0.5-cm increments until the distal sensor is located in the high-pressure zone of the LES.

5. Tape the catheter in place, and record the LES resting pressure.

6. Give the patient a 5-cc bolus of room-temperature water. Observe the relaxation as the pressure falls from resting pressure and the sphincter contracts following the passage of the bolus. Once the relaxation is complete, allow a 20- to 30-second interval before giving the patient another swallow of water. Continue in this manner until 10 relaxations have taken place (Fig. 40.3).

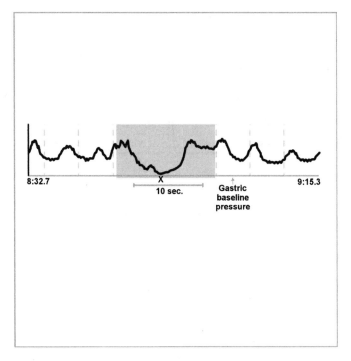

**Fig. 40.3.** Normal swallow-induced LES relaxation showing measurement of residual pressure at the X.

## Measurement of the Body of the Esophagus

1. The study of the body of the esophagus evaluates muscle response to water swallows. The muscle normally contracts beginning from the proximal (top) portion of the esophagus and progresses in an orderly peristaltic sequence to the distal (bottom) portion of the esophagus.

2. Position the catheter with the distal sensor located 3 to 5 cm above the proximal (top) border of the LES. This will position the sensors at 3 to 5, 8 to 10, and 13 to 15 cm above the LES. Most catheters have sensors or ports 5-cm apart allowing assessment of esophageal peristalsis. Some catheters will include an additional one to two sensors spaced at 5-cm intervals.

3. Once the catheter has been properly positioned and taped in place, allow a period of 10 to 15 seconds to establish the esophageal resting pressure as a baseline or reference point for assessing body contractions.

4. Give a series of 5-cc boluses of room-temperature water with a 20- to 30-second wait between swallows (Fig. 40.4). This

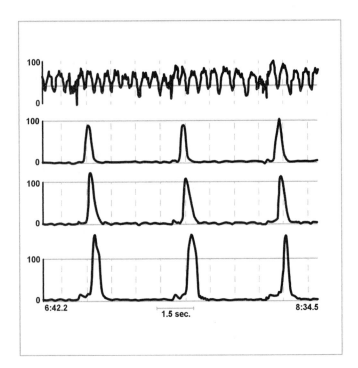

**Fig. 40.4. Esophageal body contractions.**

allows time for the smooth muscle to repolarize. Each swallow should be annotated using computer keys designated for a swallow. If a strip chart is used, mark the swallow in the graph to distinguish the water swallow from a dry swallow.

5.  Continue in this manner until 10 wet swallows have taken place. **Note:** if the software allows viewing both the LES and esophageal body on the same screen, only 10 complete wet swallows are needed with the distal sensor stationed in the LES.

**Measurement of Upper Esophageal Sphincter**

1.  The final portion of the study involves assessment of the UES. Like the LES, the UES is a sphincter which is tonically contracted and relaxes with swallowing. Unlike the LES, the UES and pharynx are made up of striated muscle.

2.  Contractions in the pharynx and UES are very rapid and require the use of the solid-state catheter to properly assess function. The response time of a low-compliance infusion system is not sufficient to capture the pharyngeal contractions.

3.  With the patient in a stable sitting position, begin by establishing a baseline or reference point in the body of the esophagus.

4. Then pull the catheter through the UES until the distal sensor shows an increase in pressure.

5. Similar to the LES pull-through, the catheter pulls are then slowed to 0.5-cm increments with a wait of 10 to 15 seconds between pulls. This allows the pressure to settle down to a true resting pressure after a catheter pull. The UES tends to grab the catheter when it is pulled, resulting in an artificial pressure spike. As the catheter is pulled through the UES, the pressure will continue to rise until the sensor passes into the high-pressure zone.

6. To properly assess UES relaxation, position the sensor above or proximal to the high-pressure zone of the UES. The UES moves up onto the sensor when the patient swallows. The UES will then relax and upon closure (return to resting pressure) will move distally off the sensor. This movement will produce an "M" configuration if the sensor has been properly positioned (Fig. 40.5).

7. Once a swallow is completed, give the next one as soon as the patient is ready. There is no reason to wait between the swallows since the area being assessed is in the striated muscle, which has rapid repolarization.

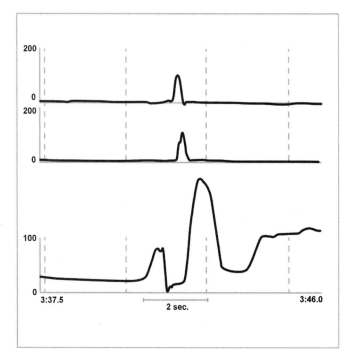

**Fig. 40.5. M configuration of UES relaxation.**

8. Continue in that manner until six wet swallows have taken place.

## POSTPROCEDURE

1. Extubate the patient.

2. Give any discharge instructions regarding follow-up.

3. There are no required postprocedure dietary or activity restrictions.

## COMPLICATIONS

1. Epistaxis

2. There have been no reports of perforation with the catheter in the literature.

## CPT Codes

**91010 –** Esophageal motility (manometric study of the esophagus and/or gastroesophageal junction) study.

## SUGGESTED READINGS

Castell DO, Diederich LL, Castell JA. Esophageal Manometry Procedure. In: Diederich L, ed. *Esophageal Motility & pH Testing.* Colorado: Sandhill Scientific, Inc, 2000:41–56.

Freeman J, Hila A. Esophageal Manometry. In: Castell DO, Richter JE, eds. *The Esophagus*, 4th ed. Philadelphia: Lippincott Williams & Wilkins, 2004:114–134.

# Ambulatory 24-Hour Esophageal pH Monitoring

Ronnie Fass, Leslie Eidelman, and Wilder Garcia-Calderon

Ambulatory 24-hour esophageal pH monitoring is a study in which continuous esophageal intraluminal pH measurement allows the detection of changes in pH caused by gastroesophageal reflux disease (GERD) episodes. Acid reflux episodes are defined as pH drops to below four in the distal esophagus, and reflux time is the elapsed time until the pH exceeds four. Normal subjects do experience reflux episodes primarily after meals, but they are not associated with GERD symptoms. A physiological range of esophageal acid exposure has been established in normal subjects. Prolonged ambulatory 24-hour esophageal pH monitoring enables identification of both symptomatic and asymptomatic reflux events in physiologic conditions.

The value of the test lies in its ability to diagnose GERD in patients with normal endoscopic findings, atypical and extraesophageal symptoms, and poor response to medical, surgical, or endoscopic therapy, as well as in identifying patients who have an increased risk for a complicated outcome (prolonged nocturnal reflux, significant asymptomatic reflux).

Development of thinner pH probes and a wireless pH-sensitive capsule have made the procedure more acceptable to patients, allowing for data collection while patients pursue their everyday activities.

Multiple pH sensor probes allow the assessment of high reflux episodes, involving the proximal esophagus and pharynx, as well as the simultaneous measurement of gastric pH if needed.

## INDICATIONS

1. Patients with nonerosive reflux disease who are being considered for surgical antireflux repair

2. Patients after antireflux surgery who continue to be symptomatic or are suspected to have ongoing abnormal acid reflux

3. Patients who continue to have GERD-related symptoms despite proton pump inhibitor (PPI) therapy administered at least twice daily (the test is performed on treatment)

4. Patients with noncardiac chest pain who failed the PPI test or an empirical trial with a PPI administered at least twice daily (the test is performed on treatment)

5. Patients with suspected otolaryngologic manifestations of gastroesophageal reflux disease who failed an empirical trial of PPI therapy administered at least twice daily (the test is performed on treatment)

6. Patients with adult-onset, nonallergic, refractory asthma who failed PPI therapy administered at least twice daily (the test is performed on treatment)

## CONTRAINDICATIONS

1. Naso-esophageal obstruction or upper esophageal obstruction

2. Severe maxillofacial trauma and/or basilar skull fracture

3. Patients who are unable to cooperate or are high risk for pulling out the pH probe

4. For the wireless pH system the test is also contraindicated in patients with coagulopathy, severe erosive esophagitis, esophageal ulceration, tight esophageal ring or a stricture, tumor (benign or malignant), varices, any obstruction in the gastrointestinal tract, pacemaker, or implanted cardiac defibrillator.

## PREPARATION

1. Inform the patient of the nature of the examination and that it entails two visits within 24 hours or 48 hours for the wireless pH system.

2. Discontinue food and liquids 6 hours prior to the study.

3. If the pH study is done off antireflux treatment, confirm that PPIs have been discontinued for at least a week. Prokinetics, $H_2$ blockers, and smooth muscle relaxants should be stopped for 2 to 3 days prior to the test. Antacids are allowed until a day prior to the test. In contrast, if the test is used to monitor treatment response, the patient should continue all medications.

4. Obtain informed consent.

## EQUIPMENT

1. Standard manometry equipment or LES locator (a pressure sensor added to the pH probe)

2. Flexible pH microelectrode with reference electrode or wireless pH capsule (mounted on a delivery device)

3. Dual sensor catheter that permits assessment of proximal esophageal acid exposure in addition to distal esophageal acid exposure

4. Standard buffer solutions for calibration (pH 7.0 and pH 1.0)

5. Reference electrode (incorporated into the capsule in the wireless pH system)

6. Ambulatory data logger powered by a battery (9V). For the wireless pH system, an external recorder device receives data signal via radiofrequency telemetry.

7. Computer software for data transfer and analysis

8. For the wireless pH system a custom-made vacuum unit capable of generating 600 mm Hg vacuum pressure to the well in the capsule, via the delivery system

**PROCEDURE**

**Catheter pH System**

1. Calibrate the pH electrode according to the supplier's instruction manual. If using a dual sensor pH probe, immerse both sensors in the buffer solution during calibration. Zero the data logger using the software program. Connect the electrode to the data logger, and place it into the 7.0 pH buffer solution for 3 minutes (also place the external reference electrode if you are using a catheter with external reference). The device should read close to 7.0. Rinse the electrode(s) and repeat the procedure with the standard buffer solution at pH 1.0.

2. Locate the LES either by standard manometry (see Chapter 40) or by using LES locator.

3. If utilizing an LES locator, use the LES identification accessory kit. It consists of a pressurized water bag connected through a tubing system to the pH catheter and to a pressure transducer. Adjust the baseline pressure to gastric pressure, and withdraw one centimeter at a time. Checking pressure changes with respiration is helpful (increasing below the diaphragm and decreasing above). A sudden rise in resting pressure identifies the LES. After a swallow there will be a relaxation followed by a pressure wave.

4. Apply a local anesthetic to the patient's nostril (gel or liquid). After a few minutes the catheter can be introduced via the nares into the stomach. After gently reaching the pharynx, flex the patient's head. Sipping water during insertion may help. To confirm that catheter is in the stomach and not curled in the esophagus, verify that the reading on the data logger is pH < 4.

5. Withdraw the pH catheter to 5 cm above the proximal margin of the previously identified LES. Fix the catheter by taping it to the cheek and passing it behind the ear. Connect the reference electrode (if external) to the skin of the chest (the area over the manubrium sterni).

6. Connect the catheter to the portable data logger.

**Wireless pH System**

1. If the pH capsule is delivered after an upper endoscopy then the proper location of placement is 6 cm above the gastroesophageal junction. If the capsule is placed transnasally or per-orally then identification of the LES is done by esophageal manometry.

2. Activate the capsule by the magnetic switch and calibrate in buffer solutions of pH 7.0 and 1.68.

3. Advance the delivery system with the capsule to 5 cm above the proximal margin of the LES. Connect the external vacuum pump to the delivery system. Apply suction by the vacuum pump for 30 seconds. Successful suction of the esophageal mucosa is achieved when the vacuum gauge on the pump stabilizes at a value > 510 mm Hg for 10 seconds.

Remove the plastic safety guard on the handle, and then press the activation button. Subsequently, twist clockwise 90 degrees the activation button and then re-extend to release the delivery device from the attached capsule. Remove the delivery system.

## PATIENT INSTRUCTIONS

1. Encourage patients to pursue their everyday activities.

2. Encourage patients to consume their regular diets. Most centers today do not apply diet restrictions on patients undergoing 24-hour esophageal pH monitoring.

3. Patients are allowed to smoke and drink alcohol.

4. Instruct the patient to keep a diary during the monitoring period. Data loggers display event buttons (markers) to record symptoms or other events. However, it is advisable that a written record be kept as well. A diary should include the following:
   a. Upright or recumbent time (awake or asleep)
   b. Meals and snacks (time of onset and ending)
   c. Exact time of symptoms of interest

5. Instruct patient to avoid getting the recorder device wet. Patients undergoing assessment with the wireless pH capsule can shower or sleep without the data receiver as long as it is kept at a range of 3 to 5 ft from the patient.

## POSTPROCEDURE

1. Remove the catheter while the patient blows out through the nose. There is no need for the patient to fast for catheter removal.

2. Go over the symptom diary with the patient.

3. The patient can resume normal activities and restart discontinued medications.

4. Download the recorded data into the computer.

5. Wireless capsules usually self-detach within 7 to 10 days after placement. In rare cases, endoscopic removal is needed. Chest x-ray is a simple test that can help to determine the status of the capsule in patients with persistent chest discomfort suspected to be caused by the capsule. Avoid magnetic resonance imaging for 30 days after placement of the pH capsule.

## INTERPRETATION

1. A completed test should last 24 hours. Short duration examinations are sometimes performed but must include at least one postprandial and nighttime (supine) period.

2. Computer software analyzes the presence of pathologic esophageal acid exposure. Most commercially available software packages analyze data for the following variables:
   a. Percent total time pH $< 4$
   b. Percent upright time pH $< 4$

    c.  Percent supine time pH < 4

    d.  Number of reflux episodes

    e.  Number of reflux episodes ≥ 5 minutes

    f.  Longest single episode of reflux

3.  The Johnson and DeMeester composite score which is calculated based on the aforementioned variables

4.  Percent total time pH < 4 is the most reliable and reproducible parameter and consequently widely accepted criteria to define an abnormal study.

5.  Commonly used reference values (see Table 41.1)

6.  Three main measurements have been created in an attempt to correlate episodes of acid reflux with symptoms. Those measurements are discussed below. Symptom correlation is particularly important in patients with atypical or extra-esophageal manifestations of GERD.

7.  Interpretation of symptom correlation: Symptoms are considered to be related to an acid reflux event when they occur in the 2- to 5-minute window following a reflux episode.

    a.  Symptom Index (SI): Percentage of symptoms reported during the study period that is associated with acid reflux event. If the value is > 50% then the symptom index is considered positive (the symptoms are due to acid reflux).

$$\text{Symptom Index} = \frac{\text{Number of symptoms related to reflux} \times 100\%}{\text{Total number of symptoms}}$$

    b.  Symptom Sensitivity Index (SSI): Percentage of reflux episodes that is associated with GERD-related symptoms.

**Table 41.1. Commonly used reference values**

|  | Catheter pH system | Wireless pH capsule (36-48 recording time) |
| --- | --- | --- |
| Percent total time pH < 4 | < 4.2 | < 5.3 |
| Percent upright time pH < 4 | < 6.3 | < 6.9 |
| Percent supine time pH < 4 | < 1.2 | < 6.7 |
| Number of reflux episodes | < 50.0 | < 36.8 (± 20.1) |
| Number of reflux episodes (≥ 5 min) | < 3.0 | < 1.2 (± 0.55) |
| Longest reflux episode (min) | < 9.2 | – |
| DeMeester & Johnson composite score | < 14.7 | – |

This parameter quantifies a patient's sensitivity to acid reflux. A positive SSI results if the value is > 10%.

$$\text{Symptom Sensitivity Index} = \frac{\text{Number of symptomatic acid reflux events} \times 100\%}{\text{Total number of acid reflux events}}$$

c. **Symptom Association Probability (SAP):** calculates the probability that symptoms and acid reflux events are truly associated. Positive SAP (positive association) is determined if the calculated value is > 95%. Calculating SAP requires a statistical program.

## SIDE EFFECTS AND COMPLICATIONS

1. Catheter pH electrode: trauma to nasopharynx, epistaxis, throat pain/discomfort, nose pain, chest pain/discomfort, cough, and dysphagia. Catheter misplacement owing to bending or rolling has been reported in less than 5% of patients within the esophagus or pharynx. Generally, the pH test has been demonstrated to significantly affect patient's lifestyle (diet, activities, sleep, etc.).

2. Wireless pH capsule: nosebleed (transnasal placement), chest discomfort/pain, and premature or failure of capsule detachment.

## CPT Codes

**91032** – Esophagus, acid reflux test, with intraluminal pH electrode for detection of gastroesophageal reflux.

**91033** – Esophagus, acid reflux test, with intraluminal pH electrode for detection of gastroesophageal reflux; prolonged recording.

**91034** – Esophagus, gastroesophageal reflux test; with nasal catheter pH electrode(s) placement, recording, analysis and interpretation, for gastroesophageal reflux testing.

**91035** – Esophagus, gastroesophageal reflux test; with mucosal attached telemetry pH electrode placement, recording, analysis and interpretation, for scenarios in which the physician performs a gastroesophageal reflux test with a Bravo probe.

## SUGGESTED READINGS

American Gastroenterological Association Medical Position Statement: Guidelines on the use of esophageal pH recording. *Gastroenterology* 1996;110(6):1981–1996.

Breumelhof R, Smout AJ. The symptom sensitivity index: a valuable additional parameter in 24-hour esophageal pH recording. *Am J Gastroenterol* 1991;86(2):160–164.

Dhiman RK, Saraswat VA, Mishra A, Naik SR. Inclusion of supine period in short-duration pH monitoring is essential in diagnosis of gastroesophageal reflux disease. *Dig Dis Sci* 1996;41(4):764–772.

Fass R, Hell R, Sampliner RE, et al. The effect of ambulatory 24-hour esophageal pH monitoring on reflux provoking activities. *Dig Dis Sci* 1999;44:2263–2269.

Johnson PE, Koufman JA, Nowak LJ, et al. Ambulatory 24-hour double-probe pH monitoring: the importance of manometry. *Laryngoscope* 2001;111:1970–1975.

Pandolfino JE, Richter JE, Ours T, et al. Ambulatory esophageal pH monitoring using a wireless system. *Am J Gastroenterol* 2003;98(4):740–749.

Streets CG, DeMeester TR. Ambulatory 24-hour esophageal pH monitoring: why, when, and what to do. *J Clin Gastroenterol* 2003;37(1):14–22.

Weusten BL, Roelofs JM, Akkermans LM, et al. The symptom-association probability: an improved method for symptom analysis of 24-hour esophageal pH data. *Gastroenterology* 1994;107(6): 1741–1745.

# Gastric Secretory Testing

## Robert S. Bulat and Roy C. Orlando

Gastric acid secretory testing is a means of quantifying basal and pentagastrin-stimulated acid production by the stomach. It has been available for well over 50 years but now is fast becoming a technique of only historical interest due to the dramatic changes in diagnosis and management of upper digestive disorders. For instance, in the past the primary reason for performing such a test was in the setting of peptic ulcer disease (PUD), a disease that is not only diminishing in frequency (in large measure due to eradication of *Helicobacter pylori* and to safer [cyclooxygenase-2 inhibitor] nonsteroidal antiinflammatory drugs) but is so effectively treated with potent acid-suppressing agents (histamine-2 antagonists, proton pump inhibitors) that the need for operative intervention has all but been eliminated. Nevertheless, clinical situations still exist in which knowledge of the capacity of the stomach to secrete acid remains important from either a qualitative or quantitative standpoint. For this reason, the techniques and interpretation of gastric secretory testing continue to be included in this work.

The principal and standard means for measurement of gastric acid secretion is by collection of gastric contents by nasogastric (NG) tube and subsequent titration of the collected contents with sodium hydroxide solution to quantitate basal and stimulated acid secretion (as described below). Other tests that may be useful to determine gastric acidity generally lack quantification and so are only applicable in selected situations. For instance, a spot check of gastric pH can be determined at the time of esophagogastroduodenoscopy (EGD) by suctioning up gastric juice and application of pH paper or pH meter to the fluid and, if acidic, pernicious anemia (PA), which requires the presence of achlorhydria, can be ruled out as a cause for hypergastrinemia. Also, Feldman and Barnett have shown that a spot check of fasting pH using gastric juice obtained by NG tube may be useful in establishing the existence of hypochlorhydria; the latter is reasonably reliable if pH is > 5 in men and > 7 in women (1). An alternate method of establishing gastric acid secretory capacity is through the use of the Congo Red test at the time of EGD. This test has gained popularity as a means for determining the completeness of vagotomy. The Congo Red test is performed at EGD by spraying the dye into the stomach and observing whether it turns red; the color is indicative of functional (acid-secreting) parietal cells with the capacity to reduce gastric pH to < 3 (2).

## INDICATIONS

### Often Helpful

1. Recurrent peptic ulcer disease

   a. To rule out acid hypersecretory states (e.g., Zollinger-Ellison syndrome [ZES], retained gastric antrum)

b. To test for completeness of vagotomy following PUD surgery

2. To evaluate the cause for fasting hypergastrinemia

a. Physiologically induced due to hypochlorhydria or achlorhydria (e.g., secondary to atrophic gastritis with or without PA)

b. Pathologically induced due to ZES or antral G-cell hyperplasia

3. To assess the adequacy of acid suppressant therapy in patients with acid hypersecretory states such as ZES

**Occasionally Helpful**

1. To diagnose ZES in a patient known to secrete acid. **Note:** Basal and maximal acid output measurements are potentially valuable for the diagnosis of ZES but are not as sensitive or specific for the diagnosis as measuring fasting and secretin-stimulated gastrin levels (2,3).

2. To diagnose PA. Achlorhydria is essential for the diagnosis of PA and so its absence rules out the diagnosis. However, achlorhydria itself is insufficient for the diagnosis because it is more frequently seen in association with atrophic gastritis unrelated to PA. Therefore there is greater specificity in diagnosing PA by measuring serum B12 levels and performing a Schilling test.

**Not Helpful**

1. For the routine evaluation of PUD

2. As predictor of PUD recurrence either preoperatively or postoperatively (1,4)

3. For determining if a gastric ulcer is benign or malignant. The majority of gastric cancers occur in patients who are not achlorhydric (5), and some benign ulcers are found in conditions of low acid secretion.

4. For establishing the etiology of dyspepsia

**CONTRAINDICATIONS**

1. Contraindications to NG tube placement. Among these are presence of an esophageal stricture or diverticulum, active nasopharyngeal pathology or recent nasopharyngeal surgery, inability to cooperate with nasogastric intubation, history of cardiac arrhythmia, or vagally mediated syncope.

2. Contraindications to pentagastrin-stimulated acid secretion. Known allergy to pentagastrin, recent upper gastrointestinal bleeding due to PUD, or other lesion that can be aggravated by acid secretion.

3. Gastric outlet obstruction. This is not an absolute contraindication but its presence will yield falsely elevated levels of acid secretion due to antral distension-induced increases in serum gastrin levels.

## PREPARATION

Explain the nature of the procedure to the patient.

1. Obtain written, informed consent.

2. Discontinue all medications that may affect acid secretion, e.g., $H_2$ blockers, antihistamines, cholinergics, anticholinergics, tranquilizers, antidepressants, and carbonic anhydrase inhibitors at least 24 hours before the procedure. Proton pump inhibitors should be stopped for 5 days prior to the test. Antacids are allowed for dyspepsia as needed up to 12 hours before the procedure.

3. Allow the patient nothing to eat or drink after midnight.

## EQUIPMENT

1. A 14- to 18-Fr NG tube, preferably double-lumen (vented)

2. Supplies for passing the NG tube (see details in Chapter 19)

3. A 50-cc or 60-cc "catheter-tip" syringe

4. Injectable pentagastrin, 6 μg/kg

5. Intermittent suction pump

6. Eight 120-cc collection containers for gastric fluid

7. A pH meter, graduated burette, small beakers, and 0.1 N NaOH for acid titration

## PROCEDURE

1. With the patient sitting, pass the NG tube via the nose into the stomach (see detailed technique in Chapter 19).

2. With the patient sitting or lying comfortably on his or her side, advance tip of the NG tube to the most dependent portion of the stomach. Verify tube position fluoroscopically or by the "water-recovery test" (6,7). The water-recovery test is performed by introducing 50 mL of water into the stomach via the NG tube and then aspirating the water back via the NG tube. Recovery of ≥ 90% of the water indicates adequate tube placement.

3. Intermittently aspirate gastric contents manually or via suction machine to collect gastric juice. Cancel the test if food particles are present or if > 200 mL of gastric juice is aspirated. Possible reasons for the large gastric volume include the presence of gastroparesis or gastric outlet obstruction or the recent ingestion of a meal.

4. Check NG tube patency periodically by injection of small amounts of air.

5. Note the presence of blood or bile in each of the aspirates. Accuracy of aspirates containing these materials may be erroneously low because blood is a buffer and bile is a marker indicating alkaline duodenogastric reflux.

6. Sputum may be swallowed by the patient during the study without significantly compromising the results because of low total acid buffering capacity.

7. Perform basal acid output (BAO) collection. Four consecutive 15-minute collections of gastric juice are performed prior to the injection of pentagastrin.

8. Following gastric collections for BAO determination, pentagastrin (6 μg/kg) is injected subcutaneously to maximally stimulate acid production (8,9). Possible side effects the patient may note include transient flushing, nausea, abdominal pain, dizziness, palpitations, and faintness.

9. Perform maximum acid output (MAO) or peak acid output (PAO) collection. Four consecutive 15-minute collections of gastric juice are performed immediately after pentagastrin injection.

## POSTPROCEDURE

1. Repeat the water-recovery test to verify that correct tube placement has been maintained throughout the study.

2. Aspirate any residual gastric fluid.

3. Remove the NG tube.

4. Resume regular diet and medications.

## DETERMINATION OF BAO, MAO, AND PAO

1. Centrifuge all samples to remove any visible particulate matter.

2. Record the volume of each of the eight 15-minute collections (four for the BAO and four for the PAO). (**Note:** Fig. 42.1 is a representative worksheet for the calculation of the BAO and PAO from the data.) (10).

3. Using 0.1 N NaOH, titrate to pH 7.0 a 5-cc aliquot from each of the 15-minute collections and record the volume of titrant.

4. Total acid content of each 15-minute collection is calculated as follows:

    a. The volume in mL of NaOH to titrate 5 cc of gastric juice to pH 7.0 multiplied by 0.1 (molarity) = mmol $H^+$ in the 5 cc of aliquot

    b. Total mmol $H^+$ in a 15-minute collection = collection volume ÷ 5 multiplied by the mmol $H^+$ in the 5 cc of aliquot

5. BAO (mmol $H^+$/hr) = sum of acid content in each of the first four 15-minute collections.

6. MAO (mmol $H^+$/hr) = sum of acid content in each of the four 15-minute collections following pentagastrin administration. The MAO and PAO (see below) are measures of total gastric acid secretory capacity, but the PAO, which is an estimate of greatest possible acid secretory capacity, is more reproducible and so is used more often clinically (8).

7. PAO (mmol $H^+$/hr) = sum of acid content in each of the two consecutive 15-minute postpentagastrin collections with the highest values multiplied by 2.

## Gastric Secretory Testing: Worksheet

Patient's name ________________ Patient # ________________

Weight __________ kg __________ Date ________________

Indication ________________

**I. FIRST HOUR – BAO**

| Sample No. | Scheduled Time (mins.) | Actual Clock Time (0-2400) Start | End | Appearance | (a) Vol. (mls) | (b) pH | (c) ml 0.1 N NaOH Sample (5ml aliquot) | (d) meq $H^2$ /ml Sample (c-50) | (e) meq $H^2$ / total Sample (axd) |
|---|---|---|---|---|---|---|---|---|---|
| 1 | 0 – 15 | | | | | | | | |
| 2 | 15 – 30 | | | | | | | | |
| 3 | 30 – 45 | | | | | | | | |
| 4 | 45 – 60 | | | | | | | | |

BAO = Σe = ________ meq $H^2$ / hr.

**II. FIRST HOUR – PAO and MAO**

Pentagastin injection (6 ug/kg: ________ ug (________ ml) Time of injection ________ (0-2400)

| Sample No. | Scheduled Time (mins.) | Actual Clock Time (0-2400) Start | End | Appearance | (a) Vol. (mls) | (b) pH | (c) ml 0.1 N NaOH Sample (5ml aliquot) | (d) meq $H^2$ /ml Sample (c-50) | (e) meq $H^2$ / total Sample (axd) |
|---|---|---|---|---|---|---|---|---|---|
| 1 | 0 – 15 | | | | | | | | |
| 2 | 15 – 30 | | | | | | | | |
| 3 | 30 – 45 | | | | | | | | |
| 4 | 45 – 60 | | | | | | | | |

PAO = Two highest adjacent (e) column values x 2 = ________ meq $H^2$ /hr.

MAO = Σe = ________ meq $H^2$ / hr.

________________
Signature

**Fig. 42.1. Gastric secretory testing worksheet.**

**INTERPRETATION**

1. Representative values for BAO, MAO, and PAO for males and females in health and disease are shown in Table 42.1. Note that there are overlapping ranges of acid secretory values between health and disease for the various categories, i.e., BAO, MAO, and PAO.

2. Males, in general, have greater values for acid secretion than females in both health and disease.

3. Values for gastric acid secretion are lower in those with gastric ulcers than with duodenal ulcers.

4. Patients with ZES have characteristically high BAO values compared to healthy subjects and subjects with PUD. This is due to high serum gastrin levels derived from tumor-secreted gastrin-driving gastric acid secretion. Furthermore, and just as important diagnostically, pentagastrin patients with ZES have a lower percentage rise in MAO or PAO over BAO than healthy or PUD subjects. This is because BAO in ZES is already being driven by high gastrin levels, and so pentagastrin injection has a more limited effect in driving the BAO to the PAO or MAO level than observed in healthy or PUD subjects.

5. Patients with achlorhydria following pentagastrin have complete gastric atrophy, a finding compatible with but not

**Table 42.1. Typical values of gastric acid secretion**

|  | BAO (mmol $H^+$/hr) | | MAO (mmol $H^+$/hr) | | PAO (mmol $H^+$/hr) | |
|---|---|---|---|---|---|---|
|  | Average | Range | Average | Range | Average | Range |
| Normal subjects |  |  |  |  |  |  |
| Males | 2.5 | 0–10 | 25 | 7–50 | 35 | 10–60 |
| Females | 1.5 | 0–6 | 15 | 5–30 | 25 | 8–40 |
| Duodenal ulcer |  |  |  |  |  |  |
| Males | 5.0 | 0.1–15 | 40 | 15–60 | 45 | 15–70 |
| Females | 3.0 | 0.1–15 | 30 | 10–45 | 35 | 15–55 |
| Gastric ulcer |  |  |  |  |  |  |
| Males | 1.5 | 0–8 | 20 | 5–40 |  |  |
| Females | 1.0 | 0–5 | 12 | 3–25 |  |  |
| Zollinger-Ellison syndrome |  |  |  |  |  |  |
| both sexes | 40 | 10–90 | 65 | 30–120 |  |  |

Source: Klein, K. Gastric Secretory testing. In: Drossman DA, ed. *Manual of Gastroenterologic Procedures*, 2nd edition. New York: Raven Press, 1987.

diagnostic of PA. The presence of pentagastrin-stimulated gastric acid secretion is, however, incompatible with a diagnosis of PA.

## REFERENCES

1. Feldman M, Barnett C. Fasting gastric pH and its relationship to true hypochlorhydria in humans. *Dig Dis Sci* 1991;36: 866–869.
2. Peetsalu A, Peetsalu M. Interpretation of postvagotomy endoscopic Congo Red test results in relation to ulcer recurrence 5 to 12 years after operation. *Am J Surg* 1998;175: 472–476.
3. Malagelada JR, Davis CS, O'Fallon WM, Go VLW. Laboratory diagnosis of gastrinoma: I. a prospective evaluation of gastric analysis and fasting serum gastrin levels. *Mayo Clin Proc* 1982;57:211–218.
4. Malagelada JR, Glanzman SC, Go VLW. Laboratory diagnosis of gastrinoma: II. a prospective study of gastrin challenge tests. *Mayo Clin Proc* 1982;57:219–226.
5. Johnston D, Pickford IR, Walker BE, Goligher JC. Highly selective vagotomy for duodenal ulcer: Do hypersecretors need antrectomy? *Br Med J* 1975;1:716–718.
6. Baron JH. Gastric ulcer and carcinoma. In: Drossman DA, ed. *Clinical Tests of Gastric Secretion: History, Methodology, and Interpretation.* New York: Oxford University Press, 1979:86–97.
7. Hassan MA, Hobsley M. Positioning of subject and of nasogastric tube during a gastric secretory study. *Br Med J* 1970;1: 458–460.
8. Findlay JM, Prescott RJ, Sircus W. Comparative evaluation of water recovery test and fluoroscopic screening in positioning a nasogastric tube during gastric secretory studies. *Br Med J* 1972;4:458–461.
9. Baron JH. Maximal stimuli. In: Baron JH, ed. *Clinical Tests of Gastric Secretion: History, Methodology, and Interpretation.* New York: Oxford University Press, 1979:25–35.
10. Klein K. Gastric secretory testing. In: Drossman DA, ed. *Manual of Gastroenterological Procedures*, 2nd edition. New York: Raven Press, 1987:59–63.

# Secretin Test

## Alphonso Brown

Chronic pancreatitis is distinguished from acute pancreatitis by the development of changes in the pancreatic ductular architecture. These ductular changes are easy to detect in severe and end-stage chronic pancreatitis; however, they may be extremely subtle in early chronic pancreatitis. In recent years improvements in radiological and endoscopic imaging techniques have facilitated the early diagnosis of chronic pancreatitis. Despite the increased sensitivity of these imaging modalities, diagnosis of early chronic pancreatitis is still very difficult. The secretin test is the most sensitive and specific test for detecting abnormalities in pancreatic exocrine function. Prior data have shown that abnormalities in the secretin test correspond to changes found on histological sections of the same pancreas. Thus, the secretin test is extremely useful in the diagnosis of chronic pancreatitis and assessment of pancreatic exocrine function. The traditional secretin test has recently been modified by obtaining pancreatic juice at endoscopy or via direct aspiration of pancreatic juice from the pancreatic duct at endoscopic retrograde cholangiopancreatography.

### INDICATIONS
1. The secretin test is used to evaluate individuals with abdominal pain, weight loss, steatorrhea, or recurrent pancreatitis in whom the diagnosis of chronic pancreatitis is suspected.

### CONTRAINDICATIONS
1. Acute pancreatitis
2. Uncooperative patients
3. Allergy to secretin

### PREPARATION
1. Give nothing by mouth after midnight.
2. Obtain informed, written consent.

### EQUIPMENT
1. A Dreiling tube (Davol Rubber Company [see Fig. 43.1]), which is a double-lumen tube with one set of aspiration ports positioned for retrieving gastric contents and the other for aspirating duodenal contents
2. Synthetic porcine secretin (SecreFlo, Repligen)
3. Collection bottles for gastric and duodenal secretions
4. Basin with ice
5. Two 50-cc catheter-tipped syringes for aspirating gastric and duodenal juice and one 10-cc syringe for administering secretin

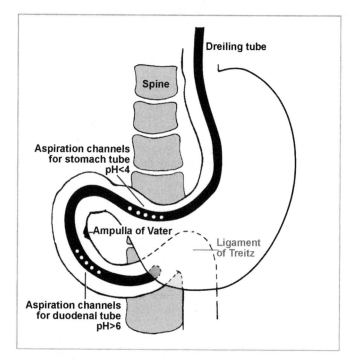

**Fig. 43.1. Schematic representation of a Dreiling tube properly positioned for performance of the secretin test. Note:** All gastric aspiration ports are within the stomach, and all duodenal ports are distal to the phylorus such that they only aspirate duodenal contents.

6. pH paper

7. No. 21 gauge needle and tubing

8. Wall suction

9. Fluoroscopy unit

**PROCEDURE**

1. Pass the Dreiling tube via the oropharynx into the esophagus and then the stomach. Using fluoroscopic guidance, maneuver and position the tube into the duodenum just beyond the ligament of Treitz.

2. With the patient supine and the tube in proper position (Fig. 43.1), aspirate juice from the duodenal and gastric channels using different 50-cc syringes. Confirm that the gastric aspirate is acidic by checking for the appropriate color change on the pH paper.

3.  After verifying that the tube is properly positioned, tape it to the nose and aspirate gastric contents until there is no return. The subject is now ready to have the baseline assessment performed.

4.  Collection of the baseline sample is as follows:

    a.  Connect both the gastric and duodenal channels to a suction unit for continuous low suctioning (25 to 40 mm Hg) for 10 to 20 minutes.
    b.  Discard the gastric juice.
    c.  Measure the volume of the baseline sample of duodenal juice, and then take the samples for cytology and $HCO_3^-$ levels. Cytology is obtained if pancreatic cancer is suspected.

5.  Administer a small test dose of the secretin (SecreFlo 0.2 mcg) in order to test for the possibility of an allergy. If there is no reaction after 1 minute, then administer the full dose of 0.2 mcg/kg body weight intravenously over 1 minute.

6.  Collection of the postsecretin infusion samples is performed as follows:

    a.  Immediately after completion of the injection of secretin, collect one sample of aspirated duodenal fluid every 20 minutes. This step will be repeated three more times in order to obtain a total of four samples.
    b.  Measure the total volume for each sample before placing a part of the sample into a collection tube for bicarbonate ($HCO_3^-$) determination.
    c.  Place the tube on ice.
    d.  Repeat Steps b and c until all four of the collected samples are completed.
    e.  Pool the remaining fluid from each sample, and place it in a beaker on ice in order to perform cytological analysis.
    f.  After completion of the sample collection, slowly remove the Dreiling tube.
    g.  After appropriately labeling the samples, send the sample to the lab for bicarbonate concentration and cytology.

**Table 43.1. Secretin test results for diagnosing chronic pancreatitis and pancreatic cancer**

|  | Diagnosis | |
|---|---|---|
|  | Chronic pancreatitis | Pancreatic cancer |
| Cytology | Negative | Positive (60% of all cases) |
| $HCO_3^-$ | < 90 mEq/L in all samples | ≥ 90 mEq/L in one or more samples |
| Total volume[a] | ≥ 2 mL/kg | < 2 mL/kg |

[a]Sum of all sample volumes after secretin divided by weight in kilograms

h.   Table 43.1 lists the cutoff values on the secretin test, which are useful in the diagnosis of chronic pancreatitis and pancreatic cancer.

## POSTPROCEDURE

Most subjects are free to resume normal activities immediately after their procedures.

## INTERPRETATION

1.   Table 43.1 lists the reference values for utilization of the secretin test in the identification of chronic pancreatitis. A bicarbonate level less than 90 mEq/L in all samples is consistent with the presence of chronic pancreatitis. If the total aspirated volume of duodenal secretion is < 2 mL/kg after the administration of secretin then this is also consistent with chronic pancreatitis or, rarely, obstruction.

## COMPLICATIONS

1.   Perforation
2.   Bleeding
3.   Allergic reactions to the secretin

## CPT Codes

**83986 –** Pathology pH, body fluid, except blood.

## REFERENCES

1.   Dreiling DA. Pancreatic secretory testing. *Gut* 1975;16:653–657.
2.   Somogyi L, Cintron M, Toskes P. Synthetic porcine secretin is highly accurate in pancreatic function testing in individuals with chronic pancreatitis. *Pancreas* 2000;21:262.
3.   Bozkurt T, Braun U, et al. Comparison of pancreatic morphology and exocrine functional impairment in patients with chronic pancreatitis. *Gut* 1994;35:1132.

# Sphincter of Oddi Manometry

Daniel J. Geenen

The sphincter of Oddi (SO) is a bundle of muscles that surrounds the ampulla of Vater, the distal common bile duct, and the distal pancreatic duct. Biliary manometry is a manometry test used to diagnose physiologic or anatomical abnormalities of the sphincter. Dysfunction of the sphincter may contribute to biliary-type pain or recurrent acute pancreatitis. Treatment with endoscopic sphincterotomy may relieve these symptoms. Performing sphincter of Oddi manometry takes patience, good communication between endoscopist and technician, and skill in interpretation.

## SPHINCTER OF ODDI MANOMETRY
## INDICATIONS

1. Diagnosis of sphincter of Oddi dysfunction
2. Biliary pain of unexplained origin
3. Postcholecystectomy upper abdominal pain
4. Idiopathic recurrent pancreatitis

## CONTRAINDICATIONS

1. Same as endoscopic retrograde cholangiopancreatography (ERCP)
2. Acute pancreatitis
3. Uncooperative patients (consider general anesthesia)

## PREPARATION OF PATIENT

1. Same as ERCP
2. Cautions about drugs for sedation
    a. No morphine
    b. No anticholinergics
    c. No glucagon
    d. No muscle relaxants

## EQUIPMENT

1. Side-viewing duodenoscope
2. Microtransducers or perfusion setup
3. Recording system
    a. Dynograph or
    b. Computerized/Solid State
4. SOM triple-lumen catheter
    a. 1.7 outer diameter
    b. 3 lumens, 0.5 mm each

    c.   Lateral orifice 0.5 mm

    d.   Black marks at 2-mm intervals

5.   Pneumohydraulic perfusion pump

    a.   Water rate 0.25 mm/minute

    b.   Reservoir pressure 375 mg Hg

6.   Standardize/calibrate entire system prior to study

7.   Transducers

    a.   Free of air bubbles

    b.   Placed at the height of the papilla

8.   An additional catheter may be taped to the outside of the scope to record duodenal pressures.

## PREPARATION OF EQUIPMENT

1.   Use approximately 500 cc of sterile water. Fill the reservoir of the pump and seal it tightly.

2.   Open the nitrogen tank valve of the perfusion machine to a PSI of 100. Open the low pressure valve to a PSI of 7.

3.   Remove any air from the transducer dome by tapping the top.

4.   Attach transducers to connecting catheters and connecting catheters to triple-lumen catheters.

5.   Turn on the perfusion valve, and prime the triple-lumen and duodenal catheters. Make sure the perfusion system is free of air bubbles. Perfuse for at least 15 minutes prior to the procedure.

6.   Standardize catheters and transducers to a baseline of 0.

## PROCEDURE

1.   Perform an ERCP with cholangiogram to rule out other causes of pain (including stone, stricture). See Chapter 7.

2.   Place the 0.018-in. guidewire into the common bile duct. Place the triple-lumen catheter over the guidewire and advance the down scope.

3.   Hold the tip of the catheter in the duodenum. Record briefly. Readings should be equal in all channels.

4.   Insert the catheter into the mid common bile duct (CBD), significantly above the sphincter of Oddi zone. Take a reading of the intraductal pressure.

5.   Perform a pull-through of the catheter through the sphincter zone, stopping sequentially at each of the black marks on the catheter. Watch for phasic waves. Record phasics and the basal pressure of the sphincter. Record pressures at each different black mark for 2 to 5 minutes.

6.   There must be continual communication between the endoscopist and technician with regard to the following:

    a.   Position of catheter

    b.   Number of black marks visible

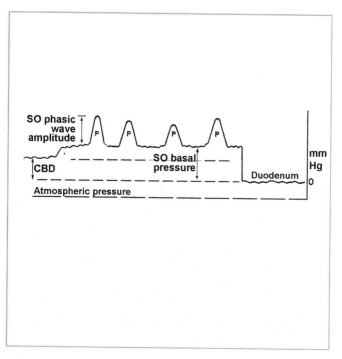

**Fig. 44.1 SO manometry interpretations**

    c.   Duodenal contractions
    d.   Patient activity

7.  There must be continual communication between the technician and endoscopist with regard to the following (Fig. 44.1):
    a.   Average baseline pressure
    b.   Phasic waves
    c.   Evidence of interference

## SPHINCTER OF ODDI MANOMETRY INTERPRETATIONS (TABLE 44.1)

### Important Measurements

1.  Duodenal pressure: Average the recorded values of all three lumens while the triple-lumen catheter is sitting within the duodenum. (The reading from the regular catheter wrapped on the endoscope is not included in these values but simply serves to establish continuous intraluminal duodenal pressures. This helps the interpreter in differentiating between SO phasic activity, duodenal contractions, and artifacts caused by breathing, retching, etc.)

2.  Common bile duct pressure: Measure the pressure observed with the triple-lumen catheter placed freely in the common bile duct, well above the sphincter zone. Again,

**Table 44.1. SO Manometry**

| Sphincter of Oddi | Abnormal |
| --- | --- |
| Basal pressure | > 40 mm Hg |
| Phasic wave activity | |
| Amplitude | > 350 mm Hg |
| Frequency | > 8 per minute |
| Propagation retrograde sequence | > 50% of total |

average the three readings to obtain the resultant value. Normal CBD pressure is approximately 15 mm Hg above duodenal pressure.

3. Gradient pressure: Gradient pressure is determined by the pressure difference between duodenal and CBD pressures. Normal CBD gradient pressure is 5 to 15 mm Hg.

4. Basal CBD SO pressure: The basal pressure is obtained during the pull-through sequence on the tracing when no phasic activity is apparent (again, the average value of all three lumens). Basal pressure is the measured difference calculated when duodenal pressure is subtracted from the baseline SO pressure between phasic waves. The normal basal pressure range is 5 to 25 mm Hg. Reproducible basal SO pressure above 40 mm Hg is compatible with SO dysfunction.

5. The frequency of phasic waves should be recorded. The normal frequency of phasic waves is three to four per minute. Phasic wave frequency of greater than eight per minute is consistent with SO dyskinesia.

6. Retrograde, simultaneous, or antegrade phasic wave propagation is important. Retrograde phasics are initiated at the distal portion of the duct, while antegrade phasics are initiated at the proximal portion of the duct. When contractions occur at the same time, the phasic waves are simultaneous. If greater than 30% of phasic waves are retrograde in origin, SO dysfunction should be considered.

7. Measure and record the average phasic wave duration. The normal range of phasic wave duration is 2.8 to 5.8 seconds. Phasic waves should be less than 300 mm Hg.

8. If there is evidence of sphincter of Oddi dysfunction, then a biliary sphincterotomy is performed (see Chapter 28).

9. In the appropriate clinical setting, manometry of the pancreatic sphincter and pancreatic sphincterotomy may be indicated.

10. During pancreatic manometry, the distal catheter channel is attached to a 10- to 20-cc syringe and intermittently aspirated (gently) to reduce the risk of pancreatitis.

11. Temporary pancreatic duct stents are placed in most patients to reduce the incidence of post-ERCP pancreatitis.

## POSTPROCEDURE

1. Monitor vital signs.
2. Admit the patient to the hospital with appropriate orders for the length of procedures or pain postprocedure
   a. Intravenous (IV) fluids at 150 to 200 cc/hour overnight (less for elderly patients and patients with history of CHP)
   b. NPO except medication until the morning
   c. IV pain medication if needed

## COMPLICATIONS

1. Pancreatitis: 3% to 30%
2. Cholangitis
3. Duodenal perforation
4. Bleeding

## CPT Codes

**43263 –** Endoscopic retrograde cholangiopancreatography (ERCP); with pressure measurement of sphincter of Oddi (pancreatic duct or common bile duct).

## SUGGESTED READINGS

Geenen JE, Hogan WJ, Dodds WJ, et al. Intraluminal pressure recording from the human sphincter of Oddi. *Gastroenterology* 1980;78:317–324.

Geenen JE, Hogan WJ. The value of sphincter of Oddi manometry. *Endosc Rev* 1987; July/August:40–46.

Johnson DA, Cattau EL Jr, Winters CW Jr. Biliary dyskinesia with associated high amplitude esophageal peristaltic contractions. *Am J Gastroenterol* 1986; 81:254–256.

Tanaka M, Ikeda S. SOM: Comparison of microtransducer and perfusion methods. *Endoscopy* 1988;20:184–188.

Thatcher BS, Sivak MV, Tedesco FJ, et al. Endoscopic sphincterotomy for suspected dysfunction of the sphincter of Oddi. *Gastrointest Endosc* 1987;33(2): 91–95.

Touli J. What is Sphincter of Oddi dysfunction? *Gut* 1989;30: 753–761.

# Small Bowel Motility and the Role of Scintigraphy in Small Bowel Motility

Jonathan Gonenne and Michael Camilleri

If a patient's small bowel motility is in question after standard evaluation and imaging (plain films or barium studies), scintigraphy and manometry are the main tools to assess small bowel motor function. These are complementary studies. Scintigraphy allows for the noninvasive assessment of the transit and propulsion of chyme. In cases of abnormal small bowel transit scintigraphy, manometry is often recommended. Manometry measures intraluminal pressure changes caused by occlusive contractions of the bowel wall, an indirect measure of contractile activity.

This chapter will focus on the "stationary techniques" of manometry performed in the lab. Prolonging a stationary fasting study to 6 hours provides the same accuracy as the ambulatory 24-hour studies in more than 90% of patients, and it also provides accurate manometric information about the antrum. If a lengthier recording or nocturnal study is needed, "ambulatory systems" are available. While the same theoretical concepts apply, a modification of catheter system and equipment is needed, as will be briefly discussed.

## INDICATIONS (1)

1. To assess for causes of gastric or small bowel stasis such as neuropathy, myopathy, or obstruction not identified on contrast or tomographic imaging

2. To assess unexplained nausea, vomiting, or other symptoms suggestive of upper gastrointestinal (GI) dysmotility

3. To distinguish generalized from localized dysmotility in patients with dysmotility elsewhere (i.e., chronic constipation, gastroesophageal reflux)

4. To diagnose suspected chronic intestinal pseudoobstruction (CIP) when the diagnosis is unclear

5. To determine the optimal approach to feeding CIP patients (oral, gastric, jejunal, total parenteral nutrition [TPN])

6. To assess unexplained abdominal pain when features of irritable bowel syndrome (IBS) are absent

7. To assess therapeutic response to a medical intervention or medication

8. To exclude GI motor dysfunction with an entirely normal study

**CONTRAINDICATIONS**

1. Those associated with esophogogastroduodenoscopy (EGD)

2. Massively dilated small bowel is a relative contraindication due to risk of perforation.

3. Known multiple jejunal diverticulosis

**PREPARATION**

1. A 12-hour fast is required (clear liquids for the evening meal on the day before).

2. Allow no medications affecting motility for 48 hours (including narcotics, tricyclic antidepressants, macrolides, anticholinergics, adrenergics). If diabetic, ensure the patient's blood glucose is < 200 mg/dL at the start of test or give half the patient's usual morning dose of insulin.

3. If the patient is on TPN, discontinue 8 hours before the study.

4. If sedation is necessary, a short-acting benzodiazepine followed by a waiting period of at least an hour is recommended prior to proceeding with measurements to avoid possible drug-induced motility effects.

**EQUIPMENT**

1. Catheters

   - Stationary systems: multilumen polyvinyl water-perfused catheter with side-holes, where water perfused side-holes serve as "sensors" (Fig. 45.1). The catheter is continuously perfused with water by means of an infusion pump at a low rate (0.1 mL/minute or less) and connected to external pressure transducers and recorders. Adequate dynamic performance of each catheter and transducer needs to be demonstrated at regular intervals, such as once per month.
   - Ambulatory systems: Teflon catheters with "solid-state" pressure transducers or impedance sensors combine solid-state miniaturized tube-mounted strain gauges with data loggers/recorders, similar to outpatient 24-hour pH monitoring (2).

2. Stationary pneumohydraulic system connected to the water-perfused catheter:

   Degassed water in a reservoir is maintained at a high constant pressure (15 psi) by nitrogen oxide, and is then reduced to atmospheric level by capillary tubing (providing high resistance) by the time the water enters the manometric assembly. Optimal perfusion rates of 0.05 to 0.1 mL/minute can be achieved either with a pneumohydraulic perfusion system and incorporation of steel capillary or other tubes that control rate of flow, or by use of commercially available external transducers that have a set flow rate (e.g., Baxter Pressure Monitoring Kit, model PX-MK099, Baxter Inc., Irvine, CA).

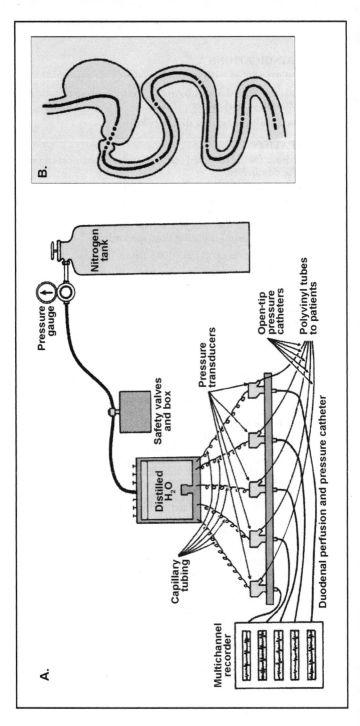

3.  Data acquisition

    *   A variety of computer-based systems are available with their own specifications. For example, for some computer software, the calibrations for pressure can be selected at 50 mm Hg or 100 mm Hg for small bowel contractions and 100 mm Hg for antral contractions. Typically the screen display is set up for a time window of 15 minutes.

4.  Standard fluoroscopy equipment

5.  Standard upper endoscope

6.  Transmucosal potential difference (TMPD) electrodes or Dent sleeve

    *   Aids the evaluation of motor activity in sphincteric regions. This consists of two saline-perfused intraluminal catheter channels, connected to an electrometer, placed on either side of the pylorus. An electrode is placed subcutaneously (ideally) or on the skin, and transmucosal potential differences are obtained. The device facilitates correct placement of pressure sensors in the terminal portion of the antrum by maintaining the potential difference between gastric and duodenal mucosa. To date, Dent sleeves have not been used extensively to evaluate the pylorus.

## PROCEDURE

1.  Prepare the system for use. Connect each multilumen perfusion tube to strain gauges and flush with distilled water; set pressure in the tank drum of the pneumohydraulic system at 10 psi (nitrogen gas); connect tubing to the water tank; and label the tracing with patient information. The external strain gauges linked to the manometric assembly should be approximately at the same height above the floor as the sensors within the gut for accurate pressure determinations. This is easily achieved by having the patient lie on a bed that can be moved vertically up or down, with the head at a 45-degree angle.

2.  Calibrate the equipment. Calibration of each strain gauge should precede every study. Before and during each study, the tracing needs to be monitored for uniformity of rate of

◄

**Fig. 45.1. Small bowel manometry.**
**A: Pneumohydraulic perfusion system, linked to a multilumen manometric catheter via interposed strain gauges. B: The catheter placement involves at least 5 side-holes spaced a few mm to 1 cm apart within the gastric portion of the tube, and two to three side-holes placed 10 cm apart in the small bowel, with the midsensor placed at the level of the angle of Treitz to ensure that a segment of jejunum can be assessed with the distal sensor. Reproduced by permission from Malagelada J-R, Camilleri M, Stanghellini V.** *Manometric Diagnosis of Gastrointestinal Motility Disorders.* **Thieme Publishers: New York, 1986, p. 41.**

rise of pressure peaks. A slow rate of rise of waves mandates review of that sensor for potential blockage or air bubbles and flushing of the system with a bolus of degassed water.

3. Position the catheter under fluoroscopy to ensure that the sensors across the antroduodenal junction are in place (see below). Radiation safety regulations at some centers recommend a maximum of 5 minutes of fluoroscopy time.

4. Place the catheter. The catheter can be placed either nonendoscopically or endoscopically.

   a. Nonendoscopic catheter placement
      - Pass the catheter with pressure sensor/transducer through the nose or mouth, guiding it beyond the pylorus into the duodenum. One can use a steerable Teflon catheter with the aid of fluoroscopy. If the nonendoscopic, routine placement does not achieve appropriate guidewire or catheter placement within 4 minutes of fluoroscopy time, an upper GI endoscopy with or without sedation should be performed to secure proper placement of the guidewire. This leaves sufficient fluoroscopy time to ensure proper positioning of the recording catheter. Currently, most centers place these tubes endoscopically.
   b. Endoscopic catheter placement
      - Place a guidewire into the small intestine by inserting the endoscope into the third portion of the duodenum and then introducing the guidewire. Advance the catheter into the upper gut over the guidewire, so that the tip is beyond the angle of Treitz.

5. Position the sensors. The sensors should be spaced from the pylorus to the proximal jejunum, starting 3 to 5 cm proximal to the pylorus (see Fig. 45.1). The pylorus can be located manometrically by identifying one of the three following patterns:

   a. A combination of distal antral peaks (duration > 5 seconds and higher amplitude, typically > 20 mm Hg, with a maximum frequency of 3 per minute) and duodenal peaks (duration < 3 seconds and lower amplitude, typically < 20 mm Hg, with a maximum frequency of 12 per minute)
   b. The presence of a high-pressure zone ("tone")
   c. The lack of contractions in the tracing from the sensor adjacent to clear antral contractions, indicating "quiescence" recorded from a large diameter duodenal bulb

6. Complete the recording phase. Some labs continue this until an activity front (or clear-cut abnormalities) is recorded; other labs focus on a 3-hour fasting and a 2-hour postprandial period.

   a. Step 1: 3 hours fasting
      i. The "pyloric" tracing should be kept in the center of the array of recordings from the antroduodenal

junction sensors; this is more easily achieved by having at least three but preferably five or more closely spaced sensors across the antroduodenal junction.

ii.  The location of the pyloric recording helps facilitate proper assessment of distal antral contractility. Careful monitoring of the waveforms is essential for optimal recordings; on average, a stationary (laboratory-based) study requires an average of five adjustments of tube location in the postprandial period to ensure accurate distal antral recordings. If this cannot be achieved by monitoring the waveforms, it is essential to repeat fluoroscopy briefly to reposition the tube correctly. Alternatively, incorporating the transmucosal potential difference apparatus into the tube assembly allows the operator to keep the tube at the pylorus by recording the difference in mucosal voltage between antral and duodenal bulb mucosa.

b.  Step 2: meal phase, then 2 hours postprandial

i.  Make certain there is no migrating motor complex (MMC) activity starting just before you feed the patient.

ii.  Advance the tube (up to 7 cm) depending upon position within the stomach, with the patient seated almost upright.

iii.  The test meal should contain at least 400 kcal to ensure a postprandial small intestinal response lasting at least 2 hours. The solid-liquid meal should be balanced and typical of the average US diet with 20% to 25% fat, 20% to 25% protein, and 50% to 55% carbohydrate. The caloric content is important because a 2-hour duration of the intestinal fed response is critical to assess the possibility of extrinsic neuropathy. The latter results in return of MMCs before the end of 2 hours postprandially (see below for details). The meal should be consumed in 30 minutes or less, with at least half of the solid meal consumed in 15 minutes. If the patient is unable to complete the solid meal, supplement with a malt shake to ensure a calorie intake ≥ 400 kcal.

iv.  The above describes the stationary system. In ambulatory manometry, the solid-state catheter is placed, obviating the need for pneumohydraulic perfusion or pressure systems/tubing. Once the patient has left the lab/medical center, the patient is instructed on meals/overnight fasting, but no adjustment to the catheter system is made. Even when the tube incorporates antral recording sites, it is not guaranteed that these will be at the right place during and after meals.

## POSTPROCEDURE

1.  Remove the stationary tube. Some labs perform a screening esophageal motility study pull-through technique (1 cm per wet swallow).

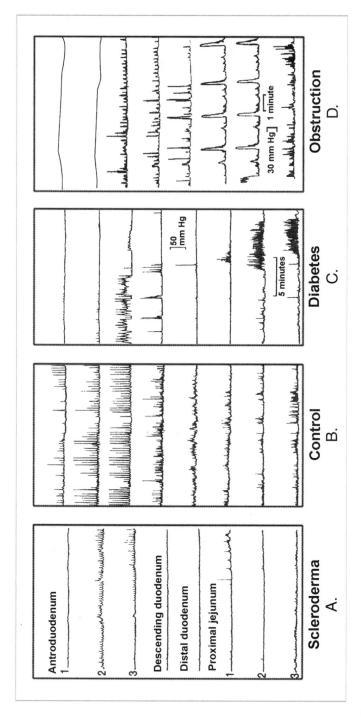

2. Turn off the pressure tank, and disconnect the tubing from the tank.

3. Clean the tube with Endozime cleaner, flush all channels, soak in high-level disinfection solution, and force air-dry all channels.

4. Print results from the computer system. Set options time for 0.25 mm/second. For esophageal motility recording phase, print at 2 mm/second.

## INTERPRETATION (SEE FIG. 45.2)

Assess the small intestine's functional integrity by analyzing the MMC, the presence/nature of the motor response to the meal, and recognized abnormal patterns (2).

### Normal (1)

1. At least one complete MMC per 24 hours, demonstrating clearly identifiable Phase 1 (quiescence), Phase II (intermittent, irregular phasic pressure activity unassociated with significant baseline elevations), and Phase III (burst of propagated, rhythmic contractions) complexes. If the fasting recording is 6 hours or less, it may not be abnormal if there are no migrating motor complexes.

   a. Conversion to the fed pattern after a 400 kcal meal without return of MMC for at least 2 hours.

   b. Postprandial pattern is induced 5 to 10 minutes after meal ingestion, peaking in 10 to 20 minutes.

   c. Distal postprandial antral contractility (antral amplitude < 40 mm Hg suggests a myopathic process; a frequency < 1 per minute during the first postprandial hour suggests a neuropathic process) (3).

   d. Small intestinal contractions exceeding 20 mm Hg, with average > 10 mm Hg; lower average amplitude may be observed in dilated intestines with normal motility.

### Abnormal Patterns

1. Neuropathic (4)

   a. Definition: The contractile response pattern is disorganized, while the actual amplitudes are normal.

   b. Variations: Antral hypomotility, abnormal propagation of phase III of the MMC, hypercontractility ("bursts" of phasic activity or sustained uncoordinated pressure activity), and failure of the fasting to be converted to a fed response.

◄────────────────────────────────────

Fig. 45.2. Examples of classical gastroduodenal manometry tracings during the postprandial period. A: Low amplitude contractions, a myopathic pattern. B: Control tracing-normal postprandial fed pattern. C: Normal amplitude but premature MMC activity in the postprandial period, a neuropathic pattern. Note the absence of antral contractions. D: Simultaneous long-duration contractions above the level of the obstruction, and a normal fed pattern below the proximal jejunum.

    c. "Bursts" are defined as groups of contractions occurring at the typical frequency of phase III, lasting at least 2 minutes, and associated with tonic elevation of baseline pressure. They have been reported in extrinsic neuropathies and in chronic intestinal pseudoobstruction.

    d. With regard to a finding of "decreased frequency" of MMCs, only the complete absence of MMCs over 24 hours is abnormal.

    e. The frequency of intestinal MMCs is increased (more than three per 3 hours) in extrinsic vagal neuropathy/vagotomy.

    f. Differential diagnosis: Bacterial overgrowth shows hypomotility with rare phase III activity, weak and disorganized contractions (4). Rumination has a characteristic pattern with an artifactual increase in intraabdominal pressure at all levels of the upper gut, typically postprandially.

    g. Examples of neuropathy in small bowel dysmotility include diabetes mellitus, paraneoplastic, medications, Chagas' disease, chronic idiopathic intestinal pseudoobstruction, viral infections, Von Recklinghausen's disease, spinal cord injury, and Parkinson's (5).

    h. Although often displaying a myopathic pattern, amyloidosis, dermatomyositis, and systemic sclerosis may also exhibit neuropathic characteristics, which may reflect the earlier stage of the disease affecting the gut.

2. Myopathic

    a. Definition: Small bowel demonstrates low-amplitude contractions (average < 10 mm Hg) with or without decreased frequency of contractions at the sites affected. There is often a poor response to enteric feeding (4).

    b. Differential diagnosis: Because the sensitivity of the sensors depends on luminal diameter, they may show low-amplitude contractions because of nonspecific dilatation as in extreme aerophagia or mechanical obstruction.

    c. Examples of myopathy in small bowel dysmotility include scleroderma, amyloidosis, hollow visceral myopathy, mitochondrial cytopathy, familial visceral myopathy I–III; muscular dystrophy, dermatomyositis, and chronic intestinal pseudoobstruction (5).

3. Mechanical obstruction

    a. Prolonged intestinal contractions, lasting > 8 seconds, which are simultaneous or very rapidly propagated. Synonymous terms for these contractions are giant migrating contractions, prolonged propagating contractions, or power contractions.

    b. Postprandial clustered contractions (> 30 minutes duration) separated by quiescence (> 1 minute). This pattern is less predictive than the prolonged simultaneous contractions.

**COMPLICATIONS**

If placing catheters endoscopically, the same risks as EGD.

**ROLE OF SCINTIGRAPHY IN SMALL BOWEL MOTILITY**

**Indications (1)**

1. Noninvasive method measuring upper GI transit and assessing the existence of a motor disorder. This is often used as a screening test prior to manometry.

2. Evaluate persistent symptoms suggestive of "gastroparesis" (i.e., nausea, early satiety).

3. Evaluate suspected pseudoobstruction.

4. Evaluate chronic diarrhea or constipation when the traditional workup is negative or there is suspicion of a vagal nerve injury.

5. Assess therapeutic response to a medical intervention or medication.

**Contraindications**

Pregnancy. Women of childbearing age should undergo a pregnancy test (6).

**Preparation**

Patients fast for 12 hours and must be off medications (including anticholinergics, macrolides, and tricyclic antidepressants) affecting motility for at least 48 hours.

**Equipment**

1. Radiolabeled solids or liquids. Examples are $^{99m}$Tc-sulfur colloid labeled solid food particles and indium-111-diethylenetriamine petaacetic acid (DTPA) in water (7,8).

2. A large field-of-view gamma camera with a dedicated computer for analysis to detect field of interest (1)

**Procedure**

1. The radiolabeled material is mixed with food and ingested by the patient.

2. The patient lies on a tilt table at 45° to the horizontal or else stands (see below).

3. Anterior and posterior images with the large field-of-view gamma camera are obtained while the patient is standing. Imaging is performed immediately after ingestion of a radiolabeled meal, and after 2, 4, and 6 hours for gastric and small bowel transit.

**Postprocedure**

1. For the small intestine, the proportion of $^{99m}$Tc reaching the colon at 6 hours is used as a surrogate marker for small bowel transit (9).

2. Standard corrections for depth (geometric mean of anterior and posterior counts), isotope decay, tissue attenuation, and Compton scattering are necessary (6,10).

## Interpretation

1. The definitions of fast and slow small bowel transit are colonic filling at 6 hours of < 26.6% and > 97.9%, respectively, though there may be marked intraindividual variance (11).

2. Results may be altered by colonic dysfunction or obstruction to defecation.

3. There is not always concordance between symptoms and transit disorders (1).

## REFERENCES

1. Camilleri M, Hasler WL, Parkman HP, et al. Measurement of gastrointestinal motility in the GI laboratory. *Gastroenterology* 1998;115:747–762.
2. Kellow JE. Principles of motility and sensation testing. *Gastroenterol Clin North Am* 2003;32:733–750, ix.
3. Weston S, Thumshirn M, Wiste J, Camilleri M. Clinical and upper gastrointestinal motility features in systemic sclerosis and related disorders. *Am J Gastroenterol* 1998;93:1085–1089.
4. Hansen MB. Small intestinal manometry. *Physiol Res* 2002; 51:541–556.
5. Coulie B, Camilleri M. Intestinal pseudo-obstruction. *Ann Rev Med* 1999;50:37–55.
6. von der Ohe MR, Camilleri M. Measurement of small bowel and colonic transit: indications and methods. *Mayo Clin Proc* 1992;67:1169–1179.
7. Charles F, Camilleri M, Phillips SF, et al. Scintography of the whole gut: clinical evaluation of transit disorders. *Mayo Clin Proc* 1995;70:113–118.
8. Bonapace ES, Maurer AH, Davidoff S, et al. Whole gut transit scintigraphy in the clinical evaluation of patients with upper and lower gastrointestinal symptoms. *Am J Gastroenterol* 2000; 95:2838–2847.
9. Camilleri M, Zinsmeister AR, Greydanus MP, et al. Towards a less costly but accurate test of gastric emptying and small bowel transit. *Dig Dis Sci* 1991;36:609–615.
10. Camilleri M, Zinsmeister AR. Towards a relatively inexpensive, noninvasive, accurate test for colonic motility disorders. *Gastroenterology* 1992;103:36–42.
11. Cremonini F, Mullan BP, Camilleri M, et al. Performance characteristics of scintigraphic transit measurements for studies of experimental therapies. *Aliment Pharmacol Ther* 2002;16: 1781–1790.

# Breath Hydrogen Tests for Lactose Intolerance and Bacterial Overgrowth

Syed I.M. Thiwan and William E. Whitehead

The breath hydrogen test is a simple, safe, and noninvasive study. Although it was originally designed for carbohydrate intolerance and bacterial overgrowth, its scope has been extended to other areas in recent years. The test is moderately sensitive but much more specific in the diagnosis of these disorders than alternative techniques. As this test can sometimes detect carbohydrate malabsorption or bacterial overgrowth even in asymptomatic patients, it should be interpreted in the context of the clinical setting. Discordance often exists between the patient's self-claim of intolerance and test results (1,2).

The usual symptoms of carbohydrate malabsorption are diarrhea, abdominal pain, bloating, and flatulence. Occasionally it can present with vomiting and nausea. Small bowel bacterial overgrowth is characterized by the presence of an abnormally high number of bacteria in the upper gastrointestinal tract with attendant nutrient malabsorption. It is commonly associated with abnormal gastrointestinal (GI) transit due to mechanical factors (e.g., surgically defunctionalized loops) or abnormal motility secondary to a systemic disorder such as diabetes or changes in gastric acid (postgastrectomy). The usual symptoms are diarrhea, steatorrhea, weight loss, bloating, and macrocytic anemia.

The principal gases in the GI tract are carbon dioxide ($CO_2$), hydrogen ($H_2$), methane ($CH_4$), nitrogen ($N_2$), and oxygen ($O_2$). While $N_2$ and $O_2$ are derived from swallowed air, $H_2$ and $CH_4$ are primarily produced by bacterial metabolism. The bacteria in the normal colon break down the nonabsorbable but fermentable substrates such as lactulose and sorbitol or malabsorbed carbohydrates that reach the colon and give off hydrogen, carbon dioxide, and trace gases in the process. When bacteria are present at abnormally high levels in the small intestine, these bacteria may digest food before it can be absorbed and liberate the same gases.

A fraction of the gases liberated in the lumen of the bowel by bacterial action is absorbed into the circulation and is carried to the lungs and expired. Thus, the amount of $H_2$, $CO_2$, and $CH_4$ in the breath can be used to estimate the amount of these gases in the gut. The assumption behind these tests is that the amount of hydrogen excretion after a carbohydrate load in maldigesting or malabsorbing patients will be elevated. By controlling the diet the day before the test, one can bring the hydrogen excretion to close to zero at baseline. When a patient with carbohydrate malabsorption consumes that particular carbohydrate, there is an increase in $H_2$ excretion in the expired air. The timing of this peak and the magnitude of the peak help to identify whether it is carbohydrate malabsorption (peaks after 60 minutes) or small bowel bacterial overgrowth (peaks before 60 minutes). This forms the basis for breath hydrogen tests.

## INDICATIONS

1. Diagnosis of lactose intolerance or other carbohydrate malabsorption
2. Diagnosis of small bowel bacterial overgrowth

## CONTRAINDICATIONS

None. Consider using nonabsorbable sugar such as lactulose for patients with diabetes mellitus for testing of small bowel bacterial overgrowth.

## PREPARATION

1. Avoid oral antibiotics and lactulose (Chronulac) for at least 2 weeks prior to testing.
2. Avoid taking drugs that affect the motility or the transit of the gut (e.g., tricyclic antidepressants, calcium channel blockers, laxatives, and prokinetic agents) for at least 4 days before the test.
3. Avoid nonfermentable carbohydrates (pasta, breads, and fiber cereals) the night before the test (3).
4. Take nothing by mouth overnight (a minimum of 4 to 6 hours in infants).
5. Avoid candy and chewing gums at least an hour before the test.
6. Avoid smoking (increases $H_2$ level) and physical exercise (decreases $H_2$ level) for 2 hours before testing and during testing.
7. Avoid sleeping during the study since it can falsely elevate the hydrogen level because of hypoventilation.

## EQUIPMENT

1. Breath analyzers: There are several types of breath analyzers available. One (QuinTron) is based on solid-state technology and others (such as LactoFAN, Micro-$H_2$) are based on fuel cell technology. Fuel cell-based analyzers are portable but have the disadvantage of cross-sensitivity with carbon monoxide (CO), and they only measure $H_2$. Among all the breath analyzers, QuinTron-model SC, which also measures methane, is the only analyzer that has the ability to detect and correct for contamination of the sample with room air or dead space air during the collection procedure by measuring $CO_2$.
2. Breath collection devices: The accuracy and reliability of breath testing depends on obtaining a reliable sample of alveolar air. This is accomplished by collecting an end-expiratory air sample as it most closely represents the alveolar air. For adults and young children who can follow

directions, it is not very hard to coordinate the timing of collection with the end of expiration. A modified Haldane-Priestly device is commonly used in the collection process (4,5).

It is often difficult to obtain a reliable sample of alveolar air from neonates and children who are too young to follow the directions. Pediatric face masks, nasal prongs, and nasopharyngeal or oropharyngeal catheters have been used in these settings, with nasal prongs being the most widely used. Commonly available devices for pediatric use are Kid sampler, and Baby sampler from QuinTron, which are similar to the standard adult device but smaller in size.

3. Breath hydrogen test substrates

   a. Lactose 25 to 50 g for tests of lactose malabsorption. Higher doses may increase sensitivity but may bring on the symptoms of intolerance. Fructose is sometimes used for the diagnosis of fructose malabsorption in 25- to 50-g doses. The fructose test may not correlate with the clinical condition as fructose is absorbed by facilitative diffusion, and so its absorptive capacity is limited in most people.

   b. Lactulose 10 to 12 g for small bowel bacterial overgrowth or measurement of small bowel transit time. One study (6) used a higher dose and found a lower frequency (27% with 12 g versus 14% with 20 g) of low $H_2$ producers (either no rise or less than 20 ppm increase over baseline breath $H_2$ level with lactulose).

   c. Glucose 50 to 80 g (1 to 2 g/kg), sucrose 50 g, and xylose 15 to 25 g for small bowel bacterial overgrowth.

## PROCEDURE

A baseline breath sample at end expiration is collected before administering the test meal.

1. Place the mouthpiece in the patient's mouth, and ask him or her to form a tight seal around it with his or her lips.

2. Ask the patient to exhale through the mouth normally into the sampling device after a normal inspiration. The discard bag collects the first portion of expired air, and when it is full, the one-way valve in the T-piece and the collection bag will open, and the end-expiratory air will flow into the collection bag.

3. When both bags are full, tell the patient to stop expiring and remove the mouthpiece. Sometimes a nose clip may be needed, or the patient can pinch his or her nose to make sure all the expired air goes through the mouth. An alternative method is to aspirate 3 to 5 mL of the expired air from nasal prongs at the end of expiration while observing the patient's breathing pattern. The nasal prongs are held at the nose by either the patient or the examiner. The breath samples can be stored in these bags for up to 48 hours without significant loss of these gases.

4. Ask the patient to drink a specified amount (1 to 2 g/kg, max 50 g in most cases) of a substrate in a 10% to 20% aqueous

solution. The test solution should preferably be at room temperature. Since all the carbohydrates used for testing yield hydrogen when digested by bacteria, theoretically any substrate can be used with the hydrogen test for the diagnosis of small bowel bacterial overgrowth. To diagnose a particular carbohydrate malabsorption, that particular sugar is used for the breath $H_2$ test.

5. Breath sample collection: Different protocols exist specifically for different purposes of the breath $H_2$ test. For the diagnosis of carbohydrate malabsorption, breath samples are collected every 30 minutes for a total of 3 to 4 hours or until a positive response is seen. If an aqueous solution was used for the sugar, 3 hours is probably enough, but if milk is used as a substrate, a minimum of 4 hours of testing is needed because of the effect of the fat in milk on gastric emptying (5). For small bowel bacterial overgrowth, breath samples are collected every 15 to 20 minutes for at least 2 hours or until a positive response is seen. If lactulose is used for the diagnosis of bacterial overgrowth, it is important to extend the test for an additional hour or two to capture the second peak caused by the colonic fermentation (5). For transit study, breath samples are collected every 10 minutes beginning 30 minutes after lactulose for the initial 2 hours and then every 20 minutes after first 2 hours until a rise of 3 ppm over the immediate preceding level is recorded three times consecutively (5). A minimum of two consecutive samples should be measured.

**POSTPROCEDURE**

Instruct the patient to return to previous activities.

**COMPLICATIONS**

1. Diarrhea
2. Bloating
3. Abdominal pain (may occur in patients with a positive test)

**INTERPRETATION**

The result is usually expressed as the concentration of hydrogen excreted in breath in parts per million (ppm). Hydrogen levels usually go down in the fasting state unless the subject has extremely slow transit. Thus the baseline value can be assumed to be the lowest value recorded at any sampling time. The difference between the peak and the baseline value is delta ppm. The fasting breath hydrogen concentration in healthy children and adults is in the range of 2.1 to 12.1 ppm. One percent of those people had $H_2$ concentration of more than 30 ppm, and none exceeded 42 ppm (3).

**Carbohydrate Intolerance (Lactose and Fructose)**

1. A rise in $H_2$ above baseline of greater than 20 ppm is considered abnormal at 2 to 3 hours (1,6,7). Measuring methane also increases the accuracy of the $H_2$ breath test since it detects non-$H_2$ producers (8,9,10) who produce methane instead of $H_2$ or in addition to $H_2$.

2.  An increase in methane by 12 ppm is interpreted as a positive test even in the absence of a rise in $H_2$ (5). Some studies have used either percentage (at least 100%) increase in breath $CH_4$ concentration or the area under the curve for $CH_4$ for interpretation of the breath test when low $H_2$ production was encountered.

3.  In the case of both $H_2$ and $CH_4$ production, it is prudent to add the increases of both $H_2$ and $CH_4$ levels to determine the degree of malabsorption. A sum of both levels of $H_2$ and $CH_4$ of more than 15 to 20 ppm can be considered as a positive test, although it is probably an underestimate as two molecules of $H_2$ are needed to form one molecule of methane (5).

**Small Bowel Bacterial Overgrowth**

1.  Any increase in breath $H_2$ above a predefined threshold (a rise of either 10 or 12 ppm) that occurs within the first 60 minutes is considered abnormal and indicative of small bowel bacterial overgrowth (3,11). Any peak in the concentration of $H_2$ exceeding baseline by a predetermined amount is abnormal with the glucose breath $H_2$ test no matter when the peak occurs because glucose should be readily absorbed in the small intestine (11).

2.  In some laboratories a peak in breath $H_2$ above a predefined threshold that occurs more than 60 minutes after ingestion of lactulose is considered abnormal and indicative of a positive test if it is followed by a second peak indicating entry of the sugar into the cecum. These two peaks should be clearly separable, and the first peak (small bowel) should precede the second or colonic peak by at least 15 minutes. Often the first peak is at least 10 ppm, and the second colonic peak is at least 20 ppm of breath $H_2$ level over the baseline. The rationale is that an early peak indicates bacterial overgrowth in the proximal small bowel and that a late peak is indicative of small bowel bacterial overgrowth in the distal small bowel.

3.  Different laboratories have used different criteria for what constitutes an abnormal increase in breath $H_2$ over baseline. Some laboratories use the mean fasting $H_2$ level plus two standard deviations to define the fasting $H_2$ value for that laboratory, while others require a rise of 10 or 20 ppm over baseline. A fasting breath $H_2$ of greater than 20 ppm is considered abnormal (3,11) and is probably indicative of small bowel bacterial overgrowth, although a baseline level of breath $H_2$ above 40 ppm is more definitive. A baseline $H_2$ concentration above 20 ppm occurs in approximately one third of the patients with bacterial overgrowth.

**LIMITATIONS**

1.  Some patients will have a flat hydrogen breath test (no rise in breath $H_2$). This could be present in 5% to 27% of normal people (6,8–10). Flat response to lactulose could be from methane production, altered bacterial flora secondary to antibiotic use, recent severe diarrhea, use of laxatives or

enemas, colonic pH, and extremely slow transit. To overcome these problems the following measures are suggested:

  a. The methane level should be simultaneously measured with every test, or it should be subsequently measured after a flat test (8–10). Another option is to readminister the breath test on a different day using a nonabsorbable sugar such as lactulose, which is definitely known to reach the colon. This will prove whether the patient is capable of producing $H_2$ or not.

  b. Since colonic pH alters bacterial activity, a low colonic pH may result in a false negative study. Chronic use of lactose in intolerant patients can result in lower colonic pH causing a false negative study. A trial of magnesium sulfate (5 g dissolved in tap water, given orally twice on the day before repeating the breath test) can be given to raise colonic pH (12).

  c. Surreptitious use of antibiotics or recent use of antibiotics can result in a false negative study.

  d. A transit study may identify the patients with extremely slow transit, or one can extend the duration of study to 8 hours in patients suspected of having a slow transit.

2. Intestinal transit could alter the result. Fast transit could give a false positive result with lactulose breath test for small bowel bacterial overgrowth while slow transit can cause a false negative test. If a false negative test is suspected on clinical grounds, see number 1(d) above.

3. The breath test is difficult to interpret in patients with lung disorders. Hyperventilation may artificially lower the concentration of $H_2$ or methane in the breath.

4. With lactulose it may be difficult to discriminate distal small bowel bacterial overgrowth from a normal colonic $H_2$ peak. Interpreter reliability of the lactulose breath test is lower than the glucose or lactose breath test because it requires a double peak, one peak from the small intestine and the other from the colon, whereas the glucose test produces a single peak (7) that is always abnormal. However, the glucose breath test is insensitive to small bowel bacterial overgrowth that is restricted to the distal small bowel.

5. There is a high degree of positivity of breath $H_2$ tests for small bowel bacterial overgrowth in elderly patients. This is attributed to the presence of high duodenal bacterial levels, possibly secondary to the high prevalence of achlorhydria; however, not all of these patients have significant symptoms clinically.

6. Infants and small children may give false negative studies because the breath sample is contaminated with room air. The best control for this is to test all samples for $CO_2$ and to repeat any samples for which the $CO_2$ level is very low.

7. Improper preparation for the test or improper performance of the test such as nonadherence to the dietary advice on the

part of patient, sleeping, and smoking by the patient or by anybody in the vicinity of breath analyzer may result in a false positive test.

## OTHER USES FOR THIS TECHNIQUE

1. Measurement of intestinal transit time, i.e., orocecal transit time with lactulose (13): This method of testing orocecal transit time has the advantage of involving no radioisotopes or barium. However, error of measurement is introduced by the fact that the observed transit time is influenced by where in the cycle of migrating motor complexes the test meal is ingested, and lactulose itself has an accelerating effect on gut motility.

2. Testing for mucosal integrity/intestinal malabsorption with the xylose breath $H_2$ test, because xylose is minimally metabolized This may be useful in the follow-up of celiac disease patients treated with dietary therapy.

3. Verifying whether or not the bowel preparation has cleared combustible $H_2$ and $CH_4$ from the colon before colonoscopy with polypectomy, as there is a risk of explosion with these gases.

4. Other uses are for identification of intestinal gas syndromes with specific foods and indirect measurement of gastric acid secretion.

## CPT Codes

**91065** – Breath hydrogen test (e.g., for detection of lactase deficiency).

## REFERENCES

1. Newcomer AD, McGill DB, Thomas PJ, Hofmann AF. Prospective comparison of indirect methods for detecting lactase deficiency. *N Engl J Med* 1975;293:1232.
2. Suraez FL, Savaiano DA, Levitt MD. A comparison of symptoms after the consumption of milk or lactose-hydrolyzed milk by people with self-reported severe lactose intolerance. *N Engl J Med* 1995;333:1.
3. Perman JA, Modler S, Barr RG, et al. Fasting breath hydrogen concentration: normal values and clinical application. *Gastroenterology* 1984; 87:1358.
4. Thompson DG, Binfield P, De Belder A, et al. Extraintestinal influences on exhaled breath hydrogen measurements during the investigation of gastrointestinal disease. *Gut* 1985;26(12): 1349–1352.
5. Hamilton LH. *Breath Tests & Gastroenterology*, 2nd ed. Milwaukee, WI: QuinTron Instrument Company, 1998.
6. Corazza G, Strocchi A, Sorge M, et al. Prevalence and consistency of low breath $H_2$ excretion following lactulose ingestion. Possible implications for the clinical use of the $H_2$ breath test. *Dig Dis Sci* 1993;38(11):2010–2016.
7. Corazza GR, Menozzi MG, Strocchi A, et al. The diagnosis of small bowel bacterial overgrowth. *Gastroenterology* 1990; 98:302.

8. Montes RG, Saavedra JM, Perman JA. Relationship between methane production and breath hydrogen excretion in lactose-malabsorbing individuals. *Dig Dis Sci* 1993;38:445.

9. Corazza GR, Benati G, Strocchi A, et al. The possible role of breath measurement in detecting carbohydrate malabsorption. *J Lab Clin Med* 1994;124(5):695–700.

10. Rumessen JJ, Nordgaard-Anderson I, Gudmand-Hoyer E. Carbohydrate malabsorption: quantification by methane and hydrogen breath tests. *Scand J Gastroenterol* 1994;29(9): 826–832.

11. Kerlin P, Wong L. Breath hydrogen testing in bacterial overgrowth of the small intestine. *Gastroenterology* 1988;95: 982–988.

12. Vogelsang H, Ferenci P, Frotz S, et al. Acidic colonic microclimate—possible reason for false negative hydrogen breath tests. *Gut* 1988;29:21–26.

13. Miller MA, Parkman HP, Urbain JC, et al. Comparison of scintigraphy and lactulose breath hydrogen test for assessment of orocecal transit. Lactulose accelerates small bowel transit. *Dig Dis Sci* 1997;42:1.

# Anorectal Manometry and Biofeedback

Yolanda V. Scarlett

Rectal manometry is a test of anorectal function that can provide useful information about disorders that affect defecation and continence. There are various methods of performing the studies (1,2), and minimum standards of performance have been recommended (3). The equipment used to perform anorectal manometry may also be used to provide biofeedback training for patients with constipation due to obstructed defecation and for those with fecal incontinence due to various causes. Before performing anorectal manometry or biofeedback, one should obtain hands-on instruction and supervision from someone experienced in manometry. Manometry training programs are available through some of the companies marketing manometric equipment (Medtronic, Minneapolis, Minnesota; Sandhill Scientific, Highlands Ranch, Colorado).

## INDICATIONS
1. Constipation
2. Fecal incontinence
3. Evaluation prior to biofeedback training for pelvic floor dyssynergia
4. Evaluation prior to biofeedback training for continence strategies
5. Preoperative evaluation before procedures involving the anus and or rectum such as creation of a pouch, ileoanal anastomosis, and elective sphincteroplasty

## CONTRAINDICATIONS
Use of latex balloons in individuals with latex allergy.

## PREPARATION
In general, no preparation is required. If a large amount of stool is anticipated or present, a rectal enema may be administered. Patients may continue on their usual medications, and dietary modification is not required. Informed consent must be obtained.

The procedure should be explained to the patient. Afterwards, the patient should be asked to change into a hospital gown.

## EQUIPMENT
Required equipment includes the following:
1. A probe. Both water-perfused and solid-state probes or catheters are commercially available for rectal manometry. Pressure-sensitive transducers are arranged radially along

the probe and spaced several centimeters apart. Reusable and disposable probes are available (Andorfer Medical Specialties, Inc., Greendale, Wisconsin; Gaeltec Ltd., Isle of Skye, Scotland; Medtronic, Minneapolis, Minnesota; Mui Scientific, Mississauga, Ontario, Canada; Sandhill Scientific, Highlands Ranch, Colorado).

2. A manometric recording device, a computerized recorder and storage device compatible with commercially available software, is recommended. A computerized recorder and storage device compatible with commercially available software, is recommended. A monitor, which may be a portable notebook or laptop, is desirable for the computerized systems. Software programs are designed to perform study interpretation, but editing is required to ensure accuracy.

3. A system to display the recording

4. A device to store the data

5. A sterile disposable needle

6. Surgical tape

7. 4-in. × 4-in. gauze or washcloths

8. Gloves

9. Water-soluble lubricant

10. Hospital gown

**PROCEDURE**

Before performing anorectal manometry, the equipment should be assembled and the probe and recorder calibrated according to the manufacturer's instructions.

1. Inflate the rectal balloon with 50 cc of air for 30 seconds. All of the air should be withdrawn from the balloon. If less than 50 cc of air is recovered, the balloon should be tested for leaks by reinflating the balloon under water.

2. Lubricate the balloon with a water-soluble lubricant.

3. Position the patient on the left side with knees flexed. Inspect the buttocks, perineum, and the perianal area. Check the sensation to pinprick in anterior, posterior, and bilateral positions with a sterile, disposable needle. The presence or absence of anal wink should be documented.

4. A careful digital rectal exam should be performed with notation made of the anal sphincter tone at rest, anal sphincter tone with squeezing, contraction of the puborectalis muscle, and perineal descent with Valsalva maneuver.

5. Gently insert the catheter 10 to 15 cm into the rectum (Fig. 47.1).

6. Allow the patient to rest for 3 to 5 minutes to give the patient time to adjust to the catheter and to allow the sphincter pressure to return to resting levels.

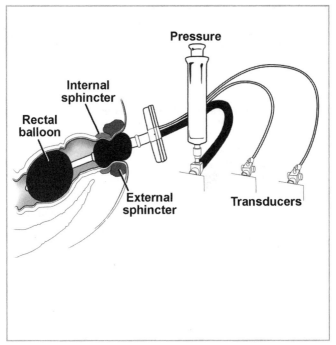

**Fig. 47.1. The apparatus used for rectal manometry is shown in position. Each balloon is linked to a separate pressure transducer. Distention of the rectal balloon with air elicits the rectosphincteric response.**

7. Identify the high-pressure zone with the continuous pull-through technique. The pressure will increase as the transducers enter the anal sphincter zone. Document the location, length, and pressure of the sphincter zone. The pressure will decrease as the transducers are pulled past the sphincter zone. Repeat the continuous pull-through twice, each time documenting the location, length, and pressure of the sphincter zone.

8. Allow the probe to remain undisturbed for 3 to 5 minutes to allow equilibration. Use the station pull-through technique to withdraw the probe into the high-pressure zone. The probe should be withdrawn 0.5 to 1.0 cm and the pressure recorded. Thirty seconds should be allowed before the pressure is recorded at each station.

9. Repeat the station pull-through technique to confirm the location and pressure of the high-pressure zone. Once the location of the high-pressure zone is confirmed, secure the probe with surgical tape.

10.   Instruct the patient to perform a squeeze and hold maneu-
      ver by contracting the external anal sphincter as intensely
      as possible and holding the contraction for 60 seconds.
      Allow a 30-second rest period, then repeat the squeeze and
      hold maneuver twice.

11.   Rapidly inflate the balloon with 60 mL of air to assess the
      relaxation of the internal anal sphincter. If reflex relax-
      ation is not seen, the position of the probe should be con-
      firmed and the rapid inflation repeated. If absence of the
      sphincter relaxation is noted, a higher volume of air may be
      used (Fig. 47.2).

12.   Determine the lowest threshold of rectal sensation by rap-
      idly inflating the rectal balloon with 60 mL of air and ask-
      ing if the patient detects the distention. Instruct the
      patient to inform you when the sensation of rectal disten-
      tion is experienced. Withdraw the air from the balloon.
      Rapidly inflate the balloon with 55 mL of air, and docu-
      ment the presence or absence of the sensation of rectal dis-
      tention. The rate of balloon inflation should be consistent
      as the sensory threshold is affected by the rate of balloon

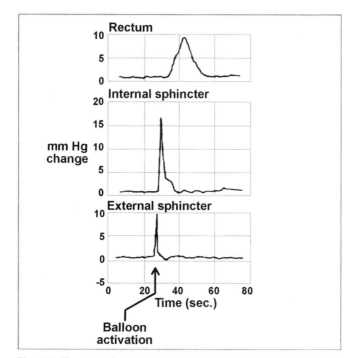

Fig. 47.2. The normal response to transient rectal distention is
shown. The resting pressure of each balloon is assigned a value of
zero with relaxation of the internal sphincter and contraction of the
external sphincter.

inflation. Continue decreasing the volume of air by increments of 5 mL, and document the lowest volume of distention detected as the first sensation threshold. Patients should be able to perceive 10 cc or less of rectal distention. Also, record the smallest volume of air associated with relaxation of the internal anal sphincter.

13. The urge threshold is the volume of rectal distention that produces a sustained urge to defecate. This is determined by cumulative distention of the rectal balloon in 20-mL increments. Allow at least 30 seconds between cumulative inflation. After the urge threshold is documented, continue to add air to the balloon in 20-mL increments until a sensation of intense urge is experienced and sustained. This volume should be recorded as the maximum volume tolerated. The balloon should be deflated and the amount of air recovered from the balloon noted to confirm accuracy.

14. Ask the patient to strain as if trying to defecate to test for pelvic floor dyssynergia. A normal response is a decrease in the pressure at the anal sphincter.

15. Ask the patient to cough. A normal response is a reflex increase in the anal sphincter pressure as the intraabdominal pressure increases.

16. After recording data, the balloon should be deflated and removed from the rectum.

**AUXILIARY TESTS**

1. The balloon expulsion test may be performed independently or at the time of anorectal manometry. This test evaluates whether the patient is able to evacuate a simulated stool. A lubricated balloon secured to a small diameter catheter is placed into the rectum.

    a. The balloon is inflated with 50 mL of air or warm water.

    b. The patient is asked to sit on a commode and expel the balloon in privacy. The individual is given 3 minutes to expel the balloon.

    c. If expulsion is not successful, the balloon is deflated and removed.

2. Additional information may be obtained from the external anal sphincter electromyography (EMG). A surface EMG sensor may be placed directly into the anal canal or skin pads placed adjacent to the anus. Surface sensors do not provide information from the puborectalis muscle. Concentric needle EMG provides data from the external anal sphincter or puborectalis but requires placement of a needle directly into the external anal sphincter or puborectalis muscle. Additional equipment including an oscilloscope is needed for concentric needle EMG.

**POSTPROCEDURE**

1. Wash the balloon and probe in warm, soapy water to remove fecal debris.

2. Disposable balloons and probes should be placed into appropriate waste receptacles.

3. Reusable equipment should be sterilized according to the manufacturer's guidelines.

4. Dry equipment thoroughly and store appropriately.

## INTERPRETATION

### Normal Sphincter Pressures

There is a range of normal pressures for the internal and external anal sphincter. Values need to be standardized for the laboratory and patient population. Suggested normals include the following:

1. In adults, the resting sphincter pressure is 40 to 90 mm Hg above the rectal intraluminal pressure. This is calculated by taking the mean of the three highest values obtained from the anal canal using the pull-through technique.

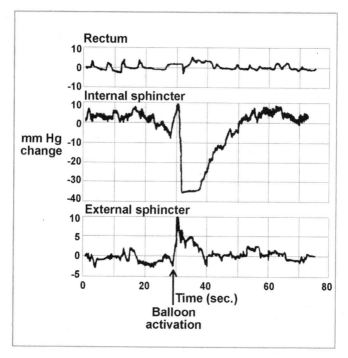

**Fig. 47.3. Manometry response in a patient with Hirschsprung's disease. The internal sphincter contracts instead of relaxing following rectal distention. The external sphincter is normal, but a strong rectal contraction not seen in the normal follows contraction of the sphincters.**

2. The maximum squeeze pressures are normally 50% to 100% above the resting pressure. In general, squeeze pressures above 100 to 125 mm Hg are considered normal. The duration of the maximum squeeze is determined by the amount of time in seconds that the patient can maintain a squeeze pressure at or above 50% of the maximum squeeze pressure.

3. Under normal circumstances, the internal anal sphincter relaxes in response to balloon distention. The resting pressure of the internal anal sphincter will decrease down to less than 30 mm Hg for up to 15 seconds. This response, the rectoanal inhibitory reflex (RAIR), is mediated by the myenteric plexus and is typically absent in Hirschsprung's disease (Fig. 47.3).

4. Simulated defecation or response to straining should produce relaxation of the external anal sphincter and puborectalis muscle. Paradoxical contraction of the external anal sphincter and/or puborectalis muscle produces an increase in the pressure referred to as pelvic floor dyssynergia.

5. The cough reflex is an involuntary response to sudden change in the intraabdominal pressure. With an increase in the intraabdominal pressure, the anal sphincter pressure should increase.

## COMPLICATIONS

Anorectal manometry is well tolerated. Serious complications have not been reported. Potential complications include rectal bleeding and perforation.

## OTHER USES FOR THIS TECHNIQUE

Anorectal manometry provides data about the anus and rectum that is useful for biofeedback. Biofeedback training involves conditioning muscle responses to visual or auditory cues and is used in the therapeutic management of both constipation and fecal incontinence. An anorectal manometry probe or EMG sensor is used to provide visual cues to the patient as specific skills are acquired.

There is lack of standardization for biofeedback technique, but review of the literature supports effectiveness of biofeedback training for both constipation (4) and fecal incontinence (5). Biofeedback training for constipation secondary to pelvic floor dyssynergia using simulated defecation, EMG sensors or manometric probes are used to train the patient to relax the pelvic floor. Biofeedback using EMG sensors is emerging as the preferred form of biofeedback for pelvic floor dyssynergia (6). Biofeedback for fecal incontinence involves motor skills training with EMG or pressure transducers and sensory discrimination training.

## CPT Codes

**91122** – Anorectal manometry.
**90911** – Biofeedback training, anorectal, including EMG and/or manometry.

## REFERENCES

1. Diamant NE, Kamm MA, Wald A, et al. AGA technical review on anorectal testing techniques. *Gastroenterology* 1999;116:732–760.
2. Wald A. Colonic and anorectal motility testing in clinical practice. *Am J Gastroenterol* 1994; 89:2109–2115.
3. Rao SSC, Azpiroz F, Diamant N, et al. Minimum standards of anorectal manometry. *Neurogastroenterol Mot* 2002;14:553–559.
4. Heymen S, Jones KR, Scarlett Y, et al. Biofeedback treatment of constipation: a critical review. *Dis Colon Rectum* 2003; 46: 1208–1217.
5. Heymen S, Jones KR, Ringel Y, et al. Biofeedback treatment of fecal incontinence: a critical review. *Dis Colon Rectum* 2001; 44: 728–736
6. Whitehead WE, Heymen S, Schuster MM. Motility as a therapeutic modality: Biofeedback treatment of Gastrointestinal Disorders. In: Schuster MM, Crowell MD, Koch KL. *Schuster Atlas of Gastrointestinal Motility in Health and Disease*, 2nd ed. Hamilton, Ontario: Decker Inc, 2002:381–397.

# Endoscopic Ultrasound

Poonputt Chotiprasidhi and James M. Scheiman

Endoscopic ultrasound (EUS) provides high-resolution images of the wall of the gastrointestinal tract in addition to providing imaging of surrounding organs such as the mediastinum and the pancreas. Endoscopic ultrasound imaging can provide complementary information beyond that provided with ductal opacification by diagnostic endoscopic retrograde cholangiopancreatography (ERCP). It represents an excellent alternative imaging technique to avoid diagnostic ERCP in cases with a low probability of needing ERCP therapy.

Endoscopic ultrasound has revolutionized the endoscopists' diagnostic and treatment armamentarium by providing rapid and accurate diagnostic information with detailed staging information for patients with suspected or proven gastrointestinal malignancies. The purpose of this chapter is to provide an overview of diagnostic upper and lower EUS. It is not intended to be a comprehensive source of instruction. Endoscopic technique and interpretation are best taught by an experienced endosonographer, supplemented by the review of recent texts of cross-sectional anatomy and EUS that outline technique and pathology in detail.

## INDICATIONS FOR DIAGNOSTIC EUS

1. To visually characterize intrinsic gut wall abnormalities seen on upper gastrointestinal (GI) series, esophagogastroduodenoscopy (EGD), computed tomography scan, magnetic resonance imaging, or colonoscopy

2. To stage esophageal carcinoma (T and N staging) including the involvement of celiac lymph nodes (M stage)

3. To evaluate known or suspected mediastinal masses and lymph nodes. It is particularly useful for staging of non-small cell lung cancer (mediastinal lymph node involvement, i.e., subcarinal or aortopulmonary window).

4. To characterize subepithelial mass of the GI tract based upon layer origin (i.e., submucosa, muscularis propria, etc.)

5. To stage gastric malignancies including adenocarcinoma and gastric lymphoma (T and N staging)

6. To characterize the source of obstruction for the patient with obstructive jaundice

7. To stage pancreatic adenocarcinoma, especially surrounding vascular and nodal involvement (T and N staging)

8. To localize a neuroendocrine tumor of the pancreas (i.e., insulinoma, gastrinoma, etc.)

9. To assist in determining the nature of a cystic lesion in the pancreas (pseudocyst versus cystic neoplasm) by imaging;

to assess feasibility and safety of fine-needle aspiration to obtain cyst fluid for analysis (amylase, lipase, carcino-embryonic antigen [CEA], cytology)

10. To detect cholelithiasis, biliary sludge, or choledocholithiasis

11. To determine the presence and severity of chronic pancreatitis

12. To stage rectal carcinoma including iliac lymph node involvement (T and N staging)

13. To evaluate internal and external anal sphincter integrity

## CONTRAINDICATIONS

### Absolute (Similar to EGD)

1. Shock (unless immediately preoperatively to guide emergent surgical therapy)

2. Acute myocardial infarction

3. Severe dyspnea with hypoxemia

4. Coma (unless patient is intubated)

5. Seizures

6. Gastrointestinal perforation

7. Atlantoaxial subluxation

8. Inability to give a consent or permission for the procedure

9. Signs of peritonitis or mediastinitis

### Relative

1. Uncooperative patient

2. Coagulopathy
   a. Prothrombin time 3 seconds over control
   b. Partial thromboplastin time (PTT) 20 seconds over control
   c. Bleeding time > 10 minutes
   d. Platelet count < 100,000/mm$^3$

3. Zenker's diverticulum

4. Upper esophageal stricture

5. Duodenal obstruction

6. Myocardial ischemia

7. Thoracic aortic aneurysm

8. Acute colonic obstruction

## PREPARATION

1. The patient should have nothing by mouth for 6 to 8 hours prior to the procedure.

2. Review the patient's medical records with attention to risks for endoscopy such as cardiopulmonary disease and coagulopathy.

3. Review the patient's symptoms and previous diagnostic testing, including relevant imaging, prior to the procedure. Be certain the study is indicated and that the patient understands the risks and benefits and agrees to the procedure.

4. If esophageal dilation is required (such as for esophageal cancer staging), obtain informed consent and assess the need for prophylactic antibiotics.

5. Obtain written, informed consent, and start an intravenous (IV) line for conscious sedation administration.

6. For anorectal ultrasound, sedation is optional; preparation is no different than flexible sigmoidoscopy. This typically involves administration of two Fleet enemas 1 hour prior to the procedure, though some examiners prefer a complete colon preparation as for colonoscopy.

## EQUIPMENT

1. Echoendoscope of choice. Radial scanning device from either Olympus (GF-UM130, GF-UM160, or EU-M60) or Pentax (FG-38UX, FG-36U). Curvilinear array system from either Olympus (EU-C60) or Pentax (EG-3630U) may be used for diagnostic EUS if this is the sole instrument available or if a fine-needle aspiration (FNA) is planned.

2. Light source

3. Ultrasound processor appropriate to echoendoscope with capacity for permanent still image production on thermal prints and/or x-ray film.

4. Water pump to instill water into the lumen to enhance acoustic coupling for imaging

5. High-resolution VHS recorder

## PROCEDURE

### Passing the EUS Endoscope

1. Anesthetize the patient's pharynx with a topical agent.

2. Place the recumbent patient in the left lateral position with bite block in place.

3. Administer conscious sedation with fentanyl, and midazolam or diazepam IV slowly until an appropriate level of sedation is reached. Diazepam has a high incidence of phlebitis, especially when infused into a small vein of the hand, but may provide a longer duration of sedation; EUS may take longer than other endoscopic procedures. Administer sedation so that the patient is comfortable but arousable enough to assist in swallowing the large echoendoscope tip.

4. Hold the scope with the left hand on the controls and the right hand on the shaft at the 25- to 30-cm mark in a partially flexed (60-degree) configuration.

5. With the patient's neck partially flexed, pass the endoscope through the hypopharynx. Using indirect visualization and

light pressure, slowly guide the tip of the scope past the epiglottis to rest on the cricopharyngeus, which is located in the midline posterior to the larynx and between the pyriform sinuses, 15 to 18 cm from the incisors. Gently insert the endoscope into the esophageal lumen during relaxation of the cricopharyngeus as the patient swallows. Be certain to keep the scope in the midline, out of the pyriform sinuses, and posterior to the larynx to avoid perforation.

6.  Once the scope has passed the upper esophageal sphincter (20 cm), advance it under oblique vision (Olympus radial) at all times and with only enough air insufflation to permit visualization. Be aware of how the scope air/water buttons work—do not fill the balloon until you have reached the area to begin ultrasound imaging.

7.  Advance the instrument with maneuvers similar to EGD/ERCP instruments in the upper GI tract and similar to flexible sigmoidoscopy for rectal EUS.

**Visualization of Esophagus, Stomach, and Duodenum**

1.  Advance the EUS endoscope through the distal esophagus, identifying the gastroesophageal junction by the change from white to coral-colored mucosa ("Z" line) and through the lower esophageal sphincter. To evaluate gastric lesions, air in the lumen should be suctioned to avoid air interference. The water balloon can then be inflated to moderate size (1 cm).

2.  The five ultrasound layers can then be visualized with either 7.5-MHz or 12-MHz ultrasound imaging (Fig. 48.1). The important task is to identify the fourth hypoechoic layer, which is the muscularis propria, for orientation at the time of staging or for characterization of intramural lesions. Water can be used to fill up the stomach (up to 500 mL) to enhance imaging. This can provide excellent acoustic coupling, but caution is advised to prevent aspiration. Elevate the head of the bed, and use the minimum amount of water necessary to obtain adequate imaging.

3.  Insert the EUS endoscope through the pyloric channel into the duodenal bulb then into the second portion of the duodenum, typically by torquing clockwise and turning the tip posteriorly, usually down and to the right.

4.  To image the head of the pancreas, gallbladder, proximal portion of the bile duct, portal vein, and pancreatic duct in this region, slowly withdraw the scope from the second portion of the duodenum while rotating the tip and torquing the shaft from side to side. Suction should be applied throughout to reduce air artifacts.

5.  Identification of anatomic landmarks such as the portal vein, pancreatic duct, and bile ducts in the pancreatic region is essential for accurate diagnosis. Doppler ultrasound can be used if available on the instrument to help identify structures.

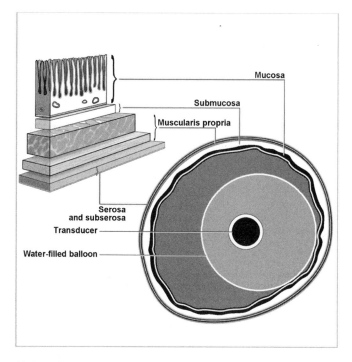

**Fig. 48.1. Wall layers of the digestive tract as seen by EUS.**

6.  Returning to the stomach, pay special attention to the body and tail of the pancreas using splenic vessels as landmarks. The celiac artery takeoff can be identified from the trunk of aorta at about 50 to 55 cm from the incisors.

7.  After thoroughly evaluating the pancreas by slowly withdrawing the scope while rotating the tip in a 360-degree fashion, remove the excess air from the stomach by suction to minimize abdominal distention.

8.  Some experts find the use of specific instrument locations, or stations to help identify relevant landmarks when imaging the pancreas (Table 48.1).

9.  When imaging a wall lesion, make sure the ultrasound beam is perpendicular to the lesion to avoid imaging artifacts. This takes considerable skill obtained through experience. Ideally the area of interest should be in the focal zone of the ultrasound probe, usually about 1.5 cm from the probe.

10. Avoid overcompression with the balloon, which can distort the intrinsic layer structure of the gut wall when imaging luminal tumors to avoid mistakes in staging.

**TABLE 48.1. Pancreas/retroperitoneum:
standard positions**

| Level | Position | Structures imaged |
|---|---|---|
| I | Descending duodenum | CBD, PD, pancreas (H), ampulla, RK |
| II | Duodenal bulb apex | Pancreas (H), PV, IVC, C, CBD,GB |
| III | Duodenal bulb | SV, pancreas (H), SMA, liver |
| IV | Antrum of stomach | Liver, pancreas (B), SV, C |
| V | Body of stomach | Pancreas (B), PD, SV, SA, CA, HA, RV |
| VI | Fundus of stomach | Pancreas (T), PD, spleen, SA, SV, LK |

H = head; B = body; T = tail; PV = portal vein; C = confluence; GB = gallbladder; SV = splenic vein; SMA = superior mesenteric artery; RK = right kidney; CBD = common bile duct; PD = pancreatic duct; SA = splenic artery; CA = celiac axis; HA = hepatic artery; RV = renal vessels; LK = left kidney. Adapted from: Catalano MF. Normal structures on endoscopic ultrasonography: Visualization measurement data and interobserver variation. *Gastrointestinal Endoscopy Clinics of North America* 1995:5:475–486.

**HELPFUL TIPS**

1. In patients with achalasia, the esophagus should be emptied of retained food prior to endoscopy using a large-diameter tube and lavage. This will permit better visualization and prevent aspiration.

2. If esophageal varices are encountered and are not clinically suspected, make sure they are documented.

3. Copies of EUS images should be attached to the procedure note to allow the referring physician to examine the findings.

**POSTPROCEDURE**

1. Complete a detailed procedure report, and write a note in the medical record.

2. Give nothing by mouth until the gag reflex and sensation in the throat returns.

3. The patient should not drive after conscious sedation. Detailed instructions should be given since many patients do not recall verbal discussions after sedation.

**INTERPRETATION**

1. Endoscopic ultrasound is a procedure in which the endosonographer is challenged to know what images must be obtained and to be sure that an adequate evaluation is

performed. For example, careful interrogation of the relationship of a pancreatic cancer to adjacent vasculature is essential, and can only be done "real-time." Postimaging evaluation by viewing videotapes or still images is key to be certain one has performed a complete examination.

2. Placing the relevant information in the context of overall patient management is essential and relies on the experience of the sonographer in the context of a multidisciplinary management team including surgeons and radiologists.

## COMPLICATIONS

Overall complication rates are in the range of 0.1% to 0.2%, with mortality in the range of 0.014% to 0.065%.

1. Sedation-related
   a. Respiratory arrest (0.07%)
   b. Phlebitis (variable)

2. Perforation (0.033% to 0.1%). The most common sites are the pharynx, upper esophagus, and stomach.

3. Bleeding (0.03%). This is from biopsies (FNA), dislodging clots from bleeding points, and Mallory-Weiss tears induced by retching during endoscopy.

4. Aspiration (0.08%). The risk can be decreased by giving the patient nothing by mouth, lavaging patients with bleeding or achalasia, and using minimum air insufflation.

5. Retropharyngeal hematomas.

### CPT Codes

**43231** – Esophagoscopy with endoscopic examination.
**43232** – Esophagoscopy with transendoscopic ultrasound-guided intramural or transmural fine needle aspiration/biopsy(s).
**43237** – Esophagoscopy with endoscopic ultrasound examination limited to the esophagus.
**43238** – Esophagoscopy with transendoscopic ultrasound-guided intramural or transmural fine needle aspiration/biopsy(s), esophagus (includes endoscopic ultrasound examination limited to the esophagus).
**43259** – Upper endoscopic ultrasound.
**45242** – Upper GI endoscopy with transendoscopic ultrasound guided intramural or transmural fine needle aspiration/biopsy(s).
**45341** – Sigmoidoscopy with endoscopic examination.
**45342** – Sigmoidoscopy with transendoscopic ultrasound guided intramural or transmural fine needle aspiration/biopsy(s).

### SUGGESTED READINGS

Anderson MA, Carpenter S, et al. Endoscopic ultrasound is highly accurate and directs management in patients with neuroendocrine tumors of the pancreas. *Am J Gastroenterol* 2000;95(9): 2271–2277.

Anderson MA, Scheiman JM. Initial experience with an electronic radial array echoendoscope: randomized comparison with a mechanical sector scanning echoendoscope in humans. *Gastrointest Endosc* 2002;56(4):573–577.

Byrne MF, Jowell PS. Gastrointestinal imaging: Endoscopic Ultrasound. *Gastroenterology* 2002;122:1631–1648.

Kochman ML, Elta GH, Bude R, et al. Utility of a linear array ultrasound endoscope in the evaluation of suspected pancreatic disease. *Gastrointest Surg* 1998;2(3): 217–222.

Rosch T, Classen M. *Gastroenterologic Endosonography*. New York: Thieme, 1992.

Scheiman JM, Carlos RC, Barnett JL, et al. Can endoscopic ultrasound or magnetic resonance cholangiopancreatography replace ERCP in patients with suspected biliary disease? A prospective trial and cost analysis. *Am J Gastroenterol* 2001;96(10): 2900–2904.

Tierney WM, Francis IR, Eckhauser F, et al. The accuracy of EUS and helical CT in the assessment of vascular invasion by peripapillary malignancy. *Gastrointest Endosc* 2001;53(2): 182–188.

Wallace MB, Hawes RH. Emerging indications for EUS. *Gastrointest Endosc* 2000;52(6 Suppl): S55–60.

# Endosonography-Guided Fine Needle Aspiration Biopsy

Maurits J. Wiersema and Michael J. Levy

Endosonography (EUS) has evolved from solely a diagnostic imaging modality to a method that allows tissue acquisition and therapeutic intervention. Endosonography-guided fine needle aspiration (EUS FNA) biopsy permits pathologic confirmation of imaging findings. The ability to biopsy lesions that are either too small to identify on conventional cross-sectional imaging (computed tomography or magnetic resonance) or inaccessible by percutaneous techniques due to surrounding vascular and/or vital structures secures the role of EUS FNA.

The safety and accuracy of EUS FNA has now been demonstrated in thousands of patients (1). Although diagnostic accuracy and risk are biopsy site-dependent, most series report sensitivity for detection of malignancy ranging from 85% to 100% with extremely infrequent complications (1–3). The recent addition of EUS-guided trucut biopsy may enhance diagnostic accuracy in stromal and hematopoetic tumors (4).

## INDICATIONS

Endosonography-guided fine needle aspiration of intramural and periintestinal structures can be readily accomplished from the esophagus, stomach, duodenum, and rectosigmoid colon. These sites afford an acoustic window to periintestinal and mediastinal lymphadenopathy; solid organs including the pancreas, liver, kidneys, and adrenal glands; and the bile duct, gallbladder, and pleural/peritoneal-based effusions. Although lesions within the colon and adjacent tissues may be accessible with EUS FNA, the experience in this setting is limited.

Indications for EUS FNA include the following:

1. Primary diagnosis of intramural or periintestinal solid and/or cystic lesions

2. Staging of regional and distant lymphadenopathy in digestive and pulmonary neoplasia

3. Evaluation of unexplained mediastinal, retroperitoneal, and/or abdominal lymphadenopathy

4. Sampling of peritoneal and/or pleural fluid

5. Prior nondiagnostic biopsy procedures (including surgical biopsy) for above described conditions

## ABSOLUTE CONTRAINDICATIONS

1. Uncorrectable coagulopathy (International Normalized Ration [INR] > 1.4)

2. Uncorrectable thrombocytopenia (Platelets < 80,000)

## RELATIVE CONTRAINDICATIONS

1. Undrained biliary obstruction
2. Bronchogenic duplication cyst
3. Mesenteric venous collaterals in needle path
4. Luminal stenosis requiring dilation
5. Lymph node biopsy in which the primary tumor is within the needle path

## PREPARATION

Endosonography-guided fine needle aspiration is best performed using the electronic curved linear array echoendoscope that permits continuous real-time visualization of the needle as it is advanced into the periluminal space. Patients require an overnight fast and a full colonoscopy prep for those undergoing examination of the rectum (or colon).

The risk for bacteremia post-EUS FNA of solid lesions biopsied from the upper intestinal tract is quite low and similar to diagnostic endoscopy, thereby not requiring antibiotics (1). However, biopsy of cystic lesions has been associated with serious infectious complications (2). It is recommended that all patients undergoing biopsy of a perirectal lesion or aspiration of a cystic lesion or fluid compartment (i.e., ascites) be given prophylactic antibiotics (quinolone) which are continued for 48 hours after the procedure. This is to prevent local infectious complications rather than the distant sequelae of bacteremia.

## EQUIPMENT

1. The electronic curved linear echoendoscope permits continuous visualization of the needle as it is advanced beyond the biopsy channel. Some instruments are equipped with an elevator that facilitates targeting of biopsy sites.

2. EUS FNA needles are available in several sizes including a 19, 22, and 25 gauge. Most published reports have used the 22-gauge needle. In pancreas masses, a diagnostic advantage was not seen with the 19- versus 22-gauge needle (unpublished data, Mayo Clinic, Rochester). Trucut needles (19 gauge) are now available (4). The stiffness of the trucut device limits biopsies to sites allowing the distal bending section of the echoendoscope to be kept relatively straight (esophagus, stomach ± duodenal bulb). Due to the cost and rigidity of the device, reserving its use for patients in whom FNA sampling and cytology is nondiagnostic or when histologic specimens are needed (i.e., lymphoma) is recommended.

3. On-site cytology support is an important component of EUS FNA. This also allows for collection of material to perform ancillary studies when the adequacy assessment suggests this may be helpful (i.e., culture, flow cytometry, histochemical analysis).

Two nurses or one registered nurse (RN) and a technician are needed when performing EUS. With the addition of FNA, a third support person (cytotechnician) is needed to assist with slide preparation and also to provide an on-site assessment of sample adequacy. The biopsy specimens are later reviewed by a cytopathologist for final interpretation. In some centers, an interpretation is performed by an on-site cytopathologist. The RN monitors the patient's response to sedation while the technician facilitates equipment needs. We routinely provide intravenous fluids during the exam to facilitate administration of medications, as the procedures require substantially more time and often sedation than conventional endoscopy.

## PROCEDURE

1. When appropriate, perform standard forward-viewing endoscopy to identify luminal abnormalities, and note their location relative to anatomic landmarks (e.g., tumor distance from incisors or anal verge).

2. When appropriate, perform radial EUS to identify intramural and periluminal abnormalities. This may not be needed for patients with pancreatic pathologies, as the imaging plane with the linear echoendoscope may be sufficient. If a malignancy is being evaluated, a complete diagnostic EUS should be initially performed to allow adequate staging.

3. Place the targeted lesion in the projected plane of the needle path. This differs among the various linear echoendoscopes. Avoid tubular structures between the transducer and target as they may represent vascular structures. Doppler examination allows easy distinction. In patients with portal hypertension, particular care must be taken in that compression of the lumen may mask intervening varices.

4. Advance the needle catheter device with the stylet in place through the biopsy channel. If the echoendoscope has an elevator, this should be in the down or fully released position. Secure the handle mechanism of the needle to the luer lock on the biopsy port after removing the rubber valve. Some FNA needles come with a short spacer device that is attached between the biopsy port and the needle hub. Prior to inserting the EUS FNA needle device through the biopsy channel, lock the needle within the fully withdrawn position.

5. The optimal degree of balloon inflation that should be present when performing EUS FNA will be gleaned from experience and personal preference but is generally less than for radial examination. Due to the nature of the linear echoendoscope, the balloon is typically left inflated with the up/down ratchet turned "up" to displace the balloon behind the transducer. Within the esophagus, duodenum, and colon, balloon inflation can help keep the echoendoscope tip in a more stable position. With the needle sheath protruding from the biopsy channel, a small pocket of air potentially is created, which diminishes acoustic coupling and impairs imaging. This can be overcome by periodically pressing the suction valve.

6.  In the United States, the EUS image typically is oriented so that the needle enters the ultrasound view from the right side of the screen and traverses toward the bottom left corner of the image. As one is gaining experience with the technique, the distance from the transducer to the center of the targeted lesion can be measured and the depth stop set at this distance (to avoid needle over-advancement). Under continuous imaging, advance the needle into the target.

7.  Once in the target, remove the stylet and apply negative pressure with a 10-mL syringe. Several manufacturers' needles are supplied with a modified syringe harboring a lock, thereby simplifying this task. Due to echoendoscopes from different manufacturers having different lengths, some needle manufacturers have developed an adjustable sheath length or spacers to accommodate the variation. Our preference is to use a needle that is made specifically for the length instrument we use, thereby avoiding the potential for inadvertent biopsy channel puncture by misjudging the proper sheath length. The degree of negative pressure may be important. In vascular tumors (e.g., neuroendocrine) or in lymph nodes, limited or no negative pressure results in a less bloody aspirate that may allow for easier cytology interpretation. The degree of negative pressure should be increased if the initial biopsies contain a sparse sample or decreased following bloody aspirates.

8.  With negative pressure applied, make five to ten gradual, to-and-fro movements within the lesion. Maintain the position of the needle within the target avoiding accidental withdrawal into the lumen when negative pressure is applied. If this occurs, the specimen may become contaminated with lumen contents and epithelium. Prior to removing the needle, release the negative pressure. With the needle fully withdrawn and the stop secured, unscrew and remove the device from the biopsy channel.

9.  Prepare slides:

    a.  Slides and glass tubes for specimen collection should be labeled individually with the patient name or identification and pass number.
    b.  Spray the material onto glass slides with subsequent fixation (air dry, spray fixed, or ethanol fixed).
    c.  Collect a saline wash through the needle for a cell block. Each pass should be collected in a separate glass tube. The stylet is cleaned with a gauze pad to remove any remaining blood. Purge the needle of residual saline with air and then reinsert the stylet.
    d.  If the needle is clogged, use the stylet to clear the device.
    e.  Collect material for culture and special studies in preservative media as recommended by pathology.
    f.  For cystic lesions, leave the entire specimen in a syringe. If biochemical analysis is planned (e.g., carcinoembryonic-antigen, amylase), do not dilute the specimen with a saline rinse.

10. When attendant cytology review is unavailable, we typically perform five passes and stop. With pancreas adenocarcinoma, this practice may reduce the rate of malignancy detection to 60% to 70%.

Several special circumstances may arise that require modification of the above technique, including the following:

1. The muscularis propria of the stomach can be difficult to penetrate. By using the elevator and a more perpendicular angle of entry with the needle as well as a swift jabbing motion, the needle can usually be advanced through the intestinal wall. In this setting, securing the needle stop to a certain depth may minimize the potential for overextension.

2. When performing EUS FNA of small lesions (< 5 mm), maximal magnification of the EUS image will facilitate targeting and confirmation of entry into the lesion. Care should be taken not to overextend the needle, which is more prone to occur when image magnification is employed.

3. Small lesions that are firm may appear to deflect the needle or be quite difficult to enter. A needle trajectory that is as close as perpendicular to the lesion surface as possible is ideal. Second, a rapid jabbing motion may facilitate entry. In some circumstances, once the intestinal wall has been traversed, an adjustment in the needle direction may be needed.

4. Occasionally the stylet can no longer be used due to bending/difficulty readvancing it through the needle. Sampling of lymph nodes and cystic pancreatic lesions is best done with a stylet to avoid contamination by luminal epithelial cells. For solid pancreas lesions and liver masses this may not be a concern.

5. After several passes, the needle will develop a curve that can result in a needle trajectory outside the plane of imaging (i.e., the needle goes right or left of the transducer). When this occurs, rotate the echoendoscope to recapture the location of the needle. If particularly troublesome, the needle should be replaced.

6. Bloody aspirates can arise from vascular lesions and/or when the patient has recently been on anticoagulant/antiplatelet agents (even with normalization of hemostatic measures). In this setting, reduction of the negative pressure may reduce blood contamination. Additionally, targeting the edge of the lesion may result in less traversal of the vascular supply.

7. Hypocellular specimens typically reflect errors in targeting, insufficient negative pressure, and/or desmoplastic lesions.

8. If a blood return can be seen entering the aspirating syringe during EUS FNA, one should place the entire specimen in a glass tube, as little of the material contained within the needle will be representative tissue.

9. Occasionally, an echopoor expanding region will arise around the biopsied lesion, which represents hemorrhage

(5). We typically apply pressure with the echoendoscope transducer at the biopsy site and observe the area for 10 to 15 minutes to ensure stability. When limited in size and in patients with normal hemostatic parameters, this does not appear to be clinically significant and does not necessitate an alteration in postprocedure care.

## POSTPROCEDURE

1. Patients are monitored in a recovery area with discharge criteria equivalent to standard endoscopic procedures.

2. We advise patients who undergo pancreas EUS FNA to take clear liquids for their first meals.

3. In patients with prolonged procedures or those requiring large doses of analgesia, provide 500 to 1000 mL of normal saline and consider a single dose of an antiemetic in recovery.

4. Patients undergoing liver biopsy are observed for 2 hours with adherence to bed rest. On their release, they are advised to minimize activity for 24 hours.

5. All patients should be advised to contact the endoscopist (rather than the referring physician) immediately for any distress (e.g., fever, abdominal pain, or nausea).

6. Those patients who undergo biopsy of a perirectal and/or cystic lesion or aspiration of a fluid compartment (e.g., ascites) are provided a prescription for an oral quinolone to be taken for 48 hours.

## COMPLICATIONS

1. Pneumoperitoneum has been reported when endoscopy closely follows EUS FNA (1).

2. Pancreatitis. Patients undergoing pancreatic EUS FNA should not undergo endoscopic retrograde cholangiopancreatography on the same day due to a potentially additive risk for pancreatitis (1). With antibiotic administration using the above criteria, the collective risk for EUS FNA is < 1% for nonpancreatic lesions. In pancreatic lesions, the risk of pancreatitis may be as high as 1%. Needle gauge and number of passes does not appear to influence this risk.

3. Portal vein thrombosis has been reported after EUS FNA of a pancreas cancer (1).

4. Perforation (typically related to dilation of malignant esophageal strictures to facilitate passage of the echoendoscope)

5. Sedation risks

6. Bleeding

7. Infection (either from the EUS FNA puncture, phlebitis related to the venous catheter, and/or aspiration)

## CPT Codes

**43242** – EGD with transendoscopic ultrasound-guided intramural or transmural fine needle aspiration biopsy.

**43232** – Esophagoscopy, rigid or flexible; with transendoscopic ultrasound-guided intramural or transmural fine needle aspiration/biopsy(s).

**43238** – Upper gastrointestinal endoscopy including esophagus, stomach, and either the duodenum and/or jejunum as appropriate; with transendoscopic ultrasound-guided intramural or transmural fine needle aspiration/biopsy(s), esophagus (includes endoscopic ultrasound examination limited to the esophagus).

**45342** – Sigmoidoscopy, flexible; with transendoscopic ultrasound guided intramural or transmural fine needle aspiration/biopsy(s).

**45392** – Colonoscopy, flexible, proximal to splenic flexure; with transendoscopic ultrasound guided intramural or transmural fine needle aspiration/biopsy(s).

## REFERENCES

1. Wiersema MJ, Norton ID. Endoscopic ultrasound-guided fine-needle aspiration biopsy UpToDate 2003, www.uptodate.com.
2. Wiersema MJ, Vilmann P, Giovannini M, et al. Endosonography-guided fine-needle aspiration biopsy: diagnostic accuracy and complication assessment. *Gastroenterology* 1997;112:1087–1095.
3. Norton ID, Wiersema MJ. Endoscopic ultrasound-guided fine-needle aspiration biopsy. In: Gress FG, Bhattacharya I, eds. *Endoscopic Ulrasound.* Qu au-where in mass? Massachusetts: Blackwell Science, 2001:136–148.
4. Wiersema MJ, Levy MJ, Harewood GC, et al. Initial experience with EUS-guided trucut needle biopsies of perigastric organs. *Gastrointest Endosc* 2002;56(2):275–278.
Affi A, Vazquez-Sequeiros E, Norton ID, et al. Acute extraluminal hemorrhage associated with EUS-guided fine needle aspiration: frequency and clinical significance. *Gastrointest Endosc* 2001;53(2):221–225.

# Endosonography-Guided Celiac Plexus Neurolysis

## Maurits J. Wiersema and Michael J. Levy

Pain resulting from unresectable pancreatic cancer represents the most common indication for celiac plexus neurolysis (CPN). In these patients, therapy with nonsteroidal antiinflammatory agents is often insufficient and employment of opioids is necessary. Although the latter are excellent at controlling pain, untoward side effects including anorexia, dry mouth, constipation, nausea, vomiting, and sedation may limit their utility. Celiac plexus neurolysis results in good to excellent pain relief in 70% to 90% of patients, which continues through the time of death (1,2). These outcomes appear to be independent of the technique for performing CPN (anterior or posterior percutaneous, surgical, and more recently, endosonography-guided).

Pain control in chronic pancreatitis can be more problematic due to the potential for addiction to pain relievers. Unfortunately, CPN is not as effective in this setting, with an initial response rate of 50% and most patients developing pain recurrence within 3 to 6 months (1).

The efficacy of CPN is diminished in persons dependent on large doses of opioids, in the presence of direct tumor infiltration of the celiac plexus region, and with repeated CPN. Although most studies have found that CPN reduces pancreatic cancer pain, it rarely eliminates pain, and nearly all patients require continued opioid use. By improving analgesia, CPN may also minimize other deleterious effects induced by pain or opioid use. Wiersema and Wiersema initially described endosonography (EUS)-guided CPN as an alternative means of accessing the celiac ganglia for purposes of neurolysis (3). Subsequent publications have supported the utility and safety of the technique (1).

## INDICATIONS/CONTRAINDICATIONS

Selection of EUS versus percutaneously guided CPN is influenced by local availability and expertise. The percutaneous approach is often favored due to lower cost. However, when EUS is performed for staging and/or biopsy, EUS CPN can be safely performed, providing additional benefit to the patient with lower overall cost. Typically, CPN is reserved for patients with upper abdominal pain that radiates into the back.

Indications for EUS CPN include (1) the following:

1. Painful unresectable pancreatic or retroperitoneal malignancy (weight of evidence is in favor of usefulness/efficacy)

2. Painful chronic pancreatitis (usefulness/efficacy is not as well established by evidence/opinion)

Contraindications for EUS CPN include the following:

1.   Uncertainty regarding the cause of the pain

2.   Uncorrectable coagulopathy (International Normalized Ratio > 1.4)

3.   Uncorrectable thrombocytopenia (platelets < 80,000)

4.   Altered anatomy that precludes access to the celiac plexus region

Some consider a history of multiple prior CPNs in patients with chronic pancreatitis a relative contraindication.

**PREPARATION**

1.   An overnight fast is adequate preparation for performing EUS CPN. Patients with delayed gastric emptying due to obstruction and/or opioid use should be placed on a clear liquid diet for 24 hours prior to the procedure to minimize the risk of retained gastric contents.

2.   Individuals on anticoagulants and/or antiplatelet agents should have these stopped with a sufficient interval to allow normalization of hemostasis prior to the procedure (typically 3 to 5 days).

3.   We do not routinely administer antibiotics prior to EUS CPN when performed with absolute ethanol as this has a bactericidal effect and infectious complications have not been described in this setting. However, when a steroid solution is used for the CPN, preprocedure antibiotics (e.g., ampicillin, sulbactam) may be warranted due to the inability to maintain sterility of the injection needle as it passes through the echoendoscope biopsy channel and gastric lumen. This risk may be even greater in patients on high-dose acid suppressive therapy (4). One series described development of a retroperitoneal abscess poststeroid EUS CPN when antibiotics were not administered (4).

4.   Typically, EUS CPN is performed on outpatients, utilizing conscious sedation and noninvasive monitoring (blood pressure, oximetry, electrocardiography).

5.   Patients are placed in the left lateral decubitus position and given 500 to 1,000 mL of normal saline intravenously during the exam to counteract the orthostasis that may arise from splanchnic blood pooling post-EUS CPN.

6.   Although fluoroscopy is not needed, it may be of help when first performing the procedure to verify needle placement. When done with fluoroscopy, a test solution of contrast can be initially injected to verify distribution and needle placement.

**EQUIPMENT**

A linear scanning echoendoscope in conjunction with a 22-gauge EUS fine needle aspiration (FNA) needle are used for performing EUS CPN. If EUS FNA is done during the exam, a new needle is used for the CPN to avoid potential malignant seeding of the celiac plexus. Medications specific for EUS CPN beyond those employed for endoscopy include the following:

1. Bupivacaine (0.25%) 20 mL (without epinephrine)

2. Dehydrated ethanol (98%) 20 mL

3. Normal saline (for flushing) 20 mL

When a steroid solution is used for EUS CPN (typically for painful chronic pancreatitis), the preference is triamcinolone suspension (80 mg in 8 mL). All syringes should be labeled, with medication drawn up prior to initiating the EUS CPN. Two 10-mL syringes should be used for the bupivacaine, ethanol, and normal saline with the steroid placed in two smaller 5-mL syringes. Larger syringes are not well suited for the procedure due to the resistance with injection.

## PROCEDURE

1. Advance the linear scanning echoendoscope into the proximal stomach, and rotate posterior to allow visualization of the aorta. This can usually be seen at the cardia and appears in a longitudinal view (Fig. 50.1).

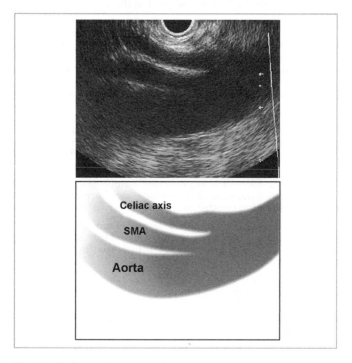

**Fig. 50.1. Endoscopic ultrasound appearance from the proximal stomach demonstrating the aorta with the takeoff of the celiac artery (right) and superior mesenteric artery (left). Cranial direction is to the right.**

2. Advance the instrument, and note the celiac artery, which is the first vessel arising from the aorta below the diaphragm. The celiac plexus is not identified as a discrete structure but is located based on its position relative to the celiac trunk.

3. Use color Doppler to confirm vascular landmarks and verify the presence of flow prior to the EUS CPN.

4. Prime a 22-gauge EUS FNA needle with saline after removing the central stylet.

5. Pass the assembly through the echoendoscope biopsy channel and secure to the luer lock assembly (biopsy valve removed).

6. Place the elevator (if the echoendoscope is so equipped) in the full down position to allow full advancement of the needle sheath assembly.

7. Under continuous, real-time EUS imaging, advance the needle immediately adjacent and anterior to the lateral aspect of the aorta at the level of the celiac trunk (Fig. 50.2). For safety, measure the distance of intended needle

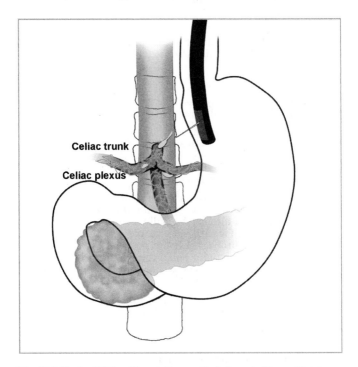

**Fig. 50.2. Under EUS guidance, the needle is inserted immediately adjacent and anterior to the lateral aspect of the aorta at the level of the celiac trunk.**

advancement on the EUS image, and then secure the depth stop on the needle hub at this level. This may prevent inadvertent entry into vascular structures.

8. Flush the needle with 3 to 5 mL of normal saline to remove any tissue from the tip that may have entered during traversal of the stomach and retroperitoneum.

9. In thin patients, inject an additional 10 to 20 mL of saline to create an echopoor space providing a larger target region in which to inject the remaining agents. This will ensure that the injection is sufficiently posterior in the retroperitoneal space.

10. Prior to each subsequent injection, aspirate from the syringe to be sure there is no entry into a blood vessel. A blood flashback may take up to 15 seconds, even when within the aorta, due to the small needle gauge and length employed.

11. For EUS CPN in malignancy, inject 10 mL of bupivacaine (0.25%) followed by 10 mL of dehydrated ethanol (98%). This produces an echogenic cloud. Bupivacaine is initially administered since injection of the ethanol may lead to patient discomfort.

12. Inject an additional 3 to 5 mL of normal saline to flush the needle of ethanol. This prevents seeding of the needle track with alcohol, and this may produce transient severe postprocedure pain.

13. Withdraw the needle.

14. Repeat the entire process after rotating the echoendoscope to image the contralateral side of the aorta.

15. Occasionally, in obese patients or those with altered anatomy, or when extensive tumor is present, one may need to inject all of the solution immediately anterior to the celiac artery trunk. The efficacy of single versus bilateral injection has not been compared.

16. In chronic pancreatitis, after administering bupivacaine, we use triamcinolone suspension (40 mg in 4 mL in each side) instead of alcohol. A small volume of ethanol can be injected (4 mL for each side) in addition to the steroid to improve the neurolysis although no published data support this practice. Due to the small volume, flushing the needle with saline postinjection is important to allow the full steroid dose to be injected.

17. Post-EUS CPN, reassess the celiac artery and aorta by Doppler to confirm continued flow.

**POSTPROCEDURE**

1. After EUS CPN and on arrival to the recovery room, check movement of all extremities immediately.

2. Monitor vital signs until the patient is fully awake with continued less intense observation through 2 hours.

3.  Before discharge, check the blood pressure in the supine and upright positions to assess for orthostasis. If a substantial fall in blood pressure is identified, administer additional intravenous normal saline, also, instruct the patient not to walk that evening (wheelchair and sitting/lying only) and hold blood pressure medications.

Most patients who respond to EUS CPN will experience improved pain control within 48 hours of the procedure. When ethanol is used, patients may have a transient increase in pain that can last for 3 to 4 days. If protracted, a computed tomography scan of the abdomen is needed to assess for complications.

## COMPLICATIONS

### Minor (1)

1.  Orthostasis (30% to 40%, transient, lasting 1 to 3 days)
2.  Diarrhea (40% to 50%, may last 1 to 7 days)
3.  Local pain (90% to 100%, 1 to 2 days)

### Major (1)

1.  Lower extremity weakness and paraesthesia
2.  Paraplegia
3.  Gastroparesis (injection occurs too far caudally and anterior)
4.  Chronic diarrhea
5.  Retroperitoneal abscess (4)

Major complications have been described in up to 1% to 2% of patients undergoing percutaneous CPN. Aside from the single report of a retroperitoneal abscess, the above major complications have not been described with EUS CPN. Neurologic complications arise from spinal cord ischemia or direct injury to the spinal cord or somatic nerves. Spinal cord ischemia may result from thrombosis or spasm of the artery of Adamkiewicz located on the left of the spine between T-8 and L-4, which perfuses the lower two-thirds of the spinal cord. Paraplegia has been reported with percutaneous (with and without imaging guidance) and surgical approaches, however not with EUS CPN. This may reflect the more limited experience and/or the more anterior distribution of the injected solution with the latter approach.

### CPT Codes

**43259** – Upper gastrointestinal endoscopy including esophagus, stomach, and either the duodenum and/or jejunum as appropriate; with endoscopic ultrasound examination.

If the block is done with a biopsy then

**43242** – EGD with transendoscopic ultrasound guided intramural or transmural fine needle aspiration biopsy(s).

**64680** – Destruction by neurolytic agent, celiac plexus, with or without radiologic monitoring.

## REFERENCES

1. Levy MJ, Wiersema MJ. EUS-guided celiac plexus neurolysis and celiac plexus block. *Gastrointest Endosc* 2003; 57(7):923–930.
2. Eisenberg E, Carr DB, Chalmers TC. Neurolytic celiac plexus block for treatment of cancer pain: a meta-analysis. [erratum appears in *Anesth Analg* 1995;(81)1:213]. *Anesth Analg* 1995; 80:290–295.
3. Wiersema MJ, Wiersema LM. Endosonography-guided celiac plexus neurolysis. *Gastrointest Endosc* 1996;44:656–662.
4. Gress F, Schmitt C, Sherman S, et al. Endoscopic ultrasound-guided celiac plexus block for managing abdominal pain associated with chronic pancreatitis: a prospective single center experience. *Am J Gastroenterol* 2001; 96:409–416.

# The Procedure Unit

Melissa C. Brennen

The operational features of every endoscopy unit are unique. Therefore, there are no strict criteria that can define an exclusive plan. This chapter offers general guidelines for the design, organization, and administration of a gastrointestinal (GI) unit.

## Location and Characteristics

1. The driving forces in developing an endoscopy unit are the number and types of procedures to be performed; this determines the number of procedure rooms needed. Units are often developed to meet immediate demands and do not adequately anticipate future growth. The universal trend is that the percentage of procedures being performed in an ambulatory setting is increasing. If an endoscopy unit is hospital-based, it should be easily accessible to outpatients.

2. Endoscopy rooms should be 200 square feet, at a minimum.

3. The minimum number of procedure rooms should be two in a hospital facility. For larger units, there should be one endoscopy room per 1,000 to 1,500 procedures annually, including radiographic and multipurpose rooms for complex and highly therapeutic procedures (1).

4. Procedure units should have physical separation between clinical areas, administrative areas, and the waiting area. Clinical areas should be subcategorized into preprocedural, intraprocedural, and postprocedural (2).

## Basic Procedure Room Equipment and Supplies

1. The procedural table, with adjustable height and positioning, should be the central focus of the room. There should be enough space around the table to move freely, to easily transport the patient, and to respond to an emergent situation.

2. An endoscopy cart with a processor and light source, and necessary equipment for data entry and photodocumentation

3. Two video monitors with unimpeded views

4. Patient monitoring equipment (blood pressure, heart rate, oxygen saturation, as well as electrocardiographic and end-expiratory carbon dioxide monitoring for high-risk patients)

5. Piped oxygen and suctioning

6.  Power outlets with back-up to an emergency energy supply

7.  Necessary computer infrastructure

8.  Ceiling tracking for intravenous (IV) hooks and curtains to maintain patient privacy

9.  Bright ceiling lighting with a dimmer switch and shades, if windows are present (2)

10. Adequate ventilation and temperature controls

11. An electrocautery unit with return electrode pads and connecting wires

12. X-ray view boxes

13. Chairs and stools, both rolling and step stools

14. Writing surfaces

15. Surfaces for collection and preparation of specimens

16. Hand-washing sink

17. Telephone and intercom systems

18. Sufficient storage for GI accessories, gloves, gowns, and masks. Endoscopic accessories should include the following: biopsy forceps, polypectomy snares, and instruments for injection therapy and thermal therapy.

19. Linen supply and hamper; containers for trash, sharps, and hazardous waste

20. Medications for sedation, (e.g., diazepam and/or midazolam). Medications for analgesia (e.g., meperidine, morphine, and/or fentanyl [sublimaze]). Reversal agents (e.g., flumazenil and naloxone).

21. Other supplies include the following: syringes, needles, IV supplies, topical anesthetics, lubricant jelly, epinephrine, sterile saline vials, absolute ethanol vials, material for tattoos (e.g., Spot), sclerosants, injectable antiemetics, and atropine.

# Equipment and Supplies Adjacent to Procedure Rooms

1.  Patient toilet facilities should be accessible from all procedure rooms and from the patient preparation and recovery areas. This facility should be equipped with a hand-washing sink, a sitting bench, handrails, and a call bell. All bathrooms should comply with American Disability Act standards (3).

2.  A patient preparation area should incorporate dressing rooms with patient lockers for personal belongings. This area should have privacy measures and should include sinks, clean linen, a hamper for dirty linen, and a gurney.

3.   A staffed recovery area should include separate bay areas for privacy. Patient monitoring equipment, a call bell, oxygen, and suction apparatus are also required.

4.   A central cleaning and disinfection area/soiled utility room is needed. This room requires a hopper for disposable wastes, large clean and dirty sinks, a gluderaldehyde soaking area, automated endoscope reprocessors, an ultrasonic cleaner, suction, and compressed air. Good ventilation is a must in this room.

5.   A storage/clean utility room is needed for storage of scopes, endoscopic accessories (e.g., bougies and balloon dilators), medications, and IV supplies. This room should include a locked narcotic box.

6.   Two small refrigerators are necessary, a clean one for storage of medications requiring refrigeration and a "dirty" refrigerator for storage of patient specimens.

7.   A storage area for the emergency crash cart and defibrillator are needed.

8.   Storage space for the travel endoscopy cart, if applicable, is necessary.

9.   A linen storage area is required.

10.   Private patient consultation room(s) is a must.

# Medical Administration Area Organization

1.   The nucleus of the management team includes a director, ideally a physician, and a nurse manager. Their offices should be located in the endoscopy unit.

2.   Other physician offices may also be located in the lab.

3.   Physician workrooms should be equipped with computers, dictation areas, telephones, and an intercom system.

4.   There should be a staff education area with textbooks, periodicals, videos and a VCR.

5.   A conference room is recommended.

6.   An area for a computer server to facilitate report generation, storage of photodocumentation, and record keeping is also important.

7.   A lounge area with a refrigerator is recommended.

8.   Staff locker rooms and bathrooms should also be included.

# Reception Area Organization and Equipment

The reception area should be at the front of the endoscopy unit and located next to the waiting room area. The waiting room should include an average of eight seats per procedure room and should include a bathroom, a television set, magazines, patient education materials, a coat rack, and possibly a pay phone. This area must be wheelchair accessible. If pediatric patients are seen, there should be a children's corner with a table and toys. The reception area itself should also include the following:

1. A designated window area for patient check-in

2. A patient identification embosser and paperwork packets for procedure documentation

3. Telephone and intercom systems

4. Computers

5. Areas for storage and filing of documents and medical records

6. Organized process for incoming and outgoing mail

7. Copier and fax machine

# Secretarial Area Organization and Equipment

In larger endoscopy units, an appointment secretary should be separated from the reception area and reception duties. There should be a designated area for this secretary with his or her own desk, phone line, computer, copier, and fax machine. His or her primary responsibility is scheduling appointments.

# Nursing Staff Responsibilities

1. Registered nurses should have at least one year of experience on a medical-surgical floor prior to working in endoscopy; some exposure to cardiovascular and respiratory disorders is particularly important. GI procedure nurses should have a minimum certification of basic life support (BLS) (4).

2. Preparing the patient for the procedure includes confirming that preprocedure requirements have been met; notifying physicians of any contraindications to performing the procedure (e.g., poor prep or patient not stopping anticoagulants); and obtaining a baseline assessment, medical, surgical, and social history, and a list of current medications.

3. The nursing staff should properly arrange and set up the procedure room and endoscopy equipment.

4. Administration of sedation per physician orders is the nurse's responsibility. All registered nurses should be extremely knowledgeable about the medications used for sedation and the use of reversal agents.

5. The nurses must ensure patient safety by monitoring the patient during the procedure, identifying any changes in his or her status and level of sedation, and providing emotional support.

6. The nursing staff will assist physicians during the procedure with patient positioning, technical support, and specimen collection and handling.

7. The patient should be monitored postprocedure to ensure that he or she is safe for discharge according to the facility's discharge criteria (e.g., Aldrete score). Educating patients and significant others based on the specific procedure and findings, and providing discharge instructions and having a significant other sign to verify understanding are also the responsibility of the nursing staff.

8. Providing proper documentation of all patient care is required.

9. Nurses must maintain competence to troubleshoot technical problems, such as equipment malfunction or computer errors.

10. The nurses should stay current with competencies and certifications by participating in continuing education, in continuous quality improvement, and in applicable research studies.

11. Ensuring proper cleaning of the endoscopy equipment and procedure rooms is necessary.

12. Communicating with GI team members and facilitating team collaboration is a nursing staff duty.

## Secretarial Staff Responsibilities

The front office staff plays a key role in the patient's visit to the endoscopy unit. They are the first contact with the patient and set the tone for the visit. Their responsibilities include the following:

1. Patient check-in and imprinting procedural documents with patient identifiers

2. Scheduling appointments and maintaining the scheduling system. This difficult task requires a thorough understanding of unit flow and staffing patterns.

3. Mailing appointment slips and preparation instructions to patients

4. Calling in prescriptions for purgatives such as GoLytely, as ordered by the physician

5. Calling patients with appointment reminders

6. Maintaining a log documenting cancellations, no-shows, and reschedules

7. Maintaining a procedure call-back system

8. Charge entry and patient billing; obtaining medical insurance information

9. Answering phone calls and directing patients and family to appropriate areas

10. Identifying and attending to patient needs in the waiting room

## Responsibilities to Patients

All endoscopy personnel are responsible for providing high quality care according to standards of patient care and professional ethics. Patient safety is a primary focus. They are also expected to educate patients and their families and to provide emotional support. Finally, patient confidentiality is a must.

## Management of Equipment (Including Reprocessing)

1. Maintaining an inventory of all equipment and accessories is necessary.

2. Handling scopes and equipment according to the manufacturer's guidelines is important. Scopes should not be bent. Special care should be given to the distal tip, where most damage occurs. An instrument repair log should be kept to identify patterns of damage.

3. Equipment should be disinfected or sterilized according to the manufacturer's guidelines. All detachable parts such as valves, buttons, and water bottles should be taken apart and cleaned and/or sterilized separately.

4. Endoscopes are cleaned using high-level disinfection. The following should always be performed: immediately after scope use, clean water should be aspirated through the suction channel, and water should be ejected through the air/water channel. Leak testing should be performed. The scope is then immersed in water and detergent and washed thoroughly. Special attention should be given to cleaning the distal end, biopsy channel, and suction ports. All channels should be brushed and suctioned. The scope is then put in the automated endoscope washer-disinfector (AEWD) where it is disinfected further. First, detergent and water perfuse the channels and outside of the scope. Then the scope and channels are immersed in disinfectant, such as gluderaldehyde or peracetic acid, for a programmed period of time. Finally, the disinfectant returns to its reservoir, and the cycle completes with a water rinse. Some AEWDs have an alcohol rinse and drying cycle. If it does not contain these processes, the scope should be taken out of the reprocessor

and dried manually. The inside channels should be dried using alcohol and/or compressed air. Moisture left in the scope can promote microorganism growth.

5. Scopes should be hung vertically, not coiled, in a well-ventilated room.

6. Accessories may be disposable or reusable. All reusable equipment should be cleaned according to manufacturer's guidelines. Sterilization is required for instruments that break mucosal barriers, such as biopsy forceps. Water bottles and bite blocks should be high-level disinfected using gluderaldehyde or peracetic acid. Blood pressure cuffs and pulse oximeters can be cleaned using low-level disinfection.

7. All endoscopy staff should adhere to regulations with regard to universal blood and body fluid precautions (5). Several organizations such as the American Society for Gastrointestinal Endoscopy (ASGE), the Joint Commission on Accreditation of Healthcare Organizations (JCAHO), the Society of Gastroenterology Nurses and Associates (SGNA), the American College of Gastroenterology (ACG), and the American Society of Colon and Rectal Surgeons (ASCRS) are committed to assisting the FDA and manufacturers in addressing infection control issues in GI device reprocessing (6).

## REFERENCES

1. Tytgat GNJ. The endoscopy unit. In: Classen M, Tytgat GNJ, Ligthdale CJ, eds. *Gastroenterological Endoscopy*. New York: Thieme, 2002:91–100.
2. Sivak MV Jr, Manoy R, Rich ME. The endoscopy unit. In: Sivak MV Jr, ed. *Gastorenterology Endoscopy*. Philadelphia: WB Saunders Co, 2000:50–78.
3. Reinhold MP. The procedure unit. In: Drossman DA, ed. *Manual of Gastroenterologic Procedures*. 3rd ed. New York: Raven Press, 1993:1–9.
4. Bowlus B, ed. *Gastroenterology Nursing. A Core Curriculum*. 2nd ed. St. Louis: Mosby, 1998.
5. American Gastroenterological Association. The American Gastroenterological Association Standards for Office-Based Gastrointestinal Endoscopy Services. *Gastroenterology* 2001;121:440–443.
6. Gastrointestinal endoscopy, infection control and hospital epidemiology. Multi-society guideline for reprocessing flexible gastrointestinal endoscopes. *Gastrointest Endosc* 2003;53:1:1–8.

# Handling of Specimens

Jason D. Conway

A. **Bacterial**

| | |
|---|---|
| Sample type: | Stool or rectal swab |
| Container: | Sterile screw-capped container |
| Preservative: | None |
| Amount: | > 10 cc |
| Processing: | Cultures should be transported to the lab and processed as soon as possible. *C. difficile* Toxin A enzyme immunoassay (EIA) specimens may be stored for up to 72 hours at 8°C if needed. Storage for > 72 hours should be at −70°C. |

B. **Viral**

| | |
|---|---|
| Sample type: | Tissue, only swabs with synthetic tips (polyester or Dacron) and plastic shafts, stool |
| Container: | Sterile screw-capped container containing freshly thawed Viral Transport Media (VTM), except Rotavirus stool samples, which should be in a sterile container with no media or preservative. Swabs should be broken off and sent in the container with VTM. |
| Processing: | Specimens should be refrigerated and processed within 2 hours. Rotavirus specimens may be stored for up to 3 days at 2°C to 8°C or −20°C for longer storage. |

C. **Fungal**

| | |
|---|---|
| Sample type: | Brushings, washings, or stool |
| Container: | Sterile screw-capped container |
| Preservative: | Sterile saline or water should be used to prevent the specimen from drying out. |
| Processing: | Specimens may be stored briefly at room temperature or refrigerated but should be transported to the lab and processed as soon as possible. |

D. **Parasites**

| | |
|---|---|
| Sample type: | Stool, tissue, duodenal aspirates |
| Container: | Sterile screw-capped container |
| Preservative: | None if specimens can be examined immediately. If stool cannot be examined within 2 hours, one specimen should be fixed in 10% formalin and another in polyvinyl alcohol. |

Amount:            > 10 cc liquid stool or > 50 g solid stool
Processing:        Specimens should be transported to the lab
                   and processed as soon as possible.

E.   Pathology

Sample type:       Tissue
Container:         Sterile screw-capped container
Preservative:      10% (v/v) Neutral Buffered Formalin or
                   other appropriate fixative. The fixative vol-
                   ume should be at least ten times the volume
                   of the specimen
Processing:        Specimens may be stored for several weeks
                   at room temperature.

F.   Cytology

Sample type:       Brushings or washings
Container:         Sterile screw-capped container
Preservative:      ThinPrep General Cytology Fixative or
                   other appropriate fixative
Processing:        If slides are made, they should not be
                   allowed to dry prior to fixation. Specimens
                   may be stored for several weeks at room
                   temperature.

## SUGGESTED READINGS

Cibas ES, Ducatman BS, eds. *Cytology: Diagnostic Principles and Clinical Correlates*. Philadelphia: W.B. Saunders Co, 1996.

Manual of Pathology and Laboratory Medicine Clinical Services. University of North Carolina Hospitals McLendon Clinical Laboratories, 2003: http://www.pathology.med.unc.edu/path/labs/

McClatchey KD, ed. *Clinical Laboratory Medicine*. Philadelphia: Lippincott Williams & Wilkins, 2002.

# Doses of Common GI Drugs Used in GI Procedures

Sanjib P. Mohanty

| Medication name | Starting dosage | Increment value | Comments |
| --- | --- | --- | --- |
| 2% viscous lidocaine | 15 mL | 15 | Maximum dose: 4.5 mg/kg for topical anesthesia |
| 4% lidocaine HCl | 7.5 mL | 7.5 | Maximum dose: 4.5 mg/kg for topical anesthesia |
| 98% denatured alcohol | 0.1 mL | 0.1 | Maximum dose: 1 mL for ulcer hemostasis |
| Acetaminophen | 500 mg | 500 | Premedication for contrast allergies |
| Atropine | 0.4 mg | 0.2 | Maximum dose: 2 mg for tachycardia |
| Benzocaine 20% spray | 1 spray | 1 | For topical anesthesia for anal fissures, achalasia |
| Botulinum toxin type A | 80 to 100 units | 100 | 20 units × 4 quadrants for anal fissures, achalasia |
| Bupivacaine 0.25% | 20 mL | 20 | See Chapter 50 |
| Cholecystokinin | 0.2 mg/kg | 0.2 | For bile collection and crystal analysis |
| Diazepam | 5 mg | 2.5 | Total dose varies for sedation |
| Diphenhydramine | 25 mg | 12.5 | Premedication for contrast allergies |
| Droperidol | 1.25 mg | 1.25 | Obtain preprocedure EKG to measure $QT_c$ interval |
| Fentanyl | 50 mcg | 25 | Total dose varies for analgesia/anesthesia |
| Flumazenil | 0.2 mg | 0.2 | Maximum dose: 3 mg To reverse benzodiazepine effects |
| Glucagon | 0.2 mg | 0.2 | For decreasing duodenal peristalsis |

| Glycopyrrolate | 0.2 mg/mL | 0.2 | To decrease duodenal peristalsis |
|---|---|---|---|
| Meperidine | 25 mg | 12.5 | Total dose varies for analgesia/sedation |
| Methylpred-nisolone | 40 mg | 10 | Premedication for contrast allergies |
| Midazolam | 1 mg | 0.5 to 1.0 | Total dose varies for sedation |
| Morphine sulfate | 2 mg | 1 | For analgesia/sedation |
| Morrhuate sodium | 50 mg/mL | 1 to 2 mL | Maximum dose: ≤ 20 mL |
| Naloxone | 0.2 mg | 0.2 | Maximum dose: 4 mg To reverse narcotic effects |
| Promethazine | 25 mg | 12.5 | For nausea |
| Secretin | 0.2 mcg/kg | 2 | To stimulate pancreatic secretions |
| Sucralfate | 1 gm po | 1 | For gastric ulcers and varices |
| Triamcinolone 30 mL | 40 mg | 40 | Maximum dose: 5 to 10 mg |
| Triamcinolone diacetate | 40 mg | 20 | See Chapter 50 |

# Guidelines for Endoscopic Screening and Surveillance

Jason D. Conway

## Definitions

Screening: Endoscopy performed on average risk, asymptomatic individuals to detect cancerous or precancerous lesions.

Surveillance: Endoscopy performed on individuals already known to be at increased risk of cancer due to a previously detected structural abnormality (e.g., previous polyps or inflammatory bowel disease [IBD]), to detect a cancerous or precancerous lesion.

A.  Colorectal Cancer Screening for Patients at Average Risk

Average-risk individuals are those over 50 who do not have a personal history of colorectal cancer or adenomatous polyp, IBD or genetic polyposis syndrome, or first-degree family member with colorectal cancer or adenomatous polyp. All men and women over the age of 50 at average risk should be offered colorectal cancer screening. Clinicians should review the effectiveness and risks of each of the below strategies with the patient.

Screening regimens based on modality chosen

Fecal occult blood test (FOBT)

| | |
|---|---|
| Screening interval: | 1 year |
| Test specifics: | Two samples from three consecutive stools should be examined using a guaiac-based test. The samples should not be rehydrated. Patient should follow dietary restrictions prior to sampling stools. |
| Positive test: | If any sample is positive for occult blood, proceed to colonoscopy. |

Flexible Sigmoidoscopy

| | |
|---|---|
| Screening interval: | 5 years |
| Test specifics: | Exam should be performed by trained examiner. Prep should be adequate and colon examined to or near splenic flexure. |
| Positive test: | If neoplasm is seen, proceed to colonoscopy. |

**Combined Fecal Occult Blood Test and Flexible Sigmoidoscopy**

| | |
|---|---|
| Screening interval: | 1 year for FOBT, 5 years for sigmoidoscopy |
| Test specifics: | As per recommendations for individual tests above. |
| Positive test: | If any sample is positive for occult blood or neoplasm seen on sigmoidoscopy, proceed to colonoscopy. |

**Colonoscopy**

| | |
|---|---|
| Screening interval: | 10 years |
| Test specifics: | Exam should be performed by trained examiner. Prep should be adequate and entire colon examined. |
| Positive test: | If neoplasms are seen and removed, see "Postpolypectomy Surveillance" guidelines below. |

**Double-Contrast Barium Enema**

| | |
|---|---|
| Screening interval: | 5 years |
| Test specifics: | Exam should be performed by trained radiologist. Prep should be adequate and entire colon visualized. |
| Positive test: | Abnormalities should be followed up with colonoscopy. |

B. **Postpolypectomy Surveillance**

Colorectal cancer risk

Colorectal cancer risk should be defined by the initial or baseline colonoscopy and then refined with each subsequent examination. The patient's age, comorbidities, family history, and quality of the prep should all be considered when determining the interval of follow-up colonoscopy. The following guidelines are for patients who, prior to first colonoscopy, have no more than average risk for developing colorectal cancer (i.e., not those patients with a history of IBD, colorectal cancer, significant family history, or genetic polyposis syndrome).

Surveillance intervals based on risk
Very low risk

| | |
|---|---|
| Definition: | No polyps or only hyperplastic polyps |
| Follow-up colonoscopy: | 10 years |

Low risk

| | |
|---|---|
| Definition: | 1 or 2 adenomas < 1 cm each |
| Follow-up colonoscopy: | 5 years until one negative exam, then every 10 years |

Intermediate risk

| | |
|---|---|
| Definition: | 3 or 4 adenomas < 1 cm each, or at least one adenoma ≥ 1 cm |
| Follow-up colonoscopy: | 3 years until two negative exams, then every 10 years |

High risk

| | |
|---|---|
| Definition: | ≥ 5 adenomas, or ≥ 3 adenomas at least one of which ≥ 1 cm |
| Follow-up colonoscopy: | 1 year, then every 3 years |

Very high risk

| | |
|---|---|
| Definition: | Large sessile polyp ≥ 2 cm, or malignant polyp with good prognostic features defined as complete excision with margins free of involvement, not poorly differentiated, and no vascular or lymphatic involvement. |
| Follow-up colonoscopy: | 3 months until site is free of abnormal tissue, then every 3 years |

Malignant polyps with poor prognostic features or very large polyps that cannot be completely resected endoscopically should be referred for surgery.

C. Colorectal Cancer Screening and Surveillance for Patients with IBD

Colorectal cancer risk in patients with IBD

Patients with uclerative colitis and Crohn's colitis are at increased risk of developing colorectal cancer. This risk may be modified by disease severity, extent, and duration. Screening and surveillance guidelines are based on duration and extent of disease, although randomized controlled data are lacking.

Screening and surveillance interval

Left-sided colitis only

| | |
|---|---|
| First screening: | 15 years after onset of disease |
| Surveillance interval: | 1 to 2 years |

Pancolitis

| | |
|---|---|
| First screening: | 8 years after onset of disease |
| Surveillance interval: | 1 to 2 years |

Indeterminate extent of disease

| | |
|---|---|
| First screening: | 8 to 10 years after onset of disease |
| Surveillance interval: | 1 to 2 years |

Biopsy technique

Expert opinion suggests that four quadrant biopsies be taken at 10-cm intervals throughout the entire colon. Strictures and mass lesions (excluding pseudopolyps) should be extensively biopsied. If a polyp is removed, adjacent flat mucosa should also be biopsied.

Recommendations based on pathology

All pathologic specimens should be evaluated by a pathologist experienced with dysplasia in IBD. Active inflammation may lead to false positive results. The following recommendations are again based on expert opinion only. The decision to proceed to colectomy should be individualized, and take into consideration patient age, comorbidities, severity of disease, life expectancy, family history of colorectal cancer, and history of primary sclerosing cholangitis.

Flat mucosa

| | |
|---|---|
| Dysplasia grade: | High, multifocal low, or unifocal low* |
| Recommendation: | Colectomy |

Mass lesion or stricture

| | |
|---|---|
| Dysplasia grade: | Any |
| Recommendation: | Colectomy |

*Unifocal low-grade dysplasia in flat mucosa should prompt consideration of colectomy, although there is less consensus among experts compared to high or multifocal low-grade dysplasia.

D. Barrett's Esophagus Surveillance

Who should be surveyed?

Patients with biopsy-proven Barrett's esophagus (intestinal metaplasia in the esophagus) should be considered for surveillance only if therapeutic intervention for early cancer would prolong life expectancy. The grade of dysplasia determines the time interval of surveillance.

Biopsy technique

Active esophageal inflammation should be treated prior to biopsy as this may be misinterpreted as dysplasia. Four-quadrant biopsies should be taken every 2 cm of the Barrett's segment. Specific biopsies should focus on ulcers, erosions, nodules, strictures, or other mucosal abnormalities. For high-grade dysplasia, four-quadrant biopsies taken every 1 cm within the Barrett's segment may be considered.

Surveillance intervals based on grade of dysplasia

No dysplasia

| | |
|---|---|
| Definition: | Two consecutive EGDs with biopsies showing no dysplasia |
| Follow-up EGD: | 3 years |

Low-grade dysplasia

| | |
|---|---|
| Definition: | Low-grade dysplasia confirmed on repeat EGD |
| Follow-up EGD: | 1 year until no dysplasia |

High-grade dysplasia

| | |
|---|---|
| Definition: | Repeat EGD rules out cancer and documents high-grade dysplasia. Consider confirmation by an expert pathologist. |
| Follow-up EGD: | Focal - 3 months |
| Multifocal— | Consider surgery |
| Mucosal irregularity | Consider EMR or surgery |

## SUGGESTED READINGS

Atkin WS, Saunders BP. Surveillance guidelines after removal of colorectal adenomatous polyps. *Gut* 2002;51(Suppl V):v6–v9.

Bond JH. Polyp guideline: diagnosis, treatment, and surveillance for patients with colorectal polyps. *Am J Gastroenterol* 2000;95: 3053–3063.

Levine DS, Haggitt RC, Blount PL, et al. An endoscopic biopsy protocol can differentiate high grade dysplasia from early adenocarcinoma in Barrett's esophagus. *Gastroenterology* 1993;105:40–50.

Reid BJ, Blount P, Feng Z, et al. Optimizing endoscopic biopsy detection of early cancers in Barrett's high grade dysplasia. *Am J Gastroenterol* 2000;95:3089–3096.

Sampliner RE. Updated guidelines for the diagnosis, surveillance, and therapy of Barrett's esophagus. *Am J Gastroenterol* 2002;97: 1888–1895.

Schmitz RJ, Sharma P, Topalovski M, et al. Detection of Barrett's esophagus after endoscopic healing for erosive esophagitis. *Am J Gastroenterol* 2000;95:2433 (abstract).

Weinstein W. Erosive esophagitis impairs accurate detection of Barrett's esophagus: a prospective, randomized, double blind study. *Gastroenterology* 1999;116:A352(G1538) (abstract).

Winawer S, Fletcher R, Rex D, et al. Colorectal cancer screening and surveillance: clinical guidelines and rationale—update based on new evidence. *Gastroenterology* 2003;124:544–560.

# DDW Cards/Useful Websites

Sanjib P. Mohanty

## Patient Resources

Crohn's and Colitis Foundation of America

**http://www.ccfa.org/**

International Foundation for Functional GI Disorders

**http://www.iffgd.org**

Irritable Bowel Syndrome Support Group

**http://www.ibsgroup.org/**

GERD Support Group

**http://heartburn.about.com/cs/adultgerdsupport/**

## Endoscopy Equipment

Alveolus, Inc.

**http://www.alveolus.com/home.htm**

(704) 998-6008
401 North Tryon Street
10th Floor
Charlotte, NC 28202

Bard Endoscopic Technologies

**http://www.bardendoscopy.com/**

C. R. Bard, Inc.
(978) 663-8989
(800) 826-BARD (Customer Service)
129 Concord Road, Bldg. #3
Billerica, MA 01821

BARRx, Inc.

**http://www.barrx.com/**

BARRX Website is Under Construction
(408) 331-3185
1346 Bordeaux Drive
Sunnyvale, CA 94089

Cordis Corporation

**http://www.cordis.com/index.asp**

A Johnson & Johnson Company
(800) 327-7714
14201 N.W. 60th Avenue
Miami Lakes, FL 33014

Curon Medical, Inc.

**http://www.curonmedical.com/**

(408) 733-9910
(877) 734-2873 (Customer Service)
735 Palomar Avenue
Sunnyvale, CA 94085

Edwards Lifesciences Corporation

**http://www.edwards.com/FlashIntro.aspx**

(800) 424-3278
One Edwards Way
Irvine, CA 92614

Ethicon Endo Surgery, Inc

**http://www.ethiconendo.com/index.jsp**

Johnson & Johnson
(800) USE-ENDO (Customer Service)
4545 Creek Road
Cincinnati, OH 45242

Fujinon, Inc.

**http://www.fujinonendoscopy.com/**

Fuji Photo Optical Co., LTD
(973) 633-5600
(800) 490-0661 (Customer Service)
10 High Point Drive
Wayne, NJ 07470

Given Imaging, Inc

**http://www.givenimaging.com/Cultures/en-US/given/
english**

(770) 662-0870
5555 Oakbrook Parkway, # 355
Norcross, GA 30093

Hobbs Medical Inc.

**http://www.hobbsmedical.com**

(860) 684-5875
(800) 344-6227 (Customer Service)
8 Spring Street
P. O. Box 46
Stafford Springs, CT 06076

Horizons International Corporation

**http://www.horizonscorp.com**

(787) 842-4000
(800) 256-4716 (Customer Service)
P.O. Box 7273
Ponce, PR 00732-7273

Immersion Medical

**http://www.immersion.com/medical/**

(301) 984-3706
55 West Watkins Mill Road
Gaithersburg, MD 20878

Integrated Medical Systems

**http://www.imsservices.com/**

(800) 783-9251
1823 27th Avenue South
Birmingham, AL 35209

Karl Storz Endoscopy

**http://www.karlstorz.com/**

KARL STORZ Endoscopy-America, Inc.
(310) 338-8100
(800) 421-0837 (Customer Service)
600 Corporate Pointe
Culver City, CA 90230-7600

Mandel + Rupp
e-mail: manel-rupp@t-online.de
0 21 04/94 68-0
Gruitener Strabe 11
40699 Erkrath
Deutschland

Medi-Globe USA

**http://www.mediglobe.com**

Medi-Globe Group-Germany
(480) 897-2772
6202 S. Maple Ave., Suite 131
Tempe, AZ 85283

Medtronic-Gastroenterology

**http://www.medtronic.com/physician/gastroenterology
.html**

Medtronic, Inc.
(763) 514-4000
(800) 328-0810 (Customer Service)
710 Medtronic Parkway
Minneapolis, MN 55432-5604

Microvasive

**http://www.bostonscientific.com/**

Boston Scientific
(508)-650-8000
(800) 225-3226 (Customer Service)
One Boston Scientific Place
Natick, MA 01760-1537

NDO Surgical

**http://www.ndosurgical.com/**

(508) 337-8881
125 High Street, Suite 7
Mansfield, MA 02048

Olympus Medical Endoscope & Surgical Products

**http://www.olympusamerica.com/hc_section/hc_home.asp**

Olympus America Inc.
(800) 645-8160
(800) 848-9024 (Customer Service)
2 Corporate Center Drive
Melville, NY 11747

Pentax

**http://www.pentaxmedical.com**

Pentax Precision Instrument Corporation
(845) 365-0700
(800) 431-5880 (Customer Service)
Corporate Headquarters
30 Ramland Road
Orangeburg, NY 10962-2699

PriMed Instruments Inc

**http://www.primedinstruments.com**

(877) 565-0565
1080 Tristar Drive Unit 14
Mississauga, ON L5T 1P1
Canada

Sandhill Scientific, Inc.

**http://www.sandhillsci.com/**

(303) 470-7020
(800) 468-4556 (Customer Service)
9150 Commerce Center Circle, Suite 500
Highlands Ranch, CO 80126

Simbionix USA Corporation

**http://www.simbionix.com/**

(216) 229-2040
(866) 746-2466 (Customer Service)
11000 Cedar Ave., Suite 210
Cleveland, OH 44106

Smith & Nephew Endoscopy

**http://www.endoscopy1.com/US/Home.asp**

Smith & Nephew, Inc.
(800) 343-5717
150 Minuteman Road
Andover, MA 01810

Stryker Endoscopy

**http://www.strykerendo.com/site/home.nsf/home.html?
Openpage**

(408) 754-2000
(800) 624-4422 (Customer Service)
5900 Optical Court
San Jose, CA 95138

The Scope Exchange

**http://www.scopex.com**

(336) 544-2100
(888) 252-1542 (Customer Service)
4210 Tudor Lane
Greensboro, NC 27410

U. S. Endoscopy

**http://www.usendoscopy.com/**

(440) 639-4494
5976 Heisley Road
Mentor, OH 44060

U. S. Surgical

**http://www.ussurg.com/**

(203) 845-1000
(800) 722-8772 (Customer Service)
150 Glover Avenue
Norwalk, CT 06856

W. L. Gore & Associates, Inc.

**http://www.goremedical.com/HomePage**

(928) 779-2771
(800) 437-8181 (Customer Service)
P.O. Box 2400
Flagstaff, AZ 86003-2400

Wilson-Cook Medical GI Endoscopy

**http://www.cookgroup.com/wilson_cook/**

Cook Group, Incorporated
(336) 744-0157
(800) 245-4717 (Customer Service)
4900 Bethania Station Road
Winston-Salem, NC 27105

## Medications

**http://www.astrazeneca-us.com/products/ta_page.asp?ta=4**

**http://www.axcanscandipharm.com/home.aspx?lang=
en-us&n=4&m=16**

**http://www.novartis.com/products/en/product_list_ab
.shtml**

**http://www.remicade.com/**

# GI Professional Groups

American Gastroenterological Association (AGA)
**http://www.gastro.org/**

American Society for Gastrointestinal Endoscopy (ASGE)
**http://www.asge.org/**

American Association for the Study of Liver Diseases (AASLD)
**http://www.aasld.org/**

American College of Gastroenterology (ACG)
**http://www.acg.gi.org/**

# CPT Modifiers

Sanjib P. Mohanty

**22 Unusual Procedural Services:** When the service(s) provided is greater than that usually required for the listed procedure, it may be identified by adding this modifier to the usual procedure number.

**26 Professional Component:** Certain procedures are a combination of a physician component and a technical component. When the physician component is reported separately, the service may be identified by adding this modifier to the usual procedure number.

**51 Multiple Procedures:** When multiple procedures are performed at the same session by the same provider, the primary procedure or service may be reported as listed. The additional procedure(s) or service(s) may be identified by appending this modifier to the additional procedure or service code(s).

**53 Discontinued Procedure:** Under certain circumstances, the physician may elect to terminate a surgical or diagnostic procedure. Due to extenuating circumstances or those that threaten the well-being of the patient, it may be necessary to indicate that a surgical or diagnostic procedure was started but discontinued. This circumstance may be reported by adding this modifier to the code reported by the physician for the discontinued procedure.

**59 Distinct Procedural Service:** Under certain circumstances, the physician may need to indicate that a procedure or service was distinct or independent from other services performed on the same day. This modifier is used to identify procedures/services that are not normally reported together but are appropriate under the circumstances. This may represent a different session or patient encounter, different procedure or surgery, different site or organ system, separate incision/excision, separate lesion, or separate injury not ordinarily encountered or performed on the same day by the same physician. However, when another already established modifier is appropriate it should be used rather than modifier '59'.

**62 Two Surgeons:** When two surgeons work together as primary surgeons performing distinct part(s) of a procedure, each surgeon should report his/her distinct operative work by adding this modifier to the procedure code. Each surgeon should report the cosurgery once using the same procedure code.

# Complete Listing of CPT Codes

**Chapter 1 Preprocedure Assessment of Patients Undergoing Gastrointestinal Procedures**
None

**Chapter 2 Bowel Preps**
None

**Chapter 3 Analgesia and Sedation**
**99141** – Moderate (conscious) sedation.

**Chapter 4 Oral and Nasal Gastrointestinal Intubation**
**43752** – Nasogastric or orogastric tube placement, requiring physician's skill and fluoroscopic guidance (includes fluoroscopy, image documentation and report).
**44500** – Introduction of long gastrointestinal tube (eg., Miller-Abbott) (separate procedure).

**Chapter 5 Esophagogastroduodenoscopy (EGD)**
**43200** – Esophagoscopy, rigid or flexible; diagnostic, with or without collection of specimen(s) by brushing or washing (separate procedure).
**43202** – With biopsy, single or multiple.
**43215** – With removal of foreign body.
**43235** – Upper gastrointestinal endoscopy including esophagus, stomach, and either the duodenum and/or jejunum as appropriate; diagnostic, with or without collection of specimen(s) by brushing or washing (separate procedure).
**43239** – With biopsy, single or multiple.
**43241** – With transendoscopic intraluminal tube or catheter placement.
**43248** – With insertion of guidewire followed by dilation of esophagus over guidewire.
**43255** – With control of bleeding, any method.
**43258** – With ablation of tumor(s), polyp(s), or other lesion(s) not amenable to removal by hot biopsy forceps, bipolar cautery or snare technique.

**Chapter 6 Small Bowel Enteroscopy**
**44360** – Small intestinal endoscopy, enteroscopy beyond second portion of duodenum, not including ileum; diagnostic, with or without collection of specimen(s) by brushing or washing (separate procedure).
**44361** – Small intestinal endoscopy, enteroscopy beyond second portion of duodenum, not including ileum; with biopsy, single or multiple.
**44363** – Small intestinal endoscopy, enteroscopy beyond second portion of duodenum, not including ileum; with removal of foreign body.

**44364** – Small intestinal endoscopy, enteroscopy beyond second portion of duodenum, not including ileum; with removal of tumor(s), polyp(s), or other lesion(s) by snare technique.

**44365** – Small intestinal endoscopy, enteroscopy beyond second portion of duodenum, not including ileum; with removal of tumor(s), polyp(s), or other lesion(s) by hot biopsy forceps or bipolar cautery.

**44366** – Small intestinal endoscopy, enteroscopy beyond second portion of duodenum, not including ileum; with control of bleeding, any method.

**44369** – Small intestinal endoscopy, enteroscopy beyond second portion of duodenum, not including ileum; with ablation of tumor(s), polyp(s), or other lesion(s) not amenable to removal by hot biopsy forceps, bipolar cautery, or snare technique.

**44372** – Small intestinal endoscopy, enteroscopy beyond second portion of duodenum, not including ileum; with placement of percutaneous jejunostomy tube.

**44373** – Small intestinal endoscopy, enteroscopy beyond second portion of duodenum, not including ileum; with conversion of percutaneous gastrostomy tube to percutaneous jejunostomy tube.

**44376** – Small intestinal endoscopy, enteroscopy beyond second portion of duodenum, including ileum; diagnostic, with or without collection of specimen(s) by brushing or washing (separate procedure).

**44377** – Small intestinal endoscopy, enteroscopy beyond second portion of duodenum, including ileum; with biopsy, single or multiple.

**44378** – Small intestinal endoscopy, enteroscopy beyond second portion of duodenum, including ileum; with control of bleeding, any method.

**44380** – Ileoscopy, through stoma; diagnostic, with or without collection of specimen(s) by brushing or washing (separate procedure).

**44382** – Ileoscopy, through stoma; with biopsy, single or multiple.

**44385** – Endoscopic evaluation of small intestinal (abdominal or pelvic) pouch; diagnostic, with or without collection of specimen(s) by brushing or washing (separate procedure).

**44386** – Endoscopic evaluation of small intestinal (abdominal or pelvic) pouch; with biopsy, single or multiple.

## Chapter 7 Endoscopic Retrograde Pancreatography

**43260** – Endoscopic retrograde cholangiopancreatography (ERCP); diagnostic, with or without collection of specimen(s) by brushing or washing (separate procedure).

**43261** – Endoscopic retrograde cholangiopancreatography (ERCP); with biopsy, single or multiple.

## Chapter 8 Colonoscopy

**45378** – Colonoscopy, flexible, proximal to splenic flexure; diagnostic, with or without collection of specimen(s) by brushing or washing, with or without colon decompression (separate procedure).

**45380** – Colonoscopy, flexible, proximal to splenic flexure; with biopsy, single or multiple.

**45381** – Colonoscopy, flexible, proximal to splenic flexure; with directed submucosal injection(s), any substance.

**45383** – Colonoscopy, flexible, proximal to splenic flexure; with ablation of tumor(s), polyp(s), or other lesion(s) not amenable to removal by hot biopsy forceps, bipolar cautery or snare technique.

**45384** – Colonoscopy, flexible, proximal to splenic flexure; with removal of tumor(s), polyp(s), or other lesion(s) by hot biopsy forceps, bipolar cautery or snare technique.

**45385** – Colonoscopy, flexible, proximal to splenic flexure; with removal of tumor(s), polyp(s), or other lesion(s) by snare technique.

**45391** – Colonoscopy, flexible, proximal to splenic flexure; with endoscopic ultrasound examination, for colonoscopy with EUS

**45392** – Colonoscopy, flexible, proximal to splenic flexure; with transendoscopic ultrasound guided intramural or transmural fine needle aspiration/biopsy(s), for colonoscopy with fine needle aspiration.

## Chapter 9 Anoscopy and Sigmoidoscopy

**45300** – Proctosigmoidoscopy, rigid; diagnostic, with or without collection of specimen(s) by brushing or washing (separate procedure).

**45303** – Proctosigmoidoscopy, rigid; with dilation, any method.

**45305** – Proctosigmoidoscopy, rigid; with biopsy, single or multiple.

**45307** – Proctosigmoidoscopy, rigid; with removal of foreign body.

**45308** – Proctosigmoidoscopy, rigid; with removal of single tumor, polyp, or other lesion by hot biopsy forceps or bipolar cautery.

**45309** – Proctosigmoidoscopy, rigid; with removal of single tumor, polyp, or other lesion by snare technique.

**45315** – Proctosigmoidoscopy, rigid; with removal of multiple tumors, polyps, or other lesions by hot biopsy forceps, bipolar cautery or snare technique.

**45317** – Proctosigmoidoscopy, rigid; with control of bleeding, any method.

**45320** – Proctosigmoidoscopy, rigid; with ablation of tumor(s), polyp(s), or other lesion(s) not amenable to removal by hot biopsy forceps, bipolar cautery or snare technique (e.g., laser).

**45321** – Proctosigmoidoscopy, rigid; with decompression of volvulus.

**45327** – Proctosigmoidoscopy, rigid; with transendoscopic stent placement.

**46600** – Anoscopy; diagnostic, with or without collection of specimen(s) by brushing or washing (separate procedure).

**46604** – Anoscopy; with dilation, any method.

**46606** – Anoscopy; with biopsy, single or multiple.

**46608** – Anoscopy; with removal of foreign body.

**46610** – Anoscopy; with removal of single tumor, polyp, or other lesion by hot biopsy forceps or bipolar cautery.

**46611** – Anoscopy; with removal of single tumor, polyp, or other lesion by snare technique.

**46612** – Anoscopy; with removal of multiple tumors, polyps, or other lesions by hot biopsy forceps, bipolar cautery, or snare technique.

**46614** – Anoscopy; with control of bleeding, any method.

**46615** – Anoscopy; with ablation of tumor(s), polyp(s), or other lesion(s) not amenable to removal by hot biopsy forceps, bipolar cautery or snare technique.

## Chapter 10 Abdominal Paracentesis

**49080** – Peritoneocentesis, abdominal paracentesis, or peritoneal lavage (diagnostic or therapeutic); initial.

**49081** – Peritoneocentesis, abdominal paracentesis, or peritoneal lavage (diagnostic or therapeutic); subsequent.

**76942** – Ultrasonic guidance for needle placement (e.g., biopsy, aspiration, injection), imaging supervision and interpretation.

## Chapter 11 Percutaneous Liver Biopsy

**47000** – Biopsy of liver, needle; percutaneous.

**47001** – Biopsy of liver, needle, percutaneous when done for indicated purpose at time of other major procedure (List separately in addition to code for primary procedure).

**76942** – Ultrasonic guidance for needle placement (e.g., biopsy, aspiration, injection), imaging supervision and interpretation.

## Chapter 12 Injection Therapy for Hemostasis and Anal Fissures

**43236** – Upper gastrointestinal endoscopy including esophagus, stomach, and either the duodenum and/or jejunum as appropriate; diagnostic, with submucosal injection.

**43255** – Upper gastrointestinal endoscopy including esophagus, stomach, and either the duodenum and/or jejunum as appropriate; with control of bleeding, any method.

**45334** – Sigmoidoscopy, flexible; with control of bleeding, any method.

**45335** – Sigmoidoscopy, flexible; with submucosal injection.

**45381** – Colonoscopy, flexible, proximal to splenic flexure; with submucosal injection.

**45382** – Colonoscopy, flexible, proximal to splenic flexure; with control of bleeding, any method.

**64640** – Destruction by neurolytic agent; other peripheral nerve or branch.

## Chapter 13 Bipolar Electrocautery and Heater Probe

**43236** – Upper gastrointestinal endoscopy including esophagus, stomach, and either the duodenum and/or jejunum as appropriate; diagnostic, with submucosal injection.

**43255** – Upper gastrointestinal endoscopy including esophagus, stomach, and either the duodenum and/or jejunum as appropriate; with control of bleeding, any method.

**45334** – Sigmoidoscopy, flexible; with control of bleeding, any method.

**45335** – Sigmoidoscopy, flexible; with submucosal injection.

**45381** – Colonoscopy, flexible, proximal to splenic flexure; with submucosal injection.

**45382** – Colonoscopy, flexible, proximal to splenic flexure; with control of bleeding, any method.

## Chapter 14 Clips and Loops

None

## Chapter 15 Injection Therapy of Esophageal and Gastric Varices: Sclerosis and Cyanoacrylate

**43243** – Upper gastrointestinal endoscopy including esophagus, stomach, and either the duodenum and/or jejunum as appropriate; with injection sclerosis of esophageal and/or gastric varices. **Note:** Enbucrilate injection is not FDA approved.

## Chapter 16 Endoscopic Variceal Ligation

**43244** – Upper gastrointestinal endoscopy including the esophagus, stomach, and either the duodenum and/or jejunum as appropriate; with band ligation of esophageal and/or gastric varices.

## Chapter 17 Balloon Tamponade

**43460** – Esophogastric tamponade, with balloon

## Chapter 18 Polypectomy, Endoscopic Muscosal Resection, and Tattooing

**45385** – Colonoscopy, flexible, proximal to splenic flexure; with removal of tumor(s), polyp(s), or other lesion(s) by snare technique.
**45381** – with directed submucosal injection(s), any substance.

## Chapter 19 Feeding Tubes (Nasoduodenal, Nasojejunal)

**44500** – Nasoenteric tube placement.
**74340** – Nasoenteric tube placement with radiological supervision and interpretation.
**43241** – Upper GI endoscopy; diagnostic with transendoscopic intraluminal tube or catheter placement.

## Chapter 20 Percutaneous Endoscopic Gastrostomy (PEG) and Percutaneous Endoscopic Jejunostomy (PEJ)

**43246** – Upper gastrointestinal endoscopy including esophagus, stomach, and either the duodenum and/or jejunum as appropriate; with directed placement of percutaneous gastrostomy tube.
**44372** – Small intestinal endoscopy, enteroscopy beyond second portion of duodenum, not including ileum; with placement of percutaneous jejunostomy tube.
**44373** – Small intestinal endoscopy, enteroscopy beyond second portion of duodenum, not including ileum; with conversion of percutaneous gastrostomy tube to percutaneous jejunostomy tube.

## Chapter 21 Colonic Decompression

**45321** – Proctosigmoidoscopy; rigid, with decompression of volvulus.
**45337** – Flexible sigmoidoscopy; with decompression of volvulus.
**45378** – Colonoscopy; with or without decompression.
**Note:** No additional code is available if decompression tube is deployed.

## Chapter 22 Dilation of the Esophagus: Mercury-Filled Bougies (Hurst Maloney)

**43450** – Dilation of esophagus, by unguided sound or bougie, single or multiple passes.
**43456** – Dilation of esophagus, by balloon or dilator, retrograde.

## Chapter 23 Dilatation of the Esophagus: Wire-Guided Bougies (Savary and American Endoscopy)

**43248** – Upper gastrointestinal endoscopy including esophagus, stomach, and either the duodenum and/or jejunum as appropriate; with insertion of guidewire followed by dilation of esophagus over guidewire.

## Chapter 24 Pneumatic Dilation for Achalasia

**43458** – Dilation of esophagus with balloon (30-mm diameter or larger) for achalasia.

## Chapter 25 Through-the-Scope Balloon Dilation

**43220** – Esophagoscopy; with balloon dilation (less than 30-mm diameter).
**43245** – Upper gastrointestinal endoscopy; with dilation of gastric outlet obstruction (balloon, guidewire, bougie).
**43249** – Upper gastrointestinal endoscopy; with balloon dilation of the esophagus (less than 30 mm in diameter).

## Chapter 26 Stenting of Esophageal Cancers: Placement of Expandable Stents

**43219** – Esophagoscopy, rigid or flexible; with insertion of plastic tube or stent.
**47511** – Introduction of percutaneous transhepatic stent for internal and external biliary drainage.
**47555** – Biliary endoscopy, percutaneous via T-tube or other tract; with dilation of biliary duct stricture(s) without stent.
**47556** – Biliary endoscopy, percutaneous via T-tube or other tract; with dilation of biliary duct stricture(s) with stent.
**43268** – Endoscopic retrograde cholangiopancreatography (ERCP); with endoscopic retrograde insertion of tube or stent into bile or pancreatic duct.
**43269** – Endoscopic retrograde cholangiopancreatography (ERCP); with endoscopic retrograde removal of foreign body and/or change of tube or stent.

## Chapter 27 Biliary Sludge Analysis

None

## Chapter 28 Endoscopic Sphincterotomy (Including Precut)

**43262** – Endoscopic retrograde cholangiopancreatography (ERCP); with sphincterotomy/papillotomy

## Chapter 29 Management of Lithiasis: Balloon and Basket Extraction, Endoprosthesis, and Lithotripsy

**43264** – Endoscopic retrograde cholangiopancreatography (ERCP); with endoscopic retrograde removal of stone(s) from biliary and/or pancreatic ducts.
**43265** – Endoscopic retrograde cholangiopancreatography (ERCP); with endoscopic retrograde destruction, lithotripsy of stone(s), any method.
**43268** – Endoscopic retrograde cholangiopancreatography (ERCP); with endoscopic retrograde insertion of tube or stent into bile or pancreatic duct.

## Chapter 30 Management of Biliary and Pancreatic Ductal Obstruction: Endoprosthesis and Nasobiliary/Nasopancreatic Drain Placement

**43260** – Endoscopic retrograde cholangiopancreatography (ERCP); diagnostic, with or without collection of specimen(s) by brushing or washing (separate procedure).

**43261** – with biopsy, single or multiple.

**43262** – with sphincterotomy/papillotomy.

**43263** – with pressure measurement of sphincter of Oddi (pancreatic duct or common bile duct).

**43264** – with endoscopic retrograde removal of stone(s) from biliary and/or pancreatic ducts.

**43265** – with endoscopic retrograde destruction, lithotripsy of stone(s), any method.

**43267** – with endoscopic retrograde insertion of nasobiliary or nasopancreatic drainage tube.

**43268** – with endoscopic retrograde insertion of tube or stent into bile or pancreatic duct.

**43269** – with endoscopic retrograde removal of foreign body and/or change of tube or stent.

**43271** – with endoscopic retrograde balloon dilation of ampulla, biliary and/or pancreatic duct(s).

**43272** – with ablation of tumor(s), polyp(s), or other lesion(s) not amenable to removal by hot biopsy forceps, bipolar cautery or snare technique.

### Chapter 31 Management of Fluid Collections

Contingent upon concomitant ERCP and stent placement

**43262** – Endoscopic retrograde cholangiopancreatography (ERCP); with sphincterotomy/papillotomy.

**43268** – Endoscopic retrograde cholangiopancreatography (ERCP); with endoscopic retrograde insertion of tube or stent into bile or pancreatic duct.

**43240** – Upper Gastrointestinal Endoscopy with transmural drainage of pseudocyst.

### Chapter 32 Argon Plasma Coagulation

**43227** – Esophagoscopy, rigid or flexible; with control of bleeding.

**43228** – Esophagoscopy, rigid or flexible; with ablation of tumor(s), polyp(s), or other lesion(s), not amenable to removal by hot biopsy forceps, bipolar electrocautery, or snare technique.

**43255** – Esophagogastroduodenoscopy with control of bleeding, any method.

**43258** – Esophagogastroduodenoscopy with ablation of tumor(s), etc.

**43272** – ERCP with ablation of tumor(s), etc.

**44366** – Enteroscopy; with control of bleeding.

**44369** – Enteroscopy; with ablation of tumor(s), etc.

**44378** – Enteroscopy including ileum; with control of bleeding.

**44391** – Colonoscopy through stoma with control of bleeding.

**44393** – Colonoscopy through stoma with ablation of tumor(s), etc.

**45317** – Proctosigmoidoscopy, rigid; with control of bleeding

**45320** – Proctosigmoidoscopy, rigid; with ablation of tumor(s), etc.

**45334** – Sigmoidoscopy, flexible; with control of bleeding.

**45339** – Sigmoidoscopy flexible; with ablation of tumor(s), etc.

**45382** – Colonoscopy with control of bleeding.
**45383** – Colonoscopy; with ablation of tumor(s), etc.
**46614** – Anoscopy; with control of bleeding.
**46615** – Anoscopy; with ablation of tumor(s), etc.

## Chapter 33 Photodynamic Therapy for Barrett's High-Grade Dysplasia

**96570** – Photodynamic therapy by endoscopic application of light to ablate abnormal tissues via activation of photosensitive drug(s); first 30 minutes (List separately in addition to code for endoscopy or bronchoscopy procedures of lung and esophagus).
**96571** – Photodynamic therapy by endoscopic application of light to ablate abnormal tissues via activation of photosensitive drug(s); each additional 15 minutes (List separately in addition to code for endoscopy or bronchoscopy procedures of lung and esophagus).

## Chapter 34 Infrared Coagulation of Hemorrhoids

**46934** – Destruction of hemorrhoids, any method; internal.

## Chapter 35 Endoscopic Management of Foreign Bodies of the Upper Gastrointestinal Tract

**43215** – Esophagoscopy, rigid or flexible; with removal of foreign body.
**43247** – Upper gastrointestinal endoscopy including esophagus, stomach, and either the duodenum and/or jejunum as appropriate; with removal of foreign body.
**44363** – Small intestinal endoscopy, enteroscopy beyond second portion of duodenum, not including ileum; with removal of foreign body.

## Chapter 36 Capsule Endoscopy

**91110** – Gastrointestinal tract imaging, intraluminal (e.g., capsule endoscopy), esophagus through ileum, with physician interpretation and report.
The diagnosis codes associated with capsule endoscopy are dependent on the indication and findings. The most common codes are those for GI bleeding, once colonoscopy and upper endoscopy are nondiagnostic.

## Chapter 37 Stretta

**43257** – Upper gastrointestinal endoscopy including esophagus, stomach, and either the duodenum and/or jejunum as appropriate; with delivery of thermal energy to the muscle of lower esophageal sphincter and/or gastric cardia, for treatment of gastroesophageal reflux disease, for the Stretta procedure

## Chapter 38 Enteryx Injection for Gastroesophageal Reflux Disease

**C9704** – injection or insertion of intert substance for the submucosal/intramuscular injection(s) into the upper gastrointestinal tract, under fluoroscopic guidance.
**43234** – upper gastrointestinal endoscopy, simple primary examination (e.g., with small diameter flexible endoscope).

**43235** – upper gastrointestinal endoscopy including esophagus, stomach and either the duodenum and/or jejunum as appropriate; diagnostic, with or without collection(s) of specimen(s).

## Chapter 39 Endoscopic Sewing—EndoCinch
**43499** – Unlisted procedure, esophagus.

## Chapter 40 Esophageal Manometry
**91010** – Esophageal motility (manometric study of the esophagus and/or gastroesophageal junction) study.

## Chapter 41 Ambulatory 24-Hour Esophageal pH Monitoring
**91032** – Esophagus, acid reflux test, with intraluminal pH electrode for detection of gastroesophageal reflux.
**91033** – Esophagus, acid reflux test, with intraluminal pH electrode for detection of gastroesophageal reflux; prolonged recording.
**91034** – Esophagus, gastroesophageal reflux test; with nasal catheter pH electrode(s) placement, recording, analysis and interpretation, for gastroesophageal reflux testing.
**91035** – Esophagus, gastroesophageal reflux test; with mucosal attached telemetry pH electrode placement, recording, analysis and interpretation, for scenarios in which the physician performs a gastroesophageal reflux test with a Bravo probe.

## Chapter 42 Gastric Secretory Testing
None

## Chapter 43 Secretin Test
**83986** – Pathology pH, body fluid, except blood.

## Chapter 44 Sphincter of Oddi Manometry
**43263** – Endoscopic retrograde cholangiopancreatography (ERCP); with pressure measurement of sphincter of Oddi (pancreatic duct or common bile duct).

## Chapter 45 Small Bowel Motility and the Role of Scintigraphy in Small Bowel Motility
None

## Chapter 46 Breath Hydrogen Tests for Lactose Intolerance and Bacterial Overgrowth
**91065** – Breath hydrogen test (e.g., for detection of lactase deficiency).

## Chapter 47 Anorectal Manometry and Biofeedback
**91122** – Anorectal manometry.
**90911** – Biofeedback training, anorectal, including EMG and/or manometry.
**91120** – Rectal sensation, tone, and compliance test (i.e., response to graded balloon distention), for rectal sensation, tone and compliance tests.

## Chapter 48 Endoscopic Ultrasound
**43231** – Esophagoscopy with endoscopic examination.

**43232** – Esophagoscopy with transendoscopic ultrasound-guided intramural or transmural fine needle aspiration/biopsy(s).

**43237** – Esophagoscopy either endoscopic ultrasound examination limited to the esophagus.

**43238** – Esophagoscopy with transendoscopic ultrasound-guided intramural or transmural fine needle aspiration/biopsy(s), esophagus (includes endoscopic ultrasound examination limited to the esophagus).

**43259** – Upper endoscopic ultrasound.

**45242** – Upper GI endoscopy with transendoscopic ultrasound guided intramural or transmural fine needle aspiration/biopsy(s).

**45341** – Sigmoidoscopy with endoscopic examination.

**45342** – Sigmoidoscopy with transendoscopic ultrasound guided intramural or transmural fine needle aspiration/biopsy(s).

**45391** – Colonoscopy, flexible, proximal to splenic flexure; with endoscopic ultrasound examination, for colonoscopy with EUS.

**45392** – Colonoscopy, flexible, proximal to splenic flexure; with transendoscopic ultrasound guided intramural or transmural fine needle aspiration/biopsy(s), for colonoscopy with fine needle aspiration.

## Chapter 49 Endosonography-guided Fine Needle Aspiration Biopsy

**43242** – EGD with transendoscopic ultrasound-guided intramural or transmural fine needle aspiration biopsy(s).

**43232** – Esophagoscopy, rigid or flexible; with transendoscopic ultrasound-guided intramural or transmural fine needle aspiration/biopsy(s).

**43238** – Upper gastrointestinal endoscopy including esophagus, stomach, and either the duodenum and/or jejunum as appropriate; with transendoscopic ultrasound-guided intramural or transmural fine needle aspiration/biopsy(s), esophagus (includes endoscopic ultrasound examination limited to the esophagus).

**45342** – Sigmoidoscopy, flexible; with transendoscopic ultrasound guided intramural or transmural fine needle aspiration/biopsy(s).

**45391** – Colonoscopy, flexible, proximal to splenic flexure; with endoscopic ultrasound examination, for colonoscopy with EUS.

**45392** – Colonoscopy, flexible, proximal to splenic flexure; with transendoscopic ultrasound guided intramural or transmural fine needle aspiration/biopsy(s), for colonoscopy with fine needle aspiration.

## Chapter 50 Endosonography-Guided Celiac Plexus Neurolysis

**43259** – Upper gastrointestinal endoscopy including esophagus, stomach, and either the duodenum and/or jejunum as appropriate; with endoscopic ultrasound examination.

**64680** – Destruction by neurolytic agent, celiac plexus, with or without radiologic monitoring.

If the block is done with a biopsy then

**43242** – EGD with transendoscopic ultrasound guided intramural or transmural fine needle aspiration biopsy(s).

# Subject Index

Page numbers followed by f indicate figures; those followed by t indicate tables.

## A

Abdominal paracentesis
   analysis of aspirated fluid, 75–76
   complications, 77
   CPT codes, 77
   diagnostic, 73–74
   equipment, 72
   indications and contraindications, 72
   therapeutic, 74–75
Ablation, mucosal, side effects of, 244
Achalasia, pneumatic dilation for, 168–174
Acid output determination, 309
American endoscopy system, 164–167
Anal fissures
   CPT codes, 91
   injection therapy for, 89–91
Analgesia
   CPT code for sedation, 18
   for endoscopy, 13–18
Andersen-type intestinal tubes, 27–28
Anorectal manometry
   auxiliary tests, 345
   CPT codes, 347
   indications, 341
   normal sphincter pressures, 346–347
   other uses for, 347
   postprocedure, 345–346
   preparation and equipment, 341–342
   procedure, 342–345
Anoscopy
   CPT codes, 70
   examination, 67–68
   indications, 64
   positions, 66
   preparation and equipment, 65–66
   rectal biopsy, 68–69
Antibiotics, preprocedural, 7–9
Anticoagulants, preprocedure patient assessment for, 6–7

Argon plasma coagulation (APC)
   CPT codes, 238
   equipment and procedure, 235–237
   indications, 235
   other uses for, 237–238
   postprocedure and complications, 237
ASA classification of general physical status, 4t
Ascites
   diagnostic abdominal paracentesis for, 72–77
   fluid
      profiles, 76t
      testing of, 75t
Aspirin products, preprocedure patient assessment for, 7

## B

Bacteremia, after esophageal dilation, 180
Bacterial endocarditis, subacute (SBE), prophylaxis, 7–8, 35
Bacterial overgrowth, breath hydrogen test
   CPT code, 339
   equipment, 334–335
   indications, 334
   interpretation, 337
   limitations, 337–339
   other uses for, 339
   procedure, 335–336
Balloon dilation, through-the-scope (TTS), 176–181
Balloon expulsion test, 345
Balloon extraction, in management of choledocholithiasis, 204–205
Balloons
   rectal, 344f
   Stretta procedure, 271–274
   used in PDT, 240–243
Balloon tamponade
   complications, 123, 125
   contraindications, 119–120

Balloon tamponade (*contd.*)
  CPT code, 125
  efficacy, 125
  equipment, 121
  postprocedure, 122–123
  preparation, 120–121
  procedure, 121–122
Band ligation, variceal, 112–117
Barium enema, double-contrast,
    383
Barrett's esophagus
    surveillance, 385–386
Barrett's high-grade dysplasia,
    PDT for
  CPT codes, 245
  equipment and procedure,
    240–244
  follow-up after, 245
  indications, 239
  postprocedure and
    complications, 244
Basket extraction, in
    management of
    choledocholithiasis,
    202–204
Benzodiazepines, 15–16
Bile and pancreatic juice
    collection, 54
Biliary ductal obstruction
    management
  biliary stent placement,
    217–222
  CPT codes, 227
  early complications,
    224–226
  equipment, 216–217
  indications, 214–215
  late complications, 226
  nasobiliary catheter
    placement, 223–224
Biliary sludge analysis,
    191–193
Biliary sphincterotomy over
    guidewire, 198f
Biliary stents, 208–211
  placement, 217–222
  self-expanding metallic,
    215–216
Biofeedback, in rectal
    manometry, 341–347
Biopsy
  during colonoscopy, 60
  during EGD, 34
  FNA, EUS-guided, 357–363
  liver, percutaneous, 78–82

  rectal, with alligator
    forceps, 68–69
Bipolar electrocautery, 93–96
Bleeding
  endoclips and endoloops for,
    97–101
  following EMR, 136
  following polypectomy, 63
  gastrointestinal, hemostatic
    agents for, 88t
  as risk of endoscopic
    procedure, 6
  variceal, 103
    balloon tamponade for,
      119–125
Blunt objects, removal from
    upper GI, 257–258
Bougies
  mercury-filled, 160–163
  wire-guided, 164–167
Bowel preparation, 10–12
Breath hydrogen tests, for
    lactose intolerance and
    bacterial overgrowth,
    333–339
Bronchopulmonary injury,
    feeding tube-related,
    145

**C**
Cancers
  colorectal, screening and
    surveillance, 382–385
  esophageal, stenting, 183–189
Cannulation
  in ERCP, 51–54
  in ES, 196–199
  ileocecal valve, 61f
Capsule endoscopy
  complications, 268–269
  CPT code, 269
  equipment, 264–265
  indications and
    contraindications, 263
  interpretation, 266–268
  postprocedure, 266
  preparation, 10–12, 263–264
  procedure, 265–266
Carbohydrate malabsorption,
    breath hydrogen test for,
    333–339
Cardiac disease, assessment
    prior to gastrointestinal
    procedures, 4–5

Cardiopulmonary complications, of colonoscopy, 62

Catheters
nasobiliary, placement, 223–224
in small bowel manometry, 323, 326
in Stretta procedure, 271–272

Celiac plexus neurolysis (CPN), EUS-guided, 364–369

Cholangitis, 225–227

Cholecystitis, 227

Choledocholithiasis management
advanced techniques, 211–212
balloon extraction, 204–205
basket extraction, 202–204
biliary stents, 208–211
CPT codes, 213
generalizations, 201
indications and contraindications, 202
mechanical lithotripsy, 205–208

Cholesterol monohydrate crystals, 192f

Coagulation
argon plasma, 235–238
infrared, of hemorrhoids, 246–249

Code Blue tube, 27

Colonic decompression
CPT codes, 158
indications and contraindications, 156
postprocedure and complications, 158
preparation and equipment, 157
procedure, 157–158

Colonoscopy
complications, 62–63
contraindications, 57
CPT codes, 63
equipment and procedure, 58–60
indications, 56
postprocedure, 62
preparation for, 10–12, 57–58
screening and follow-up, 383–384
therapeutic, 61–62

Colorectal cancer, screening and surveillance, 382–385

Common bile duct
pressure measurement, 319
stones, 201

Corpak tube, 23–26

CPT codes
abdominal paracentesis, 77
anorectal manometry and biofeedback, 347
anoscopy, 70
APC, 238
balloon tamponade, 125
bipolar electrocautery and heater probe, 96
breath hydrogen test, 339
capsule endoscopy, 269
colonic decompression, 158
colonoscopy, 63
definition of CPT modifiers, 393
EGD, 36–37
endoscopic sewing–EndoCinch, 290
endoscopic variceal ligation, 117
Enteryx injection for GERD, 282–283
ERCP, 54
ES, 200
esophageal dilation with mercury-filled bougies, 163
wire-guided bougies, 167
esophageal pH monitoring, 24-hour ambulatory, 304
EUS, 355
EUS-guided CPN, 369
EUS-guided FNA biopsy, 363
feeding tubes, 146
gastrointestinal intubation, 28
injection therapy for hemostasis and anal fissures, 91
IRC for hemorrhoids, 249
lithiasis management, 213
management of
biliary and pancreatic ductal obstruction, 227
fluid collections, 233–234
manometry, esophageal, 298
PDT for Barrett's high-grade dysplasia, 245
PEG and PEJ, 155
percutaneous liver biopsy, 82

CPT codes (*contd.*)
  pneumatic dilation for
      achalasia, 174
  polypectomy and EMR, 137
  removal of foreign
      bodies in upper GI
      tract, 261
  rigid sigmoidoscopy, 69–70
  secretin test, 316
  for sedation, 18
  small bowel enteroscopy,
      44–45
  sphincter of Oddi manometry,
      321
  stenting of esophageal
      cancers, 189
  stoma and pouch endoscopy,
      45
  Stretta procedure, 276
  TTS balloon dilation, 181
Cytology
  during EGD, 34–35
  in ERCP, 54

**D**
Decompression, colonic,
      156–158
Decompression tubes
  gastric, 26–27
  intestinal, 27–28
Diabetes, assessment
      preprocedure, 4
Digital examination, for
      anoscopy and rigid
      sigmoidoscopy, 66–67
Dilation
  esophageal
    with mercury-filled
        bougies, 160–163
    with wire-guided bougies,
        164–167
  pneumatic, for achalasia,
      168–174
  TTS balloon, 176–181
Dobhoff tube, 23–26
Double-contrast barium enema,
      383
Dreiling tube, 313–314
Droperidol, 15
Drugs used in GI procedures,
      380–381
Duodenoscope
  in long position, 50f
  in short position, 51f

Duodenum visualization
  in EGD, 33–34
  in EUS, 352–353
Dysplasia
  Barrett's high-grade,
      photodynamic therapy
      for, 239–245
  grade of, 385–386

**E**
Echoendoscope, 358–362,
      365–368
Edlich tube, 27
Electrocautery, bipolar
  complications, 96
  CPT codes, 96
  equipment, 93–94
  indications and
      contraindications, 93
  postprocedure, 95
  procedure, 94
Electrohydraulic lithotripsy, 211
Electromyography, anal
      sphincter, 345
Embolization, of small pieces of
      glue, 110
Enbucrilate obturation of
      gastric varices
  complications, 109–110
  equipment and additional
      preparation, 107
  indications and
      contraindications, 106
  postprocedure care, 109
  preparation, 106
  procedure, 107–109
Endocarditis, subacute bacterial
      (SBE), prophylaxis, 7–8,
      35
EndoCinch, for GERD, 284–290
Endoclips
  contraindications, 98
  indications, 97
  other uses for, 101
  postprocedure, 100–101
  preparation and equipment, 98
  procedure, 98–99
Endoloops
  complications, 101
  contraindications, 98
  indications, 97–98
  postprocedure, 100–101
  preparation and equipment, 98
  procedure, 99–100

Endoprosthesis
  biliary
    occluded/migrated, 226
    plastic, 208–211, 214, 216
  pancreatic
    occluded/migrated, 226
    plastic and metallic, 215
Endoscope
  advancement techniques in
      colon, 59f
  passing of, in EUS, 351–352
Endoscopic cyst-gastrostomy/
      duodenostomy
  complications, 233
  CPT codes, 233–234
  indications and
      contraindications, 230
  postprocedure and
      interpretation, 232–233
  preparation and equipment,
      230–231
  procedure, 231–232
Endoscopic mucosal resection
      (EMR)
  complications, 136–137
  CPT codes, 137
  indications and
      contraindications,
      127–128
  interpretation, 136
  postprocedure, 135–136
  preparation and equipment,
      128–129
  procedure
    with cap, 133–134
    endoscopic tattooing, 135
    inject and cut method,
      132–133
    with ligation, 135
    piecemeal for large sessile
      polyps, 131–132
Endoscopic retrograde
      cholangiopancreatography
      (ERCP)
  adjunctive procedures, 54
  cannulation challenges, 54
  complications, 53–54
  CPT codes, 54
  equipment, 47–48
  ES component, 194–200
  indications and
      contraindications, 47
  patient preparation, 48–49
  postprocedure, 53
  procedure, 49–53

Endoscopic screening and
      surveillance, 382–386
Endoscopic sewing–EndoCinch
  breakdown following
      procedure, 288–289
  CPT codes, 290
  preprocedural preparation,
      284–285
  procedure, 286–288
  suture loading tag, 286
  troubleshooting common
      problems, 289
Endoscopic sphincterotomy
      (ES), 194–200
Endoscopic ultrasound (EUS)
  complications, 355
  contraindications, 350
  CPT codes, 355
  equipment and procedure,
      351–353
  helpful tips, 354
  indications, 349–350
  postprocedure and
      interpretation,
      354–355
  preparation, 350–351
Endoscopic ultrasound (EUS)-
      guided CPN
  complications, 369
  CPT codes, 369
  equipment, 365–366
  indications and
      contraindications,
      364–365
  postprocedure, 368–369
  preparation, 365
  procedure, 366–368
Endoscopic ultrasound (EUS)-
      guided FNA biopsy
  CPT codes, 363
  indications and
      contraindications,
      357–358
  postprocedure and
      complications, 362
  preparation and equipment,
      358–359
  procedure, 359–362
Endoscopic variceal ligation
  complications, 117
  CPT code, 117
  equipment and procedure,
      113–116
  indications and
      contraindications, 112

Endoscopic variceal ligation
    (*contd.*)
  postprocedure, 116–117
  preparation, 112–113
Endoscopy
  antibiotics prior to procedure,
    7–9
  approach to anticoagulants
    and aspirin products, 6–7
  capsule, 263–269
  equipment, websites for,
    387–391
  in management of foreign
    bodies in upper GI tract,
    251–261
  patient assessment prior to
    procedure, 3–6
  sedation and analgesia for,
    13–18
  small intestinal, CPT codes,
    44–45
  upper and capsule,
    preparation for, 10–12
Endoscopy unit
  equipment and supplies
    adjacent to procedure
      rooms, 372–373
    procedure room, 371–372
  location and characteristics,
    371
  management of equipment,
    376–377
  medical administration area
    organization, 373
  nursing staff responsibilities,
    374–375
  reception area organization
    and equipment, 373–374
  secretarial area organization
    and equipment, 374
  secretarial staff
    responsibilities, 375–376
Endosonography, *See*
    Endoscopic ultrasound
    (EUS)
Enteroscopy, small bowel, 38–45
Enteryx injection, for GERD,
    277–283
Esophageal cancers, stenting
  CPT codes, 189
  indications and
    contraindications,
    183–184
  postprocedure and
    complications, 188–189

    preparation and equipment,
      184
    procedure, 184–188
Esophageal manometry
  CPT code, 298
  equipment, 292
  indications and
    contraindications, 291
  intubation, 292
  measurement of
    body of esophagus, 295–296
    gastric baseline, 292
    lower esophageal sphincter,
      293–294
    upper esophageal sphincter,
      296–298
  postprocedure and
    complications, 298
  preparation for study, 291
Esophageal pH monitoring,
    ambulatory 24-hour
  catheter pH system, 301
  contraindications, 300
  CPT codes, 304
  indications, 299–300
  patient instructions, 302
  postprocedure and
    interpretation, 302–304
  preparation and equipment,
    300
  side effects and
    complications, 304
  wireless pH system, 301–302
Esophageal sphincter
    measurement
  lower, 293–294
  upper, 296–298
Esophageal varices,
    sclerotherapy, 104–106
Esophagogastroduodenoscopy
    (EGD)
  biopsy with, 34
  complications, 36
  CPT codes, 36–37
  cytology from, 34–35
  equipment, 32
  gastric pH check during, 306
  indications and
    contraindications, 30–31
  passing the endoscope, 32
  patient preparation for,
    31–32
  postprocedure, 35–36
  SBE prophylaxis, 35
  visualization with, 33–34

Esophagus
  body of, measurement,
      295–296
  dilation with mercury-filled
      bougies
    CPT codes, 163
    equipment and procedure,
        161–163
    indications, 160
    postprocedure and
        complications, 163
    preparation, 160–161
  dilation with wire-guided
      bougies
    CPT code, 167
    indications and
        contraindications, 164
    postprocedure and
        complications, 167
    preparation and
        equipment, 164–165
    procedure, 165–167
  visualization
    in EGD, 33–34
    in EUS, 352
Ethical issues, PEG tubes, 147
Ewald tube, 27
Expandable stent placement,
    183–189
Extracorporeal shock wave
    lithotripsy, 211–212


**F**
Fecal occult blood test, 382
Feeding tubes
  CPT codes, 146
  equipment, 140–141
  indications and
      contraindications, 138
  jejunal, 152–155
  postprocedure and
      complications, 145–146
  preparation, 139–140
  procedure, 141–145
  styleted, 23–26
  tips, 140f
Fine needle aspiration (FNA)
    biopsy, EUS-guided,
    357–363
Flexible colonoscopy, 10–12
Flexible sigmoidoscopy, 10–11,
    382–383
Fluid
  aspirated, analysis of, 75–76

pancreaticobiliary, collections,
    229–234
Fluoroscopy, in ERCP, 47
Food impaction, 253
  esophageal, 257
Foreign bodies in upper GI
    tract, endoscopic
    management
  complications, 261
  contraindications, 252
  CPT codes, 261
  equipment, 254–256
  indications, 251–252
  postprocedure, 260
  preparation, 252–254
  procedure, 256–260
Fructose intolerance, 336–337


**G**
Gastric baseline measurement,
    292
Gastric decompression tubes,
    26–27
Gastric lavage tubes, 27
Gastric secretory testing
  contraindications, 307
  determination of acid output,
      309
  indications, 306–307
  interpretation, 311–312
  postprocedure, 309
  preparation and equipment,
      308
  procedure, 308–309
Gastric varices, enbucrilate
    obturation, 106–110
Gastroesophageal reflux disease
    (GERD)
  endoscopic
      sewing–EndoCinch,
      284–290
  Enteryx injection for
    complications, 281–282
    contraindications, 277
    CPT codes, 282–283
    equipment and
        preparation, 277–279
    patient preparation, 277
    postprocedure, 281
    procedure, 279–281
  and 24-hour esophageal pH
      monitoring, 299–304
  Stretta procedure for,
      270–276

Gastroesophageal varices, endoscopic ligation, 112–117
Gastrointestinal bleeding, hemostatic agents for, 88t
Gastrointestinal intubation complications, 21–22
CPT codes, 28
equipment, 22
indications and contraindications, 21
patient preparation for, 22
specific tubes, 23–28
Gastrointestinal procedures common GI drugs used in, 380–381
preprocedure assessment for cardiac and pulmonary disease, 4–5
diabetes, 4
liver disease, 5–6
Gastrointestinal tract, upper, foreign bodies in, 251–261
Gastrostomy, percutaneous endoscopic (PEG), 147–155
prophylaxis for, 8–9
Glucagon administration, 41
GoLYTELY, 11–12, 57

**H**
Handling of specimens, 378–379
Heater probe complications, 96
CPT codes, 96
equipment, 93–94
indications and contraindications, 93
postprocedure, 95
procedure, 94–95
Heller myotomy, 168–170
Hemorrhage as complication of liver biopsy, 82
related to sphincterotomy, 224–225
Hemorrhoids, infrared coagulation complications, 249
CPT code, 249
equipment and preparation, 246–247
indications and contraindications, 246
interpretation of response, 249
postprocedure, 248
procedure, 247
Hemostasis CPT codes, 91
injection therapy for, 87–89
Hiatal hernia, dilatation with TTS balloon, 179f
High-grade dysplasia, Barrett's, PDT for, 239–245
Hurst dilator, 160–163
Hypoxia, management of, 17–18

**I**
Ileocecal valve, cannulation, 61f
Inflammatory bowel disease (IBD), 382–385
Informed consent, 3
Infrared coagulation (IRC), of hemorrhoids, 246–249
Injection therapy for anal fissures, 89–91
of esophageal and gastric varices: sclerosis and cyanoacrylate, 103–110
for hemostasis, 87–89
Internal cardioverter/ defibrillators (ICDs), deactivation preprocedure, 5
Intestinal decompression tubes, 27–28
Intraoperative enteroscopy, 43–44
Intubation for esophageal manometry, 292
oral and nasal gastrointestinal, 21–28
in retrieval of foreign bodies in upper GI tract, 256
Ischemia, spinal cord, 369

**J**
Jackknife position, with sigmoidoscopy table, 66
Jejunal feeding CPT codes, 155
equipment, 152–153
indications and contraindications, 152
procedure, 153–154

**K**

Knee-chest position, 66

**L**

Lactose intolerance, breath
    hydrogen test
    CPT code, 339
    equipment, 334–335
    indications, 334
    interpretation, 336–337
    limitations, 337–339
    other uses for, 339
    procedure, 335–336
Laser lithotripsy, 212
Lasers, used in PDT, 239
Lavage tubes, gastric, 27
Ligation
    EMR with, 135
    endoscopic variceal, 112–117
Lithiasis, management of,
    201–213
Lithotripsy
    advanced techniques, 211–212
    mechanical, 205–208
Liver biopsy, percutaneous
    complications, 82
    CPT codes, 82
    equipment and procedure,
        80–81
    indications and
        contraindications, 78–79
    preparation and special
        situations, 79
Liver disease, assessment prior
    to gastrointestinal
    procedures, 5–6
Looping, gastric and small
    bowel, 41

**M**

Malabsorption of carbohydrates,
    breath hydrogen test for,
    333–339
Maloney dilator, 160–163
Manometry
    anorectal, 341–347
    esophageal, 291–298
    small bowel, 322–331
    Sphincter of Oddi, 317–321
Mechanical lithotripsy, 205–208
Mercury-filled bougies, 160–163
Metallic pancreatic
    endoprosthesis, 215

Microlithiasis, 191–193
Migrating motor complex
    activity, 327, 329–330
Minnesota tube
    control of variceal
        hemorrhage, 119
    efficacy, 125
    flow chart for usage, 124f
Monitoring
    esophageal pH, ambulatory
        24-hour, 299–304
    oxygenation, during sedation,
        17
Mucosal ablation, side effects
    of, 244
Myotomy, Heller, 168–170

**N**

Nasobiliary catheter placement,
    223–224
Nasobiliary drain, 214
Nasoduodenal feeding tubes,
    138–146
Nasogastric intubation, 21–28
Nasojejunal feeding tubes,
    138–146
Nasopancreatic drain, 215
    placement, 224
Needles
    liver biopsy, 80
    Stretta procedure, 271–274
Neurolysis, celiac plexus (CPN),
    EUS-guided, 364–369
NSAIDs, preprocedure patient
    assessment for, 7

**O**

Obturation, enbucrilate, of
    gastric varices, 106–110
Opioids, 15–16
Overtube insertion, 256–257
Oxygenation monitoring, during
    sedation, 17

**P**

Pain
    as complication of liver
        biopsy, 82
    as indication for CPN, 364
Pancreatic duct
    leaks, 229
    sphincterotomy, 199–200

Pancreatic ductal obstruction management
  CPT codes, 227
  early complications, 224–226
  equipment, 216–217
  indications, 215
  late complications, 226–227
  nasopancreatic drain placement, 224
  pancreatic stent placement, 222–223
Pancreaticobiliary fluid collections, 229–234
Pancreatic stents, 216–217
  placement, 222–223
Pancreatitis, 224
  secretin test for, 313–316
Pancreatography, endoscopic retrograde, 47–54
Paracentesis, abdominal, 72–77
Patient assessment
  for gastrointestinal procedures, 3–6
  prior to sedation, 14
Penicillin sensitivity, and route of administration, 8t
Percutaneous endoscopic gastrostomy (PEG)
  complications, 151–152
  CPT codes, 155
  ethical issues, 147
  indications and contraindications, 147
  postprocedure, 151
  preparation and equipment, 148
  procedure, 148–151
  prophylaxis, 8–9
Percutaneous endoscopic jejunostomy (PEJ), 152–155
Perforation
  in colonoscopy, 62–63
  due to pneumatic dilation, 173–174
  from EMR and polypectomy, 136
  from heater probe or bipolar electrocautery, 96
  in management of ductal obstruction, 225
Personnel, for administration of sedatives, 16
Phasic waves, measurement in sphincter of Oddi manometry, 319–320

Phosphate of soda prep, 11–12, 57–58
Photodynamic therapy (PDT), for Barrett's high-grade dysplasia, 239–245
Physiologic studies, preparation for, 10–12
Placement
  band ligator on varix, 114f
  biliary stents, 217–222
  expandable stents, 183–189
  feeding tubes, 24–26, 140–145
  nasobiliary catheter, 223–224
  pancreatic stents, 222–223
  PEG tube, 150f
Plastic biliary endoprosthesis, 208–211, 214, 216
Plastic pancreatic endoprosthesis, 215
Pneumatic dilation for achalasia
  complications, 173–174
  CPT codes, 174
  equipment and procedure, 170–172
  indications and contraindications, 168–169
  postprocedure, 172–173
  preparation, 169–170
Polyethylene glycol, bowel prep, 11–12
Polypectomy
  postpolypectomy surveillance, 383–384
  snare, 127–131, 135–137
Porfimer sodium, 239–240
Positions, for anoscopy and rigid sigmoidoscopy, 66
Postpolypectomy syndrome, 136–137
Precut, in endoscopic sphincterotomy, 197–199
Prophylaxis
  percutaneous endoscopic gastrostomy, 8–9
  subacute bacterial endocarditis, 7–8, 35
Propofol, 15–16
Pseudocysts, pancreatic, drainage, 229–234
Pulmonary disease, assessment prior to gastrointestinal procedures, 4–5
Push enteroscopy, 38–42

## R

Rendezvous procedure, in
   lithiasis management,
   212
Resection, endoscopic mucosal
   (EMR), 127–129, 131–137
Retrieval devices, for foreign
   bodies in upper GI tract,
   254–255t
Rigid sigmoidoscopy
   contraindications, 65
   CPT codes, 69–70
   digital examination, 66–67
   examination, 68
   indications, 64
   positions, 66
   preparation and equipment,
      65–66
   rectal biopsy, 68–69

## S

Salem sump tube, 26–27
Savary-Gilliard endoscopy
   system, 164–167
Scintigraphy, role in small
   bowel motility, 331–332
Sclerotherapy of esophageal
   varices
   complications, 106
   CPT code, 110
   indications and
      contraindications, 104
   postprocedure care, 105
   preparation and equipment,
      104–105
   procedure, 105
Screening, colorectal cancer,
   382–385
Secretin test
   CPT codes, 316
   indications and
      contraindications, 313
   interpretation and
      complications, 316
   preparation and equipment,
      313–314
   procedure, 314–316
Sedation
   complications related to, 355
   CPT codes, 18
   levels of and indications
      for, 13
   moderate to deep,
      contraindications for, 14

Sedative/analgesic agents,
   15–18
Sharp objects, removal from
   upper GI, 259–260
Side effects
   esophageal pH monitoring,
      304
   mucosal ablation, 244
Sigmoidoscopy
   flexible, 10–11, 382–383
   rigid, 64–70
Sims' position, 66
Small bowel bacterial
   overgrowth, 337
Small bowel enteroscopy
   CPT codes, 44–45
   intraoperative, 43–44
   push, 38–42
   sonde, 42–43
Small bowel motility,
   manometry studies
   indications, 322
   interpretation, 329–330
   postprocedure, 327, 329
   preparation and equipment,
      323–325
   procedure, 325–327
   role of scintigraphy, 331–332
Snare polypectomy
   complications, 136–137
   CPT codes, 137
   indications and
      contraindications,
      127–128
   interpretation, 136
   postprocedure, 135–136
   preparation and equipment,
      128
   procedure
      pedunculated polyps,
         129–130
      sessile polyps, 130–131
Snares, types of, 260f
Sonde enteroscopy, 42–43
Specimen handling, 378–379
Sphincter of Oddi manometry
   CPT code, 321
   equipment, 317–318
   indications and
      contraindications, 317
   interpretations, 319–320
   postprocedure and
      complications, 321
   preparation of patient, 317
   procedure, 318–319

Sphincterotomy, endoscopic
   CPT code, 200
   equipment and procedure,
      196–200
   indications and
      contraindications,
      194–195
   postprocedure and
      complications, 200
   preparation, 195
Sphincters
   anal, normal pressures,
      346–347
   esophageal, measurement,
      293–294, 296–298
Spinal cord ischemia, 369
Stenting, esophageal cancers,
      183–189
Stents
   biliary, 208–211
      placement, 217–222
      self-expanding metallic,
         215–216
   pancreatic, 216–217
      placement, 222–223
Stoma and pouch endoscopy,
      CPT codes, 45
Stomach visualization
   in EGD, 33–34
   in EUS, 352–353
Stretta procedure
   CPT codes, 276
   indications and
      contraindications,
      270–271
   postprocedure and
      complications, 275
   preparation and equipment,
      271
   procedure, 271–275
Styleted feeding tubes, 23–26
Subacute bacterial endocarditis
      (SBE), prophylaxis, 7–8,
      35
Surveillance
   Barrett's esophagus, 385–386
   colorectal cancer for patients
      with IBD, 384–385
   postpolypectomy, 383–384
Suture loading tag, in
      endoscopic sewing, 286

**T**

Tamponade, balloon, 119–125

Tattooing, endoscopic, 127,
      135
Thromboembolism, patient risk
      for, 7t
Through-the-scope (TTS)
      balloon dilation
   complications, 180–181
   CPT codes, 181
   indications and
      contraindications,
      176–177
   postprocedure and
      interpretation, 180
   preparation and equipment,
      177–178
   procedure, 178–180
Transgastric pseudocyst
      drainage, 231f
Transmucosal potential
      difference electrodes, 325
Transmural burn syndrome,
      136–137
Troubleshooting, in endoscopic
      sewing, 289

**U**

Ulcers, as complication of APC,
      237
Ultrasound, endoscopic (EUS),
      349–355
   CPN guided by, 364–369
   FNA biopsy guided by,
      357–363
Upper endoscopy
   feeding tube placement aided
      by, 143–144
   preparation for, 10, 12

**V**

Varices
   bleeding, balloon tamponade
      for, 119–125
   esophageal, sclerotherapy,
      104–106
   gastric, enbucrilate
      obturation, 106–110
   gastroesophageal, endoscopic
      ligation, 112–117
Vessel coaptation, 95f
Video capsule, in capsule
      endoscopy, 265f
Visicol, pill-based prep for
      colonoscopy, 11–12

**W**

Websites
  endoscopy equipment,
    387–391
  GI professional groups, 392
  medications, 391–392
  patient resources, 387
Wire-guided bougies, 164–167

Worksheet, for gastric secretory
    testing, 310f
Workstation, for capsule
    endoscopy, 264–265

**X**

Xylose breath H2 test, 339